T0226661

Adult Brain Tumors

Editor

LARA A. BRANDÃO

NEUROIMAGING CLINICS
OF NORTH AMERICA

www.neuroimaging.theclinics.com

Consulting Editor
SURESH K. MUKHERJI

November 2016 • Volume 26 • Number 4

ELSEVIER

1600 John F. Kennedy Boulevard • Suite 1800 • Philadelphia, Pennsylvania, 19103-2899

http://www.neuroimaging.theclinics.com

NEUROIMAGING CLINICS OF NORTH AMERICA Volume 26, Number 4
November 2016 ISSN 1052-5149, ISBN 13: 978-0-323-47689-8

Editor: John Vassallo (j.vassallo@elsevier.com)
Developmental Editor: Casey Jackson

© **2016 Elsevier Inc. All rights reserved.**

This publication and the individual contributions contained in it are protected under copyright by Elsevier, and the following terms and conditions apply to their use:

Photocopying
Single photocopies of single articles may be made for personal use as allowed by national copyright laws. Permission of the Publisher and payment of a fee is required for all other photocopying, including multiple or systematic copying, copying for advertising or promotional purposes, resale, and all forms of document delivery. Special rates are available for educational institutions that wish to make photocopies for non-profit educational classroom use. For information on how to seek permission visit www.elsevier.com/permissions or call: (+44) 1865 843830 (UK)/(+1) 215 239 3804 (USA).

Derivative Works
Subscribers may reproduce tables of contents or prepare lists of articles including abstracts for internal circulation within their institutions. Permission of the Publisher is required for resale or distribution outside the institution. Permission of the Publisher is required for all other derivative works, including compilations and translations (please consult www.elsevier.com/permissions).

Electronic Storage or Usage
Permission of the Publisher is required to store or use electronically any material contained in this periodical, including any article or part of an article (please consult www.elsevier.com/permissions). Except as outlined above, no part of this publication may be reproduced, stored in a retrieval system or transmitted in any form or by any means, electronic, mechanical, photocopying, recording or otherwise, without prior written permission of the Publisher.

Notice
No responsibility is assumed by the Publisher for any injury and/or damage to persons or property as a matter of products liability, negligence or otherwise, or from any use or operation of any methods, products, instructions or ideas contained in the material herein. Because of rapid advances in the medical sciences, in particular, independent verification of diagnoses and drug dosages should be made.

Although all advertising material is expected to conform to ethical (medical) standards, inclusion in this publication does not constitute a guarantee or endorsement of the quality or value of such product or of the claims made of it by its manufacturer.

Neuroimaging Clinics of North America (ISSN 1052-5149) is published quarterly by Elsevier Inc., 360 Park Avenue South, New York, NY 10010-1710. Months of issue are February, May, August, and November. Business and editorial offices: 1600 John F. Kennedy Blvd., Suite 1800, Philadelphia, PA 19103-2899. Business and editorial offices: 6277 Sea Harbor Drive, Orlando, FL 32887-4800. Periodicals postage paid at New York, NY, and additional mailing offices. Subscription prices are USD 365 per year for US individuals, USD 564 per year for US institutions, USD 100 per year for US students and residents, USD 415 per year for Canadian individuals, USD 718 per year for Canadian institutions, USD 525 per year for international individuals, USD 718 per year for international institutions and USD 260 per year for Canadian and foreign students and residents. To receive student/resident rate, orders must be accompanied by name of affiliated institution, date of term, and the *signature* of program/residency coordinator on institution letterhead. Orders will be billed at individual rate until proof of status is received. Foreign air speed delivery is included in all *Clinics* subscription prices. All prices are subject to change without notice. POSTMASTER: Send address changes to *Neuroimaging Clinics of North America,* Elsevier Health Sciences Division, Subscription **Customer Service, 3251 Riverport Lane, Maryland Heights, MO 63043. Telephone: 1-800-654-2452 (U.S. and Canada); 314-447-8871 (outside U.S. and Canada). Fax: 314-447-8029. E-mail: journalscustomer service-usa@elsevier.com (for print support); journalsonlinesupport-usa@elsevier.com (for online support).**

Reprints. For copies of 100 or more of articles in this publication, please contact the Commercial Reprints Department, Elsevier Inc., 360 Park Avenue South, New York, NY 10010-1710. Tel.: 212-633-3874; Fax: 212-633-3820; E-mail: reprints@elsevier.com.

Neuroimaging Clinics of North America is covered by *Excerpta Medical/EMBASE,* the RSNA Index of Imaging Literature, *MEDLINE/PubMed (Index Medicus),* MEDLINE/MEDLARS, SciSearch, Research Alert, and Neuroscience Citation Index.

PROGRAM OBJECTIVE

The goal of *Neuroimaging Clinics of North America* is to keep practicing radiologists and radiology residents up to date with current clinical practice in radiology by providing timely articles reviewing the state of the art in patient care.

TARGET AUDIENCE

Practicing radiologists, radiology residents, and other healthcare professionals who utilize neuroimaging findings to provide patient care.

LEARNING OBJECTIVES

Upon completion of this activity, participants will be able to:
1. Review the management of lymphoma adult brain tumors.
2. Discuss pre- and post-treatment evaluation of brain gliomas.
3. Recognize advanced magnetic resonance imaging techniques for brain tumors.

ACCREDITATION

The Elsevier Office of Continuing Medical Education (EOCME) is accredited by the Accreditation Council for Continuing Medical Education (ACCME) to provide continuing medical education for physicians.

The EOCME designates this enduring material for a maximum of 15 *AMA PRA Category 1 Credit*(s)™. Physicians should claim only the credit commensurate with the extent of their participation in the activity.

All other health care professionals requesting continuing education credit for this enduring material will be issued a certificate of participation.

DISCLOSURE OF CONFLICTS OF INTEREST

The EOCME assesses conflict of interest with its instructors, faculty, planners, and other individuals who are in a position to control the content of CME activities. All relevant conflicts of interest that are identified are thoroughly vetted by EOCME for fair balance, scientific objectivity, and patient care recommendations. EOCME is committed to providing its learners with CME activities that promote improvements or quality in healthcare and not a specific proprietary business or a commercial interest.

The planning committee, staff, authors and editors listed below have identified no financial relationships or relationships to products or devices they or their spouse/life partner have with commercial interest related to the content of this CME activity:
Romy Ames, MD; Jalal B. Andre, MD; Ramon Francisco Barajas Jr, MD; Ali Borhani, MD; Lara A. Brandão, MD; Mauricio Castillo, MD; Lazaro D. Causil, MD; Soonmee Cha, MD; Mark F. Dalesandro, MD; Marta Drake-Pérez, MD; Anjali Fortna; Sakineh Kadivar, MD; Soheil Kooraki, MD; Marc C. Mabray, MD; Ali Mohammadzadeh, MD; Vahid Mohammadzadeh, MD; Maryam Mohammadzadeh, MD; Suresh K. Mukherji; Paulo Puac, MD; Bahman Rasuli, MD; Erin Scheckenbach; Madjid Shakiba, MD; Robert Y. Shih, MD; James G. Smirniotopoulos, MD; Houman Sotoudeh, MD; Karthik Subramaniam; John Vassallo.

UNAPPROVED/OFF-LABEL USE DISCLOSURE

The EOCME requires CME faculty to disclose to the participants:
1. When products or procedures being discussed are off-label, unlabelled, experimental, and/or investigational (not US Food and Drug Administration [FDA] approved); and
2. Any limitations on the information presented, such as data that are preliminary or that represent ongoing research, interim analyses, and/or unsupported opinions. Faculty may discuss information about pharmaceutical agents that is outside of FDA-approved labelling. This information is intended solely for CME and is not intended to promote off-label use of these medications. If you have any questions, contact the medical affairs department of the manufacturer for the most recent prescribing information.

TO ENROLL

To enroll in the *Neuroimaging Clinics of North America* Continuing Medical Education program, call customer service at 1-800-654-2452 or sign up online at http://www.theclinics.com/home/cme. The CME program is available to subscribers for an additional annual fee of USD 235.

METHOD OF PARTICIPATION

In order to claim credit, participants must complete the following:
1. Complete enrolment as indicated above.
2. Read the activity.
3. Complete the CME Test and Evaluation. Participants must achieve a score of 70% on the test. All CME Tests and Evaluations must be completed online.

CME INQUIRIES/SPECIAL NEEDS

For all CME inquiries or special needs, please contact elsevierCME@elsevier.com.

NEUROIMAGING CLINICS OF NORTH AMERICA

THE CLINICS ARE AVAILABLE ONLINE!
Access your subscription at:
www.theclinics.com

Contributors

CONSULTING EDITOR

SURESH K. MUKHERJI, MD, MBA, FACR
Professor and Chairman, Walter F. Patenge
Endowed Chair, Department of Radiology,
Michigan State University, Chief Medical
Officer & Director of Health Care Delivery,
Michigan State University Health Team, East
Lansing, Michigan

EDITOR

LARA A. BRANDÃO, MD
Chief of Neuroradiology, Radiologic
Department, Clínica Felippe Mattoso, Fleury
Medicina Diagnóstica; Radiologic Department,
Clínica IRM-Ressonância Magnética, Rio De
Janeiro, Rio De Janeiro, Brazil

AUTHORS

ROMY AMES, MD
Neuroradiology Research Fellow,
Neuroradiology Section, Department of
Radiology, University of North Carolina
School of Medicine, Chapel Hill,
North Carolina

JALAL B. ANDRE, MD
Director of Neurological MRI, Harborview
Medical Center; Assistant Professor,
Department of Radiology, University of
Washington, Seattle, Washington

RAMON FRANCISCO BARAJAS Jr, MD
Assistant Professor, Departments of Radiology
and Advanced Imaging Research Center,
Oregon Health and Science University,
Portland, Oregon

ALI BORHANI, MD
Senior Radiology Resident, Advanced
Diagnostic and Interventional Radiology
Research Center, Tehran University of Medical
Science, Tehran, Iran

LARA A. BRANDÃO, MD
Chief of Neuroradiology, Radiologic
Department, Clínica Felippe Mattoso, Fleury
Medicina Diagnóstica; Radiologic Department,
Clínica IRM-Ressonância Magnética, Rio De
Janeiro, Rio De Janeiro, Brazil

MAURICIO CASTILLO, MD
Chief, Division of Neuroradiology, Department
of Radiology, University of North Carolina
School of Medicine, Chapel Hill,
North Carolina

LAZARO D. CAUSIL, MD
Neuroradiology Research Fellow,
Neuroradiology Section, Department of
Radiology, University of North Carolina School
of Medicine, Chapel Hill,
North Carolina

SOONMEE CHA, MD
Departments of Neurological Surgery,
Radiology and Biomedical Imaging, University
of California–San Francisco, San Francisco,
California

MARK F. DALESANDRO, MD
Director of Neurological MRI, Harborview
Medical Center; Acting Instructor in
Neuroradiology, Department of Radiology,
University of Washington, Seattle,
Washington

MARTA DRAKE-PÉREZ, MD
Department of Radiology, Marqués de
Valdecilla University Hospital/IDIVAL,
Santander, Cantabria, Spain

SAKINEH KADIVAR, MD
Assistant Professor, Department of
Ophthalmology, Amiralmomenin Hospital,
Guilan University of Medical Sciences, Guilan,
Iran

SOHEIL KOORAKI, MD
Radiologist, Department of Radiology, Shariati
Hospital, Tehran University of Medical
Sciences, Tehran, Iran

MARC C. MABRAY, MD
Department of Radiology, University of New
Mexico School of Medicine, Albuquerque,
New Mexico

ALI MOHAMMADZADEH, MD
Assistant Professor, Department of Radiology,
Rajaie Hospital, Iran University of Medical
Sciences, Tehran, Iran

MARYAM MOHAMMADZADEH, MD
Assistant Professor, Division of
Neuroradiology, Department of Radiology,
Amiralam Hospital, Tehran University of
Medical Sciences, Tehran, Iran

VAHID MOHAMMADZADEH, MD
Senior Ophthalmology Resident, Department
of Ophthalmology, Farabi Hospital, Tehran
University of Medical Sciences, Tehran,
Iran

PAULO PUAC, MD
Neuroradiology Research Fellow,
Neuroradiology Section, Department of
Radiology, University of North Carolina School
of Medicine, Chapel Hill, North Carolina

BAHMAN RASULI, MD
Senior Radiology Resident, Advanced
Diagnostic and Interventional Radiology
Research Center, Tehran University of Medical
Science, Tehran, Iran

MADJID SHAKIBA, MD
Advanced Diagnostic and Interventional
Radiology Research Center, Tehran University
of Medical Science, Tehran, Iran

ROBERT Y. SHIH, MD
Associate Chief of Neuroradiology, American
Institute for Radiologic Pathology, Silver
Spring, Maryland

JAMES G. SMIRNIOTOPOULOS, MD
Chief Editor, MedPix, National Library of
Medicine, Bethesda, Maryland; Professorial
Lecturer, Department of Radiology, George
Washington University, Washington, DC

HOUMAN SOTOUDEH, MD
Pediatric Radiology Fellow, St Louis Children's
Hospital, Mallinckrodt Institute of Radiology,
Washington University in St Louis, St Louis,
Missouri

Contents

> In adults, the most common expansile "mass" lesion in the posterior fossa is a subacute stroke, whereas the most common neoplastic lesion in the posterior fossa is cerebellar metastasis (intra-axial) or vestibular schwannoma (extra-axial). Those diseases fall outside the scope of this article, which focuses on primary intra-axial tumors of the posterior fossa in adults. This category of tumors is uncommon and more frequently encountered in children. This article reviews tumors of the cerebellum, brainstem, and fourth ventricle that are seen in adult patients, following categories from the 2007 World Health Organization classification of central nervous system tumors.

> Primary central nervous system lymphomas are aggressive, high-cell-density tumors. There is recent increase in their incidence in immunocompetent patients. Knowledge of imaging findings on computed tomography and conventional MR imaging is important to suggest the diagnosis. Moreover, information obtained from advanced MR imaging techniques, such as diffusion-weighted imaging, diffusion tensor imaging, MR spectroscopy, perfusion-weighted imaging, and dynamic contrast-enhanced studies, increases diagnostic confidence and helps distinguish them from other aggressive intracranial tumors. This article discusses typical imaging findings of primary and secondary central nervous system lymphomas on computed tomography and conventional MR imaging, advanced MR imaging techniques, and changes related to steroid therapy.

> There are 2 types of central nervous system lymphoma: primary and secondary. Both have variable imaging features making them diagnostic challenges. Furthermore, a patient's immune status significantly alters the imaging findings. Familiarity with typical appearances, variations, and common mimics aids radiologists in appropriately considering lymphoma in the differential diagnosis. Moreover, special types of lymphoma, such as lymphomatosis cerebri, intravascular lymphoma, and lymphomatoid granulomatosis, also are found. This article discusses uncommon

Pretreatment Evaluation of Glioma 567

Ali Mohammadzadeh, Vahid Mohammadzadeh, Soheil Kooraki, Houman Sotoudeh, Sakineh Kadivar, Madjid Shakiba, Bahman Rasuli, Ali Borhani, and Maryam Mohammadzadeh

Glioma is considered the most common type of primary central nervous system (CNS) tumor. Imaging is crucial for diagnosis, characterization, grading, and therapeutic planning of CNS gliomas. Along with a brief description of conventional computed tomography and magnetic resonance imaging techniques, this article reviews the ever-developing role of modern imaging techniques in preoperative management of CNS gliomas. It discusses current clinical applications, promising features, and limitations of each imaging method.

Posttreatment Evaluation of Brain Gliomas 581

Mark F. Dalesandro and Jalal B. Andre

The imaging of treated gliomas is complicated by a variety of treatment related effects, which can falsely simulate disease improvement or progression. Distinguishing between disease progression and treatment effects is difficult with standard MR imaging pulse sequences and added specificity can be gained by the addition of advanced imaging techniques.

Metastasis in Adult Brain Tumors 601

Ramon Francisco Barajas Jr and Soonmee Cha

Metastatic cancer to the central nervous system is primarily deposited by hematogenous spread in various anatomically distinct regions: calvarial, pachymeningeal, leptomeningeal, and brain parenchyma. A patient's overall clinical status and the information needed to make treatment decisions are the primary considerations in initial imaging modality selection. Contrast-enhanced MR imaging is the preferred imaging modality. Morphologic MR imaging is limited to delineating anatomic deraignment of tissues. Dynamic susceptibility contrast-enhanced perfusion and diffusion-weighted physiology-based MR imaging sequences have been developed that complement morphologic MR imaging by providing additional diagnostic information.

Extraparenchymal Lesions in Adults 621

Marta Drake-Pérez and James G. Smirniotopoulos

This article reviews the most frequent extra-axial tumors of the central nervous system, from the most common meningioma to some uncommon conditions, like Rosai-Dorfman disease, focusing on imaging techniques, pearls, and pitfalls as well as a more practical approach.

Advanced MR Imaging Techniques in Daily Practice 647

Marc C. Mabray and Soonmee Cha

This article presents a summary of advanced MR imaging techniques and their use in the evaluation of patients with brain tumors. It reviews diffusion-weighted imaging, diffusion-tensor imaging, T2* susceptibility–sensitive imaging, MR spectroscopy, MR perfusion, and functional MR imaging, and discusses their current roles in the evaluation of patients with brain tumors.

Lazaro D. Causil, Romy Ames, Paulo Puac, and Mauricio Castillo

Some brain tumors results are interesting due to their rarity at presentation and over-whelming imaging characteristics, posing a diagnostic challenge in the eyes of any experienced neuroradiologist. This article focuses on the most important features regarding epidemiology, location, clinical presentation, histopathology, and imaging findings of cases considered "bizarre." A review of the most recent literature dealing with these unusual tumors and pseudotumors is presented, highlighting key points related to the diagnosis, treatments, outcomes, and differential diagnosis.

Foreword
Adult Brain Tumors

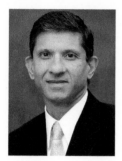

Suresh K. Mukherji, MD, MBA, FACR
Consulting Editor

Once again, it is my distinct pleasure to thank Lara Brandão for guest editing this issue of *Neuroimaging Clinics*. In this issue, Dr Brandão focuses on advanced imaging evaluation of adult brain tumors. This issue is a very nice combination of the "traditional" imaging of brain tumors and also a focus on the current "value" that advanced imaging can provide in the diagnosis and management of various intracranial neoplasms.

The range of disorders covered is extraordinary, and this is a wonderful review for neuroradiologists and radiologists who routinely interpret neuroimaging studies. It is also an excellent reference for those who will soon be taking recertification exams, like myself (sad face)! I want thank and congratulate all of the authors for their wonderful contributions. Their expertise is clearly evident by the depth of knowledge presented in each article. Your contributions are greatly appreciated by all of us.

I again thank "Superwoman!" I gave Lara that nickname in my last foreword, and my admiration and respect for her have grown even more. I am still in awe as to how she accomplishes so much with all of her other personal and professional obligations. The quality is always superb and completed in a timely manner, which make editors *very* happy. Lara, thank you again for all you do and continued success in future endeavors!

Suresh K. Mukherji, MD, MBA, FACR
Department of Radiology
Michigan State University
Michigan State University Health Team
846 Service Road
East Lansing, MI 48824, USA

E-mail address:
mukherji@rad.msu.edu

http://dx.doi.org/10.1016/j.nic.2016.08.009
1052-5149/16/© 2016 Published by Elsevier Inc.

neuroimaging.theclinics.com

Preface
Adult Brain Tumors

Imaging Characterization of Primary, Secondary, and Extraparenchymal Tumors in the Central Nervous System, Including Findings on Advanced MR Imaging Techniques as well as Treatment-Related Abnormalities

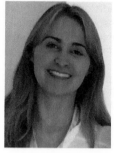

Lara A. Brandão, MD
Editor

This issue of *Neuroimaging Clinics* focuses on adult brain tumors. The most common posterior fossa tumors—metastasis and hemangioblastomas, among many differentials—are discussed in the first article, "Posterior Fossa Tumors in Adult Patients."

The next two articles address primary and secondary central nervous system (CNS) lymphomas as well as special lymphoma types, including lymphomatosis cerebri, intravascular lymphomas, and lymphomatoid granulomatosis. The article entitled, "Pretreatment Evaluation of Glioma," discusses the imaging aspects of gliomas on conventional MR imaging as well as on advanced MR imaging techniques, such as diffusion-weighted imaging, perfusion imaging, dynamic contrast-enhanced MR imaging, and MR spectroscopy, emphasizing their importance to assess presurgical grading, prognosis, and biopsy planning of CNS gliomas.

Advanced MR imaging techniques as well as PET can add specificity in differentiating treatment effects from true tumor progression in treated gliomas, as discussed in the article, "Posttreatment Evaluation of Brain Gliomas." Noninvasive imaging

techniques also play a critical role in the diagnosis and management of patients with metastatic disease to the CNS, as discussed in the article by Barajas and Cha. In this article, imaging aspects of metastasis to the calvarium, meninges, and parenchyma are discussed.

The use of physiologic MR imaging techniques as an integral part of posttreatment brain tumor imaging in metastatic disease is also addressed, since conventional MR imaging has low specificity for the diagnosis of metastatic disease progression after standard therapies.

A large and complete review of extraparenchymal tumors can be found in the article, "Extraparenchymal Lesions in Adults," with an emphasis on meningiomas and their main differentials, including nonneoplastic/inflammatory lesions, pituitary and pineal region masses, as well as cystic-appearing lesions.

The article "Advanced MR Imaging Techniques in Daily Practice," reviews the following techniques: diffusion-weighted imaging, diffusion-tensor imaging, susceptibility-weighted imaging, MRS, perfusion imaging, and fMR imaging. This article

Neuroimag Clin N Am 26 (2016) xiii–xiv
http://dx.doi.org/10.1016/j.nic.2016.08.008
1052-5149/16/© 2016 Published by Elsevier Inc.

neuroimaging.theclinics.com

emphasizes the clinical applications of these techniques as they apply to brain tumor imaging.

In this issue, we intend to offer the readers an extensive review of brain tumors in adult patients, including findings on conventional MR imaging as well as on advanced MR imaging techniques.

Recently, advanced MR imaging techniques have become an integral part of the evaluation of patients with brain tumors. These techniques are being applied to diagnose and grade tumors pre-operatively, to plan and navigate surgery intrao-peratively, to monitor and assess treatment response, and to understand the effects of treatment on the patients' brains.

The last article of this issue is a review of the most recent literature dealing with interesting rare tumors and pseudotumors is presented in the article entitled, "Adult Brain Tumors and Pseudotumors—Interesting (Bizarre) Cases," highlighting key points related to the diagnosis, treatment, outcomes, and differential diagnosis.

I would like to sincerely thank all of the authors of this issue for their invaluable contributions. I wish to express my gratitude to the consulting editor, Dr Suresh K. Mukherji, for the opportunity to lead this project. I would also like to thank the series editor, John Vassallo, developmental editor, Casey Jackson, and editorial assistant, Nicole Congleton, for their guidance and support during the preparation of this issue.

Lara A. Brandão, MD
Radiologic Department
Clínica Felippe Mattoso
Fleury Medicina Diagnóstica
Avenida das Américas 700
sala 320, Barra Da Tijuca, Rio De Janeiro
Rio De Janeiro CEP 22640-100, Brazil

Radiologic Department
Clínica IRM-Ressonância Magnética
Rua Capitão Salomão, Humaitá, Rio De Janeiro
Rio De Janeiro CEP 22271-040, Brazil

E-mail address:
larabrandao.rad@terra.com.br

Posterior Fossa Tumors in Adult Patients

 CrossMark

Robert Y. Shih, MD[a],*, James G. Smirniotopoulos, MD[b,c]

KEYWORDS

- Adult posterior fossa tumors • Cerebellum • Brainstem • Fourth ventricle

KEY POINTS

- In the adult posterior fossa, the most common "mass" is a subacute stroke, the most common tumor is a cerebellar metastasis, and the most common primary tumor is hemangioblastoma.
- Medulloblastoma and pilocytic astrocytoma can be seen in adults as well as children; low-grade and high-grade diffuse gliomas can be seen in the brainstem as well as in the cerebral hemispheres.
- Tumors of the fourth ventricle may originate from the wall (ependymoma, subependymoma, or rosette-forming glioneuronal tumor [RGNT]) or from the lumen (choroid plexus papilloma or carcinoma, meningioma, or metastasis).

OVERVIEW OF THE POSTERIOR FOSSA

The posterior fossa is the suboccipital or infratentorial compartment of the cranial vault, which extends from tentorium cerebelli superiorly to foramen magnum inferiorly, housing the cerebellum and most of the brainstem, specifically the pons and medulla. As the name indicates, the midbrain or mesencephalon is more centrally located and crosses through the tentorial incisure or notch, straddling the supratentorial and infratentorial compartments. Osseous boundaries of the posterior fossa include the clivus anteriorly, the petrous ridge of the temporal bones anterolaterally, the mastoid portion of the temporal bones laterally, and the occipital bone posteriorly-inferiorly. Overall, disease is less commonly encountered in the infratentorial than supratentorial compartment, which is partially related to volume. For example, a volumetric MR imaging analysis of adults without and with Chiari I malformation found a median posterior fossa to total intracranial volume ratio of 14% in both groups.[1]

The smaller volume of the posterior fossa also means that less mass effect is needed to produce symptoms from compression of the cerebellum, brainstem, or fourth ventricle, with the potential risk of superior vermian or inferior tonsillar herniation. In adults, the most common expansile "mass" lesion in the posterior fossa is a subacute stroke, whereas the most common neoplastic lesion in the posterior fossa is cerebellar metastasis (intra-axial) or vestibular schwannoma (extra-axial). Those diseases fall outside the scope of this article, which focuses on primary intra-axial tumors of the posterior fossa in adults. This category of tumors is uncommon and more frequently encountered in children, because infratentorial tumors predominate over supratentorial tumors after infancy and before adolescence.[2] This article reviews tumors of the cerebellum, brainstem, and fourth ventricle that are seen in adult patients, following categories from the 2007 World Health Organization (WHO) classification of central nervous system (CNS) tumors (Table 1).[3]

Disclosures: None.
[a] American Institute for Radiologic Pathology, 1100 Wayne Avenue, Suite 1020, Silver Spring, MD 20910, USA;
[b] MedPix, National Library of Medicine, 8600 Rockville Pike, Bethesda, MD 20894, USA; [c] Department of Radiology, George Washington University, 2121 Eye Street Northwest, Washington, DC 20052, USA
* Corresponding author. American Institute for Radiologic Pathology, 1100 Wayne Avenue, Suite 1020, Silver Spring, MD 20910.
E-mail address: ryshih@gmail.com

neuroimaging.theclinics.com

Table 1
Primary intra-axial tumors of the posterior fossa in adults (intra-axial = inside pia mater)

Cerebellum	Hemangioblastoma (WHO grade I)	Most common primary intra-axial tumor of the posterior fossa in adults, mesenchymal not neuroepithelial tumor, "related to the meninges" with 2007 WHO classification, hypervascular enhancing nodule ± cyst formation
	Medulloblastoma (WHO grade IV)	More common in children and younger adults (age <40), hypercellular embryonal primitive neuroepithelial tumor, lateral hemispheric mass with desmoplastic histology or SHH activation is more frequent in adults than in children
	Pilocytic astrocytoma (WHO grade I)	More common in children and younger adults (age <40), circumscribed margins, solid or mixed solid-cystic tumor, enhancement related to leaky blood-brain barrier
	Dysplastic cerebellar gangliocytoma (WHO grade I)	More common in younger adults (ages 20–40), neoplasm vs hamartoma, association with Cowden syndrome, striated cerebellar mass (usually nonenhancing)
	Cerebellar liponeurocytoma (WHO grade II)	More common in older adults (age >40), appearance is similar to medulloblastoma (look for fat density/signal), but prognosis is similar to central neurocytoma
Brainstem	Diffuse intrinsic brainstem glioma (WHO grades II–III)	More common in children and younger adults (age <40), diffuse: >50% brainstem diameter, expansile infiltrative T2 hyperintense lesion without significant enhancement, low grade in adults but high grade in children
	Malignant brainstem glioma (WHO grades III–IV)	More common in older adults (>40 y), infratentorial glioblastoma: enhancing infiltrative brainstem mass with intratumoral necrosis and peritumoral edema
	Focal tectal glioma (WHO grades I–II)	More common in children and younger adults (age <40), focal: <50% brainstem diameter, nonenhancing mass in dorsal midbrain ± obstructive hydrocephalus
Ventricle	Subependymoma (WHO grade I)	More common in older adults (>40 y), fourth ventricle > lateral ventricle > spinal cord (central canal), relatively hypovascular mass projecting into the ventricle
	Ependymoma (WHO grades II–III)	More common in children and younger adults (age <40), heterogeneous intraventricular mass with enhancement, ± extraventricular or transependymal spread
	Choroid plexus tumor (WHO grades I–III)	More common in infants and younger children, posterior fossa (fourth ventricle) is more frequently seen in adults, lobulated enhancing mass from choroid plexus
	Choroid plexus meningioma (WHO grades I–III)	More common in older adults (>40 y) and women, similar appearance to other meningiomas but centered on choroid plexus (atrium/trigone > fourth ventricle)
	RGNT of the fourth ventricle (WHO grade I)	More common in younger adults (20–40 y), thought to arise from pluripotential cells in subependymal plate, heterogeneous solid-cystic appearance often with focal enhancement, may occur outside posterior fossa

MENINGEAL TUMORS: HEMANGIOBLASTOMA (WHO GRADE I)

Hemangioblastomas are rare tumors of the central nervous system, which account for 1.0% to 2.5% of all intracranial neoplasms.[4] Nevertheless, they are the most common primary tumor of the posterior fossa in adults, due to a strong predilection for the cerebellum (also known as Lindau tumors). In one 10-year neurosurgical study of 47 treated hemangioblastomas, the vast majority were located in the cerebellum (83%), followed by the spinal cord (13%), brainstem (medulla), and pituitary stalk.[4] Most cases of hemangioblastoma are sporadic; however, approximately 25% are familial with von Hippel-Lindau syndrome (VHL) and more likely presenting with multiple hemangioblastomas and at a younger age (mean age is 29 years for VHL vs 47 years for sporadic).[4] Cerebellar hemangioblastomas frequently occur at the posterior and medial hemispheres (74% of cases), and they frequently cause symptoms like headache, ataxia, or dysmetria.[5]

Unlike the other blastomas of the CNS (eg, glioblastoma, pineoblastoma, and medulloblastoma), which are all classified as WHO grade IV neuroepithelial tumors, hemangioblastoma is classified as a WHO grade I meningeal tumor.[3] These highly vascular tumors are typically intra-axial but located at or near the pial surface of the cerebellum and spinal cord. There are rare case reports of extraaxial hemangioblastomas, for example, disseminated leptomeningeal hemangioblastomatosis in the subarachnoid space, dural-based hemangioblastoma simulating meningioma, and extradural tumors in the neural foramina and extraspinal soft tissues.[6–8] They are hypothesized to derive from embryologic multipotent stem cells (hemangioblast), which become neoplastic stromal cells with the loss of both *VHL* tumor suppressor genes and which retain the ability to differentiate into both hematopoietic and endothelial cells.[9]

The most classic radiographic appearance of a hemangioblastoma on CT or MR imaging is "a peripheral cyst in the posterior fossa with a mural nodule supplied by enlarged vessels."[10] The nodule is the tumor nidus and enhances intensely; this may be accompanied by hypervascular flow voids on spin-echo MR images (**Fig. 1**). The cyst is lined by compressed brain parenchyma with occasional reactive astrogliosis (not by tumor cells) and usually does not enhance; approximately 40% of hemangioblastomas present as solid nodules without adjacent cysts.[11] Probably all hemangioblastomas begin as solid nodules, often small and asymptomatic; vascular hyperpermeability with fluid extravasation leads to vasogenic edema followed by cyst formation, which is more likely to cause symptoms and need resection.[12,13] Surgery is also indicated when the diagnosis is uncertain; the imaging differential diagnosis includes cerebellar metastasis and pilocytic astrocytoma. On pathology, immunostains help distinguish hemangioblastoma from metastatic renal cell carcinoma.[14]

EMBRYONAL TUMORS: MEDULLOBLASTOMA (WHO GRADE IV)

Whereas the hemangioblastoma is the most common primary cerebellar tumor in adults, the medulloblastoma is the most common primary cerebellar tumor in children (age <20). In June 1924, Harvey Cushing and Percival Bailey[15] presented "spongioblastoma cerebelli" as soft embryonal tumors arising from the roof of the fourth ventricle, later renamed for a neural stem cell that has never been found (medulloblast); Cushing also reported that although medulloblastoma was often a disease of childhood (mean age 11 years), there is a different age predilection between midline vermian tumors (mean age 8 years) and lateral hemispheric tumors (mean age 31 years).[15] A quarter of cases present in adulthood, usually between 20 and 40 years old, with case reports up to 73 years old, and approximately three-quarters of these cases are lateral hemispheric, not midline vermian, which is the exact reverse of the usual pattern in childhood.[16]

The reason for this may be related to embryology and development. Modern DNA microarray gene expression analysis has shown medulloblastomas are molecularly distinct from other embryonal tumors of the CNS (primitive neuroectodermal tumor and atypical teratoid rhabdoid tumor) and are derived from cerebellar granule cell precursors, not from primitive neuroepithelial cells in the subventricular germinal matrix.[17] These cerebellar granule cell precursors migrate laterally from the rhombic lip at the roof of the fourth ventricle to the external granular layer at the surface of the cerebellar hemispheres, which may explain a more lateral preference for tumors arising later in life.[18] Due to high cellular density (small round blue cell tumor), medulloblastomas are usually hyperattenuating on CT and may be low signal intensity on T2-weighted or apparent diffusion coefficient (ADC)-weighted MR images, with circumscribed margins and variable enhancement (**Fig. 2**); peripheral tumors in adults potentially resemble meningiomas, which magnetic resonance (MR) spectroscopy can effectively distinguish (alanine peak is increased in meningiomas, $P<.001$).[19,20]

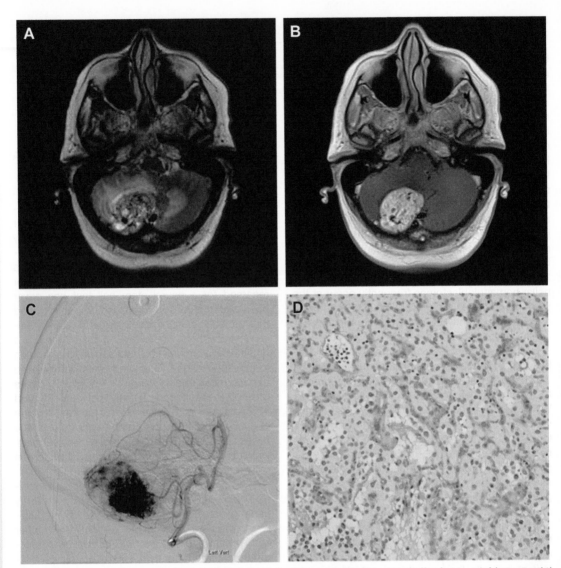

Fig. 1. A 64-year-old woman with multiple falls and shuffling gait due to a cerebellar hemangioblastoma. (*A*) Axial T2 image shows a circumscribed mass with hypervascular flow voids and vasogenic edema in the right cerebellar hemisphere. (*B*) Axial postgadolinium T1 image shows intense enhancement. (*C*) Cerebral angiography in lateral projection from left vertebral artery injection shows a hypervascular tumor blush. (*D*) Photomicrograph (H&E, original magnification ×20) shows endothelial (thin-walled vessels) and stromal components (clear vacuolated cells) in the tumor. (AIRP case contributor: Dr Paul Heideman.)

Analysis of 2037 medulloblastomas from National Cancer Institute Surveillance, Epidemiology, and End Results database found a 5-year cumulative relative survival rate of 67% in adults, lower than adolescents (69%) and children (72%) and higher than infants (42%).[21] Standard therapy is resection followed by craniospinal radiation, with metastases at presentation or recurrence conferring a worse prognosis.[22] Medulloblastoma has 4 histologic variants—the desmoplastic variant is more associated with lateral hemispheric masses in adults.[23] Medulloblastoma also has 4 molecular variants—the sonic hedgehog (SHH) pathway is activated in most adult cases.[24] These molecular subgroups have been linked to prognosis and phenotype (Fig. 3). WNT and SHH tumors have a better prognosis and localize to the cerebellar peduncles and hemispheres respectively. Groups 3 and 4 tumors have a worse prognosis and tend to be midline.[25]

ASTROCYTIC TUMORS: PILOCYTIC ASTROCYTOMA (WHO GRADE I)

Setting aside primitive embryonal tumors, primary neuroepithelial tumors of the CNS may

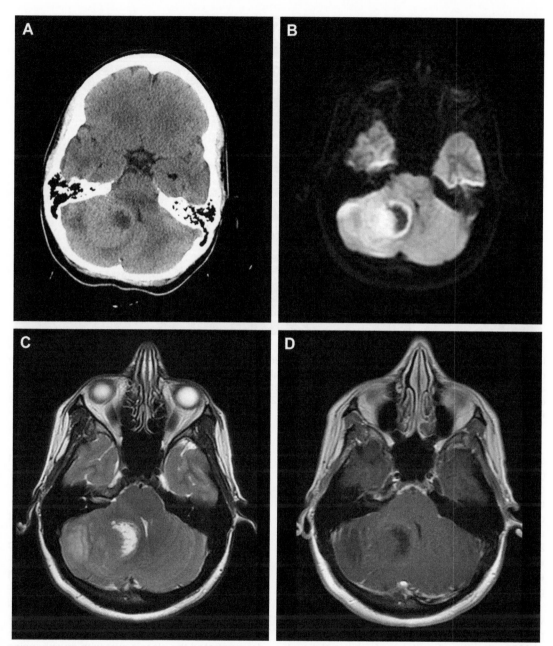

Fig. 2. A 25-year-old woman with medulloblastoma in a more lateral or hemispheric location. (A) Head CT shows a mostly hyperattenuating mass in the right cerebellum. (B) Axial DWI image shows corresponding restricted diffusion, which reflects high cellular density (small round blue cell tumor). (C) Axial T2 image shows a mostly isointense mass with cystic or necrotic changes. (D) Axial postgadolinium T1 image shows no enhancement. Medulloblastomas are more often lateral than midline in adults (opposite of children).

show glial or neuronal differentiation. With regard to gliomas, the glial cell of origin may be the astrocyte, the oligodendrocyte, the ependymal cell, or the choroid plexus epithelium. Gliomas may also be subdivided into circumscribed versus diffuse/infiltrative, based on the margins with the adjacent brain parenchyma. The classic example of a circumscribed astrocytoma is the juvenile pilocytic astrocytoma, which most commonly presents in childhood as a cerebellar or suprasellar mass, or along the optic pathways in the setting of neurofibromatosis type 1.[26] The

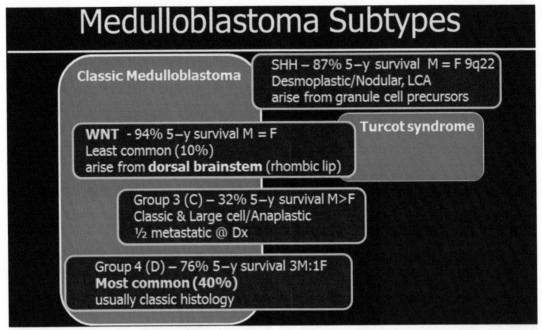

Fig. 3. Medulloblastoma has 4 histologic subtypes (classic, desmoplastic-nodular, large cell-anaplastic, and medul-loblastoma with extensive nodularity) as well as 4 molecular subtypes (WNT, SHH, group 3, and group 4). The desmoplastic-nodular histologic subtype and SHH molecular subtype are more common in adults than in children and are associated with a hemispheric location and a better prognosis. (*Data from* Molecular subgroups of medullablastoma: the current consensus. Acta Neuropathol 2012;123:465–72; and Medulloblastomics: the end of the following. Nat Rev Cancer 2012;12:818–34.)

solid component of pilocytic astrocytomas often (but not always) enhances on CT or MR imaging, due to abnormal vessels with a leaky blood-brain barrier; many demonstrate internal or neighbor cyst formation, producing a nonenhancing cyst and enhancing mural nodule appearance in 21% of cases.[27] Tumor margins tend to be well-defined with a lesser degree of peritumoral edema, compared with high-grade infiltrative gliomas.

Adult pilocytic astrocytoma is a rare diagnosis, with incidence of less than 0.1 case per 100,000 person-years in adults over age 45 years. Analysis of 3066 pilocytic astrocytomas from the National Cancer Institute Surveillance, Epidemiology, and End Results database found differences in location and prognosis between adult and pediatric patients. Although the cerebellum was the most common site in children (37%), it was slightly outnumbered by the cerebral lobes in adults (27% vs 30%). And although the cancer-specific 5-year survival rates were excellent in children (>95%), they dropped to 92%, 79%, and 64% within the 20 to 39, 40 to 59, and 60+ age groups, respectively.[28] Molecular analysis in a large series of 127 adult pilocytic astrocytomas found the BRAF-KIAA1549 fusion gene in only

20%—whereas BRAF-KIAA1549 fusion is present in greater than 60% of pediatric cases and may confer a less aggressive clinical phenotype.[29,30] Despite a higher recurrence rate in adults (30%), standard treatment is resection without adjuvant radiation.[31]

The radiologic findings are similar to pediatric pilocytic astrocytoma, with variable enhancement and cyst formation. In 1 series of 44 adult pilocytic astrocytomas, 45% were lobar (cerebral) and 27% were cerebellar, 50% were solid with variable enhancement from strong to none (**Fig. 4**), 29% were mixed solid-cystic, and 21% demonstrated the classic cyst with an enhancing mural nodule appearance.[32] A solid or mixed solid-cystic enhancing pilocytic astrocytoma can be mistaken for a high-grade glioma or metastasis in an adult patient. Elevated choline on MR spectroscopy and hypermetabolism on FDG-PET may further confuse the picture.[33] Another functional imaging technique that can be more helpful in distinguishing pilocytic from high-grade astrocytomas is diffusion-weighted imaging (DWI), with higher ADC values in pilocytic astrocytomas.[34] Anaplastic or malignant transformation (WHO grade III) is a rare phenomenon.

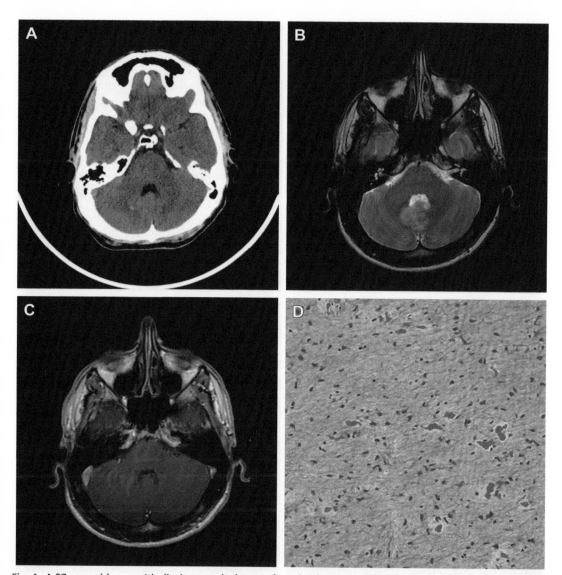

Fig. 4. A 27-year-old man with dizziness and who was found to have a cerebellar pilocytic astrocytoma. (*A*) Head CT shows a subtle isoattenuating lesion in the right medial cerebellum. (*B*) Axial T2 image shows a round circumscribed hyperintense mass. (*C*) Axial postgadolinium T1 image shows no enhancement. (*D*) Photomicrograph (H&E, original magnification ×20) shows pilocytic cells with hairlike processes plus lots of Rosenthal fibers. Although pilocytic astrocytomas often demonstrate cyst formation and contrast enhancement, they can be purely solid or nonenhancing. (AIRP case contributor: Dr Matthew Maeder.)

ASTROCYTIC/OLIGODENDROGLIAL TUMORS: DIFFUSE/INFILTRATIVE GLIOMAS (WHO GRADES II–IV)

Diffuse or infiltrative gliomas include low-grade astrocytoma or oligodendroglioma (WHO grade II), anaplastic astrocytoma or oligodendroglioma (WHO grade III), and glioblastoma (WHO grade IV). In the posterior fossa, they account for most brainstem gliomas, which are more common in children than in adults (10%–20% vs 1%–2% of

brain tumors); diffuse intrinsic brainstem gliomas (eg, pontine gliomas) comprise up to 80% of pediatric and 50% of adult brainstem gliomas.[35] They cause cranial nerve or long tract deficits and share the same imaging pattern in both populations: an expansile T2 hyperintense lesion affecting greater than 50% of the brainstem diameter, with poorly defined margins, without significant enhancement, and with elevated choline on MR spectroscopy (**Fig. 5**A).[36] Median survival is very different, approximately 9 to 12 months in children and

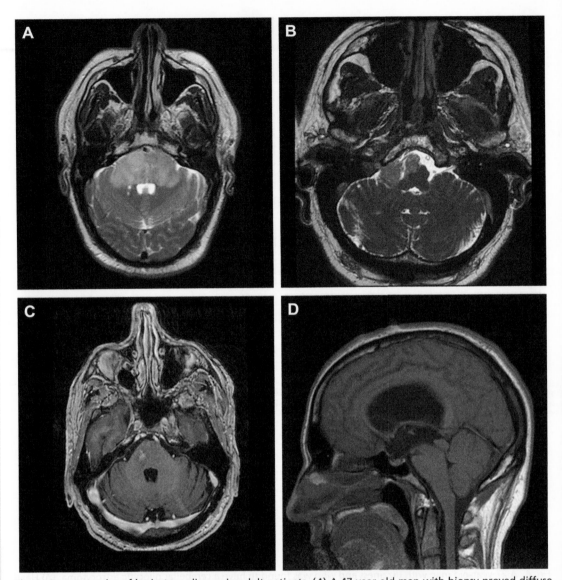

Fig. 5. Four examples of brainstem gliomas in adult patients. (A) A 47-year-old man with biopsy-proved diffuse intrinsic pontine glioma (low-grade astrocytoma) on axial T2 image (nonenhancing, not shown). (B) A 41-year-old man with biopsy-proved infiltrative brainstem glioma (anaplastic oligodendroglioma) on axial 3-D FIESTA image (exophytic growth along cranial nerves into right jugular foramen). (C) A 71-year-old man with focal enhancing malignant brainstem glioma on axial postgadolinium T1 image (diagnosis was high-grade astrocytoma at autopsy). (D) A 32-year-old man with focal tectal glioma in the dorsal midbrain (not biopsied) and severe obstructive hydrocephalus on sagittal T1 image, which was treated with shunting.

5 to 7 years in adults, because a majority of these tumors are high grade in children and low grade in adults.[37]

Although nonenhancing infiltrative brainstem gliomas tend to present in younger adults (age < 40), a second MR imaging pattern tends to present in older adults and comprises 30% of adult brainstem gliomas: a contrast-enhancing infiltrative lesion, often with intratumoral necrosis and peritumoral edema (Fig. 5C).[38] Median survival is only 11 months for these high-grade or malignant brainstem gliomas; negative prognostic factors for brainstem gliomas include age greater than 40, duration of symptoms less than 3 months, Karnofsky performance status less than 70, high-grade histology, contrast enhancement, and tumoral necrosis.[39] For both nonenhancing and enhancing adult brainstem gliomas, molecular features and clinical outcomes are similar to supratentorial IDH1 wild-type tumors for the same WHO grade.[40] Resection is not possible for infiltrative brainstem gliomas; therefore, standard treatment is stereotactic biopsy to confirm the diagnosis, followed by radiation therapy.[41]

Even though cranial nerves III–XII are peripheral nerves, glial cells (oligodendrocytes) extend to root entry/exit zones and along proximal cisternal segments, before they are replaced by Schwann cells; therefore, infiltrative brainstem gliomas can rarely involve cranial nerves (Fig. 5B).[42] Recognition of the intra-axial origin may prevent misdiagnosis as an extra-axial tumor with perineural spread, for example, nerve sheath tumor, meningioma, or carcinoma. Finally, in addition to the 2 MR imaging patterns discussed previously, there are focal tectal gliomas, which account for only 8% of brainstem gliomas in adults. These tumors are centered in the dorsal midbrain, occupying less than 50% of the brainstem diameter, and are well-defined without enhancement (Fig. 5D).[38] They have a benign and indolent natural history, with median survival of more than 10 years, and are usually low-grade when biopsied. Treatment is directed at the hydrocephalus (eg, endoscopic third ventriculostomy), rather than at the tumor.

EPENDYMAL TUMORS: SUBEPENDYMOMA AND EPENDYMOMA (WHO GRADES I–III)

The 2007 WHO classification includes 4 ependymal tumors: subependymoma (WHO grade I), myxopapillary ependymoma (WHO grade I), ependymoma (WHO grade II), and anaplastic ependymoma (WHO grade III). Subependymoma is a rare benign slow-growing neoplasm arising from glial cells in the subependymal plate, which may show astrocytic or ependymal features on histology, and which can be symptomatic or incidental (0.7% of resected brain tumors vs 0.4% of routine autopsies).[43] It has been reported from the second to ninth decades but is most common in older adults (mean age 57 years).[44] Most are intracranial and project into the fourth (50%–60%) or lateral (30%–40%) ventricles; few are intramedullary and arise around the central canal of the spinal cord.[45] On MR imaging, intracranial subependymomas tend to be completely intraventricular, with heterogeneous internal signal and often with little edema or enhancement (Fig. 6).[46]

Myxopapillary ependymoma is an intradural extramedullary tumor of the filum terminale in the lumbar spine and is not discussed further. Low-grade (WHO grade II) ependymoma and anaplastic ependymoma are thought to arise from ependymal cells lining the ventricles and central canal, or from radial glial cells in the brain parenchyma. These tumors have been reported at all ages but are most common in children, when they usually present in the fourth ventricle (10% of pediatric brain tumors). In adults, ependymoma involves the spinal cord (arising from central canal) more often than the brain (2%–6% of adult brain tumors), where it involves the supratentorial compartment (cerebral hemispheres or lateral ventricles) more often than the posterior fossa.[47] Infratentorial ependymomas account for 40% of adult intracranial ependymomas and can be midline (fourth ventricle) or lateral (cerebellopontine angles). Cerebrospinal fluid (CSF) dissemination complicates 3% to 15% of intracranial ependymomas, is more frequent in the setting of infratentorial or anaplastic tumors, and necessitates treatment with craniospinal irradiation.[48]

Like subependymoma, ependymoma often demonstrates heterogeneous internal signal on MR imaging, secondary to intratumoral calcifications, cysts, or hemorrhage (Fig. 7). Unlike subependymoma, ependymoma has a propensity to "ooze out of the foramina" of Luschka or Magendie, when located inside the fourth ventricle, and for paraventricular or transependymal invasion into the brain parenchyma.[49] Also, unlike subependymoma, ependymoma tends to be more vascular and frequently exhibits intense enhancement in the solid portions.[50] Although there is overlap and variability in the imaging appearance of both tumors, a nonenhancing and purely intraventricular mass favors subependymoma (especially in an older adult), whereas a strongly enhancing mass with transependymal invasion favors ependymoma. Maximal resection plus adjuvant radiotherapy has been shown to improve progression-free survival in adults with posterior fossa ependymomas.[51]

CHOROID PLEXUS TUMORS AND MENINGIOMA (WHO GRADES I–III)

Most tumors appearing as intraventricular arise in the brain parenchyma or ventricular wall and extend into the ventricle (eg, medulloblastoma or ependymoma). Few arise from the choroid plexus within the ventricular lumen. Except for the occipital horns and the cerebral aqueduct, choroid plexus is found inside all parts of the ventricular system and is a highly vascularized structure, responsible for CSF production via plasma filtration and active secretion (blood-CSF barrier). It is formed during embryologic development by invagination of

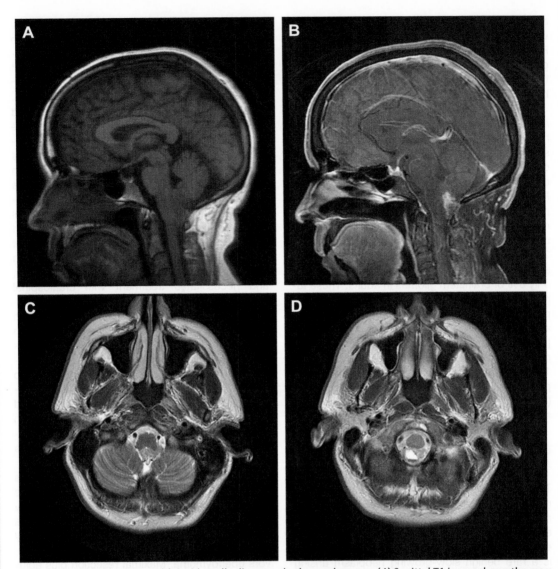

Fig. 6. A 52-year-old woman with incidentally discovered subependymoma. (*A*) Sagittal T1 image shows the mass at the inferior portion of the fourth ventricle. (*B*) Sagittal postgadolinium T1 image shows mild heterogeneous enhancement at the inferior aspect of the neoplasm. (*C*) Axial T2 image at the foramina of Luschka shows a solid component. (*D*) Axial T2 image at a slightly lower level shows a hemorrhagic or cystic component. The imaging differential diagnosis for a heterogeneous enhancing mass in the fourth ventricle includes ependymoma. Subependymoma is more likely to be hypovascular or nonenhancing.

choroidal arteries from the subarachnoid space, through leptomeninges and ependyma into the ventricles, and therefore, the choroid plexus epithelium derives from modified ependymal cells, whereas the fibrovascular stroma derives from the underlying leptomeninges. Choroid plexus is especially abundant within the atrium/trigone of the lateral ventricle (glomus choroideum); therefore, both neoplastic and non-neoplastic (eg, xanthogranuloma) pathology of the choroid plexus demonstrates a predilection for that location.[52]

Choroid plexus tumors arise from the neuroepithelial lining and include papilloma (WHO grade I), atypical papilloma (WHO grade II), and carcinoma (WHO grade III). They are rare and affect children (2%–4% of pediatric brain tumors) more frequently than adults (0.5% of adult brain tumors).[45] They are found in the lateral ventricle (43%), fourth ventricle (39%), and third ventricle (11%) as well as the cerebellopontine angle (7%), arising from small choroid tufts that normally project outside the foramen of Luschka.[53] Location is age dependent: approximately 70% of pediatric cases are

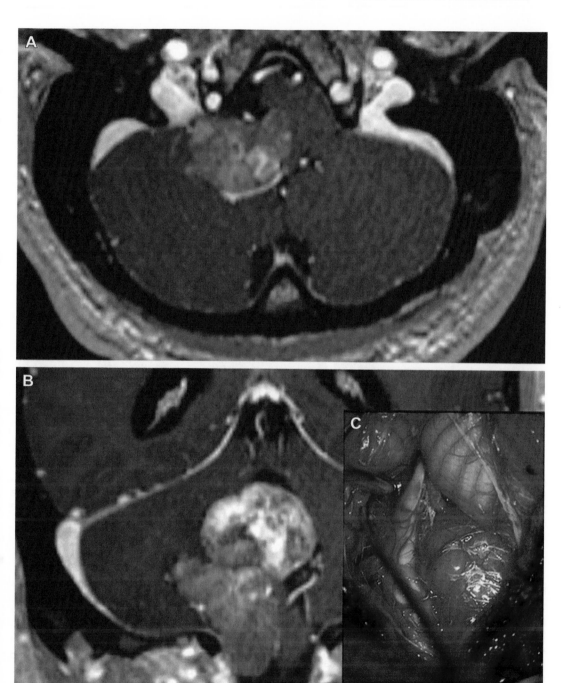

Fig. 7. A 29-year-old man with dizziness and vertigo, due to an ependymoma in the fourth ventricle. (*A*) Axial postgadolinium T1 image shows a heterogeneous enhancing mass at the right foramen of Luschka. (*B*) Coronal postgadolinium T1 image shows the mass inside the fourth ventricle. (*C*) Intraoperative photo shows a posterior view of the cerebellum and tumor. (AIRP case contributor: Dr Mohammad Shujaat.)

seen in the lateral ventricle (usually atrium or trigone); approximately 70% of adult cases are seen in the fourth ventricle.[54] Like ependymoma, choroid plexus papilloma is a circumscribed intraventricular mass with internal heterogeneity and intense enhancement; unlike ependymoma,

papilloma may show lobulated margins and hydrocephalus from CSF overproduction (**Fig. 8**).[55]

Approximately 20% of choroid plexus tumors are carcinomas, which are most common in infants and young children, but have been described in adults. They tend to be more invasive and

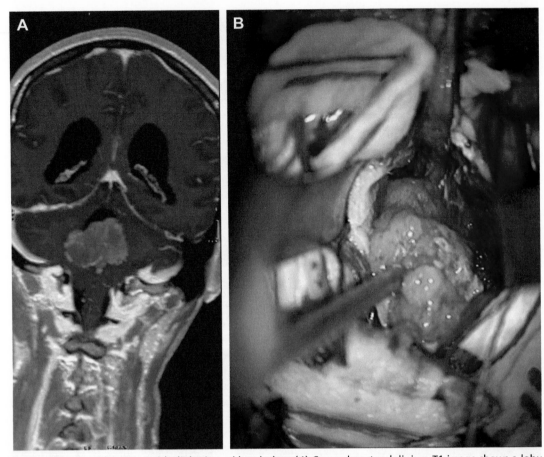

Fig. 8. A 39-year-old woman with diplopia and headaches. (*A*) Coronal postgadolinium T1 image shows a lobulated enhancing mass in the fourth ventricle with lateral ventriculomegaly. (*B*) Intraoperative photo shows a lobulated papillary mass in the fourth ventricle, which is the most common location for choroid plexus papilloma in adults (atrium or trigone of the lateral ventricles in children). (AIRP case contributor: Dr Maud Tijssen.)

hemorrhagic than papillomas; they also demonstrate higher CBF values on arterial spin-labeling perfusion-weighted imaging.[56] Nevertheless, because of significant overlap in the imaging appearance, it is acceptable to include choroid plexus tumors as a group in the differential diagnosis for an enhancing mass centered on the choroid plexus (ie, leave grading to a pathologist). Other entities that belong in the differential diagnosis include meningioma and metastasis. Meningiomas are intraventricular in less than 1% of cases, arising from meningothelial or arachnoidal cap cells in the choroid plexus stroma, usually in the atrium or trigone of the lateral ventricle and rarely in the posterior fossa.[50] Metastases account for only 6% of intraventricular neoplasms, despite the vascularity of the choroid plexus, and have been reported most commonly with renal and lung carcinoma.[57]

NEURONAL TUMORS: DYSPLASTIC CEREBELLAR GANGLIOCYTOMA (WHO GRADE I)

In 1920, Lhermitte and Duclos first reported on a cerebellar ganglion cell tumor in a 36-year-old man with progressive neurologic deficits. Dysplastic cerebellar gangliocytomas (also known as Lhermitte-Duclos disease, purkinjeoma, or granular cell hypertrophy of the cerebellum) are rare slowly growing tumors, which usually present with symptoms of local mass effect in young adults (mean age 34 years).[58] There is a classic striated cerebellum appearance on MR imaging, manifesting as alternating bands or tiger stripes of T1 hypointensity or T2 hyperintensity, which correlate with expanded or club-shaped cerebellar folia on gross pathology (Fig. 9). On histology, there is disorganized cytoarchitecture in the

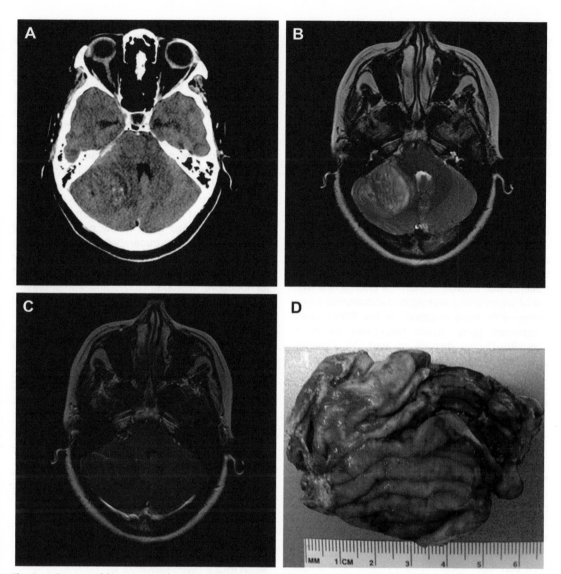

Fig. 9. A 31-year-old woman with right-sided headaches, found to have an ipsilateral cerebellar mass. (*A*) Head CT shows a heterogeneous isoattenuating mass in the right cerebellum with a few calcifications. (*B*) Axial T2 image shows a round circumscribed mass with internal striations (suggestive but not specific for Lhermitte-Duclos disease). (*C*) Axial postgadolinium T1 image shows a prominent vein without any tumor enhancement. (*D*) Gross specimen shows thickened folia in a dysplastic gangliocytoma of the cerebellum (Lhermitte-Duclos disease). (AIRP case contributor: Dr Angela Sam.)

cerebellar cortex: thickening with hypermyelination in the outer molecular layer, loss of cells in the middle Purkinje layer, and thickening with abnormally enlarged ganglion cells in the inner granular layer.[59] Radiologic-pathologic correlation suggests that the gyriform T1 and T2 signal changes may be secondary to increased intracellular water in the hypertrophied granular layer.[60]

Dysplastic gangliocytomas can have variable density on CT and may show restricted diffusion on MR imaging, due to high cellularity. There is commonly elevated rCBV on perfusion-weighted imaging and rarely gadolinium enhancement at the cortical or pial surface, due to high vascularity.[61,62] Also, hyperperfusion can be accompanied by increased uptake of thallium on single-photon emission CT or glucose on PET; therefore, Lhermitte-Duclos disease may be mistaken for high-grade tumor (eg, medulloblastoma), or vice versa, on preoperative imaging. Of the functional techniques, MR spectroscopy is most likely to be helpful because there are decreased levels of most metabolites, including choline, which would be unusual in a high-grade tumor. Elevated lactate peaks have been observed, without increased levels of lipid (no necrosis), which in conjunction with hypermetabolism on fluorodeoxyglucose (FDG)-PET, may reflect abnormally high rates of glycolysis in excess of the Krebs cycle.[63,64]

Dysplastic gangliocytoma of the cerebellum is categorized as a neuronal tumor under the 2007 WHO classification; however, there is controversy as to whether it represents a slow-growing neoplasm or hamartoma. Propensity for recurrence after subtotal resection has been used as evidence for a low-grade neoplasm.[65] On the other hand, Lhermitte-Duclos disease is associated in 40% of cases with Cowden syndrome, which is a rare autosomal dominant inherited disorder characterized by multiple hamartomas of the skin and mucosa. Patients with Cowden syndrome also have a high risk of breast (28%), thyroid, and endometrial carcinoma—80% have mutations in the PTEN tumor suppressor gene, which has been linked to Lhermitte-Duclos disease as well.[66,67] Cowden syndrome may be considered a phakomatosis with multiple neurocutaneous hamartomas and autosomal dominant inheritance (PTEN vs NF1, NF2, and VHL tumor suppressor genes).

NEURONAL TUMORS: CEREBELLAR LIPONEUROCYTOMA (WHO GRADE II)

In 1978, Bechtel and colleagues[68] reported "an unusual cerebellar tumor composed of mixed mesenchymal and neuroectodermal elements in a 44 year old man," with both well-differentiated adipose tissue and medulloblastomatous components. It has been given different names in the past (eg, lipomatous medulloblastoma) and was officially inducted as "cerebellar liponeurocytoma" in the 2000 WHO classification. There is no mesenchymal or lipomatous component; immunohistochemistry has confirmed the clusters of lipidized cells are reactive for synaptophysin and are neurocytic in origin. Although the nonlipidized neurocytes are densely packed and resemble medulloblastoma on microscopy, this neuronal or mixed neuronal-glial tumor presents in an older population (mean age 50 years) and is much less aggressive with low mitotic activity.[69] It is more similar in prognosis to central neurocytoma, a supratentorial WHO grade II neuronal tumor.[70]

Like medulloblastoma, cerebellar liponeurocytoma may involve the cerebellar hemispheres or vermis, is typically well-circumscribed with little peritumoral edema, and demonstrates heterogeneous or variable enhancement.[71] There is propensity for exophytic growth into the adjacent cerebellopontine angles or fourth ventricle; therefore, the preoperative differential diagnosis may also include ependymoma.[72] Although liponeurocytoma is ultimately a pathologic diagnosis, the visualization of macroscopic fat attenuation or signal within a cerebellar mass on CT/MR imaging should prompt consideration of this rare neoplasm.[73] Molecular analysis of gene expression profiles from cerebellar liponeurocytoma is similar to central neurocytoma but distinct from medulloblastoma; there is also significant overexpression of fatty acid binding protein 4 (FABP4), which is normally found in adipocytes or macrophages and not in normal cerebellum.[74]

There have also been a few case reports of supratentorial or extracerebellar liponeurocytomas, which are analogous to infratentorial or cerebellar liponeurocytomas on radiology (except for location), histopathology, and immunohistochemistry. Given the predilection for the lateral ventricles in younger adults, supratentorial liponeurocytomas are not currently part of the 2007 WHO classification and may be considered a rare lipidized variant of central neurocytoma.[75,76] Other case reports have described familial (an underlying germline mutation has not been identified yet) and multifocal cerebellar liponeurocytomas.[77,78] Treatment is surgical resection; however, up to 50% of patients have local recurrence on long-term follow-up. Adjuvant radiotherapy to the posterior fossa has been recommended for subtotal resections and for any liponeurocytomas with unusually aggressive histology (Ki-67 proliferation index >6%).[79]

NEURONAL TUMORS: ROSETTE-FORMING GLIONEURONAL TUMOR OF THE FOURTH VENTRICLE (WHO GRADE I)

In 2002, Komori and colleagues[80] reported "eleven cases of a distinctive tumor of the posterior fossa [with] relatively discrete, focally enhancing mass(es) primarily involving the aqueduct, fourth ventricle, and cerebellar vermis." They were mixed neuronal-glial tumors, characterized by biphasic architecture with neurocytic and astrocytic components. Similar lesions had previously been classified as dysembryoplastic neuroepithelial tumors of the cerebellum; however, there were important histopathologic differences, for example, the formation of neurocytic rosettes and perivascular pseudorosettes as well as the frequent presence of a pilocytic astrocytoma-like component. These differences led to a new entity of RGNT of the fourth ventricle, officially introduced in the most recent 2007 WHO classification "as a rare, slowly growing tumor of the fourth ventricular region that predominantly affects young adults (mean age 33)."[3]

In 1 meta-analysis of 41 patients with RGNT, the most common presenting symptoms were headaches (68%) and ataxia (39%), with frequent obstructive hydrocephalus (44%). Most are midline lesions of the posterior fossa; they are thought to arise from pluripotential cells in the subependymal plate at the ventricular wall (Fig. 10). These tumors can be solid or mixed solid-cystic and often demonstrated focal contrast enhancement (82%).[81] There is usually heterogeneous hypointensity on T1 and hyperintensity on T2 weighted images, with hypointense foci on T2* weighted images (gradient-recalled echo/susceptibility-weighted imaging) related to intratumoral calcification or hemorrhage. Both the occurrence of satellite lesions and drop metastases through CSF dissemination have been described.[82] There have also been case reports of RGNT arising outside the fourth ventricle, most commonly in the pineal region, and around

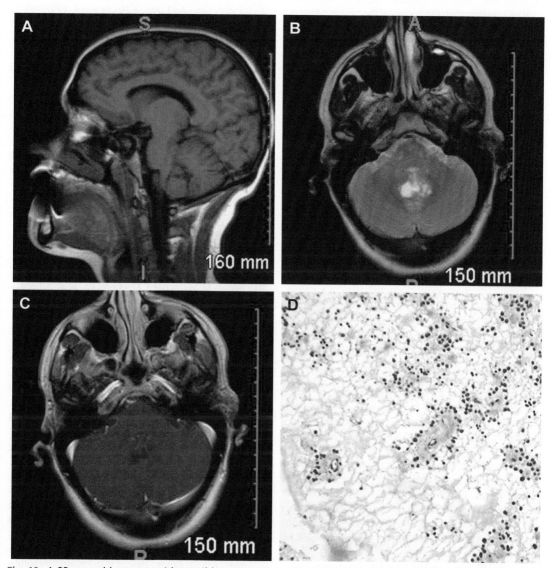

Fig. 10. A 22-year-old woman with possible seizure, found to have a lesion in the midline posterior fossa. (A) Sagittal T1 image shows a multicystic lesion involving the cerebellar vermis. (B) Axial T2 image shows a multicystic lesion at the posterior aspect of the fourth ventricle. (C) Axial postgadolinium T1 image shows no enhancement, in this particular RGNT. (D) Photomicrograph (H&E, original magnification ×20) shows a propensity to form neurocytic rosettes and perivascular pseudorosettes. (AIRP case contributor: Dr Jean Francois Mercier.)

other CSF-containing spaces from third ventricle to central canal.[83]

REFERENCES

1. Roller LA, Bruce BB, Saindane AM. Demographic confounders in volumetric MRI analysis: is the posterior fossa really small in the adult Chiari 1 malformation? AJR Am J Roentgenol 2015;204(4):835–41.
2. Barkovich J, Raybaud C. Pediatric neuroimaging. 5th edition. Philadelphia (PA): Lippincott Williams & Wilkins; 2012.
3. Louis DN, Ohgaki H, Wiestler OD, et al. The 2007 WHO classification of tumours of the central nervous system. Acta Neuropathol 2007;114(2):97–109.
4. Neumann HP, Eggert HR, Weigel K, et al. Hemangioblastomas of the central nervous system. A 10-year study with special reference to von Hippel-Lindau syndrome. J Neurosurg 1989;70(1):24–30.
5. Lonser R, Oldfield E. Hemangioblastomas. In: Winn R, editor. Youmans neurological surgery. 6th edition. Philadelphia (PA): Saunders; 2011. p. 1389–99.
6. Courcoutsakis NA, Prassopoulos PK, Patronas NJ. Aggressive leptomeningeal hemangioblastomatosis of the central nervous system in a patient with von Hippel-Lindau disease. AJNR Am J Neuroradiol 2009;30(4):758–60.
7. Kim H, Park IS, Jo KW. Meningeal supratentorial hemangioblastoma in a patient with von hippel-lindau disease mimicking angioblastic menigioma. J Korean Neurosurg Soc 2013;54(5):415–9.
8. Doyle LA, Fletcher CD. Peripheral hemangioblastoma: clinicopathologic characterization in a series of 22 cases. Am J Surg Pathol 2014;38(1):119–27.
9. Park DM, Zhuang Z, Chen L, et al. von Hippel-Lindau disease-associated hemangioblastomas are derived from embryologic multipotent cells. PLoS Med 2007;4(2):e60.
10. Lee SR, Sanches J, Mark AS, et al. Posterior fossa hemangioblastomas: MR imaging. Radiology 1989; 171(2):463–8.
11. Ho VB, Smirniotopoulos JG, Murphy FM, et al. Radiologic-pathologic correlation: hemangioblastoma. AJNR Am J Neuroradiol 1992;13(5):1343–52.
12. Lonser RR, Vortmeyer AO, Butman JA, et al. Edema is a precursor to central nervous system peritumoral cyst formation. Ann Neurol 2005;58(3):392–9.
13. Slater A, Moore NR, Huson SM. The natural history of cerebellar hemangioblastomas in von Hippel-Lindau disease. AJNR Am J Neuroradiol 2003; 24(8):1570–4.
14. Hoang MP, Amirkhan RH. Inhibin alpha distinguishes hemangioblastoma from clear cell renal cell carcinoma. Am J Surg Pathol 2003;27(8):1152–6.
15. Shonka N, Brandes A, De Groot JF. Adult medulloblastoma, from spongioblastoma cerebelli to the present day: a review of treatment and the integration of molecular markers. Oncology (Williston Park) 2012;26(11):1083–91.
16. Koeller KK, Rushing EJ. From the archives of the AFIP: medulloblastoma: a comprehensive review with radiologic-pathologic correlation. Radiographics 2003;23(6):1613–37.
17. Pomeroy SL, Tamayo P, Gaasenbeek M, et al. Prediction of central nervous system embryonal tumour outcome based on gene expression. Nature 2002; 415(6870):436–42.
18. Bourgouin PM, Tampieri D, Grahovac SZ, et al. CT and MR imaging findings in adults with cerebellar medulloblastoma: comparison with findings in children. AJR Am J Roentgenol 1992;159(3):609–12.
19. Koci TM, Chiang F, Mehringer CM, et al. Adult cerebellar medulloblastoma: imaging features with emphasis on MR findings. AJNR Am J Neuroradiol 1993;14(4):929–39.
20. Majós C, Alonso J, Aguilera C, et al. Adult primitive neuroectodermal tumor: proton MR spectroscopic findings with possible application for differential diagnosis. Radiology 2002;225(2):556–66.
21. Smoll NR. Relative survival of childhood and adult medulloblastomas and primitive neuroectodermal tumors (PNETs). Cancer 2012;118(5):1313–22.
22. Riffaud L, Saikali S, Leray E, et al. Survival and prognostic factors in a series of adults with medulloblastomas. J Neurosurg 2009;111(3):478–87.
23. Levy RA, Blaivas M, Muraszko K, et al. Desmoplastic medulloblastoma: MR findings. AJNR Am J Neuroradiol 1997;18(7):1364–6.
24. Remke M, Hielscher T, Northcott PA, et al. Adult medulloblastoma comprises three major molecular variants. J Clin Oncol 2011;29(19):2717–23.
25. Perreault S, Ramaswamy V, Achrol AS, et al. MRI surrogates for molecular subgroups of medulloblastoma. AJNR Am J Neuroradiol 2014;35(7):1263–9.
26. Lee YY, Van Tassel P, Bruner JM, et al. Juvenile pilocytic astrocytomas: CT and MR characteristics. AJR Am J Roentgenol 1989;152(6):1263–70.
27. Koeller KK, Rushing EJ. From the archives of the AFIP: pilocytic astrocytoma: radiologic-pathologic correlation. Radiographics 2004;24(6):1693–708.
28. Johnson DR, Brown PD, Galanis E, et al. Pilocytic astrocytoma survival in adults: analysis of the surveillance, epidemiology, and end results program of the National Cancer Institute. J Neurooncol 2012;108(1):187–93.
29. Theeler BJ, Ellezam B, Sadighi ZS, et al. Adult pilocytic astrocytomas: clinical features and molecular analysis. Neuro Oncol 2014;16(6):841–7.
30. Hawkins C, Walker E, Mohamed N, et al. BRAF-KIAA1549 fusion predicts better clinical outcome in pediatric low-grade astrocytoma. Clin Cancer Res 2011;17(14):4790–8.

31. Ellis JA, Waziri A, Balmaceda C, et al. Rapid recurrence and malignant transformation of pilocytic astrocytoma in adult patients. J Neurooncol 2009; 95(3):377–82.

32. Stüer C, Vilz B, Majores M, et al. Frequent recurrence and progression in pilocytic astrocytoma in adults. Cancer 2007;110(12):2799–808.

33. Fulham MJ, Melisi JW, Nishimiya J, et al. Neuroimaging of juvenile pilocytic astrocytomas: an enigma. Radiology 1993;189(1):221–5.

34. de Fatima Vasco Aragao M, Law M, Batista de Almeida D, et al. Comparison of perfusion, diffusion, and MR spectroscopy between low-grade enhancing pilocytic astrocytomas and high-grade astrocytomas. AJNR Am J Neuroradiol 2014; 35(8):1495–502.

35. Laigle-Donadey F, Doz F, Delattre JY. Brainstem gliomas in children and adults. Curr Opin Oncol 2008; 20(6):662–7.

36. Reyes-Botero G, Mokhtari K, Martin-Duverneuil N, et al. Adult brainstem gliomas. Oncologist 2012; 17(3):388–97.

37. Landolfi JC, Thaler HT, DeAngelis LM. Adult brainstem gliomas. Neurology 1998;51(4):1136–9.

38. Purohit B, Kamli AA, Kollias SS. Imaging of adult brainstem gliomas. Eur J Radiol 2015;84(4): 709–20.

39. Guillamo JS, Monjour A, Taillandier L, et al. Brainstem gliomas in adults: prognostic factors and classification. Brain 2001;124(Pt 12):2528–39.

40. Theeler BJ, Ellezam B, Melguizo-Gavilanes I, et al. Adult brainstem gliomas: correlation of clinical and molecular features. J Neurol Sci 2015; 353(1–2):92–7.

41. Reithmeier T, Kuzeawu A, Hentschel B, et al. Retrospective analysis of 104 histologically proven adult brainstem gliomas: clinical symptoms, therapeutic approaches and prognostic factors. BMC Cancer 2014;14:115.

42. Mabray MC, Glastonbury CM, Mamlouk MD, et al. Direct cranial nerve involvement by Gliomas: case series and review of the literature. AJNR Am J Neuroradiol 2015;36(7):1349–54.

43. Bi Z, Ren X, Zhang J, et al. Clinical, radiological, and pathological features in 43 cases of intracranial subependymoma. J Neurosurg 2015;122(1):49–60.

44. Yachnis A, Rivera-Zengotita M. Ependymomas and subependymoma. In: Yachnis A, Rivera-Zengotita M, editors. Neuropathology. Philadelphia (PA): Saunders; 2014. p. 99–106.

45. Smith AB, Smirniotopoulos JG, Horkanyne-Szakaly I. From the radiologic pathology archives: intraventricular neoplasms: radiologic-pathologic correlation. Radiographics 2013;33(1):21–43.

46. Hoeffel C, Boukobza M, Polivka M, et al. MR manifestations of subependymomas. AJNR Am J Neuroradiol 1995;16(10):2121–9.

47. Frazier J, Jallo G. Intracranial ependymomas in adults. In: Winn R, editor. Youmans neurological surgery. 6th edition. Philadelphia (PA): Saunders; 2011. p. 1383–8.

48. Rudà R, Gilbert M, Soffietti R. Ependymomas of the adult: molecular biology and treatment. Curr Opin Neurol 2008;21(6):754–61.

49. Spoto GP, Press GA, Hesselink JR, et al. Intracranial ependymoma and subependymoma: MR manifestations. AJR Am J Roentgenol 1990;154(4):837–45.

50. Koeller KK, Sandberg GD, Armed Forces Institute of Pathology. From the archives of the AFIP. Cerebral intraventricular neoplasms: radiologic-pathologic correlation. Radiographics 2002;22(6):1473–505.

51. Mirzadeh Z, Bina R, Kusne Y, et al. Predictors of functional recovery in adults with posterior fossa ependymomas. J Neurosurg 2014;120(5):1063–8.

52. Corbett J, Haines D, Ard M, et al. The ventricles, choroid plexus, and cerebrospinal fluid. Fundamental neuroscience for basic and clinical applications. 4th edition. Philadelphia (PA): Saunders; 2013. p. 82–94.

53. Coates TL, Hinshaw DB, Peckman N, et al. Pediatric choroid plexus neoplasms: MR, CT, and pathologic correlation. Radiology 1989;173(1):81–8.

54. Steven DA, McGinn GJ, McClarty BM. A choroid plexus papilloma arising from an incidental pineal cyst. AJNR Am J Neuroradiol 1996;17(5):939–42.

55. Milhorat TH, Hammock MK, Davis DA, et al. Choroid plexus papilloma. I. Proof of cerebrospinal fluid overproduction. Childs Brain 1976;2(5):273–89.

56. Dangouloff-Ros V, Grevent D, Pagès M, et al. Choroid plexus neoplasms: toward a distinction between carcinoma and papilloma using arterial spin-labeling. AJNR Am J Neuroradiol 2015;36(9): 1786–90.

57. Sharifi G, Bakhtevari MH, Alghasi M, et al. Bilateral choroid plexus metastasis from papillary thyroid carcinoma: case report and review of the literature. World Neurosurg 2015;84(4):1142–6.

58. Koeller KK, Henry JM. From the archives of the AFIP: superficial gliomas: radiologic-pathologic correlation. Armed Forces Institute of Pathology. Radiographics 2001;21(6):1533–56.

59. Meltzer CC, Smirniotopoulos JG, Jones RV. The striated cerebellum: an MR imaging sign in Lhermitte-Duclos disease (dysplastic gangliocytoma). Radiology 1995;194(3):699–703.

60. Smith RR, Grossman RI, Goldberg HI, et al. MR imaging of Lhermitte-Duclos disease: a case report. AJNR Am J Neuroradiol 1989;10(1):187–9.

61. Cianfoni A, Wintermark M, Piludu F, et al. Morphological and functional MR imaging of Lhermitte-Duclos disease with pathology correlate. J Neuroradiol 2008;35(5):297–300.

62. Awwad EE, Levy E, Martin DS, et al. Atypical MR appearance of Lhermitte-Duclos disease with contrast enhancement. AJNR Am J Neuroradiol 1995;16(8):1719–20.

63. Klisch J, Juengling F, Spreer J, et al. Lhermitte-Du-clos disease: assessment with MR imaging, positron emission tomography, single-photon emission CT, and MR spectroscopy. AJNR Am J Neuroradiol 2001;22(5):824–30.

64. Douglas-Akinwande AC, Payner TD, Hattab EM. Me-dulloblastoma mimicking Lhermitte-Duclos disease on MRI and CT. Clin Neurol Neurosurg 2009; 111(6):536–9.

65. Williams DW, Elster AD, Ginsberg LE, et al. Recur-rent Lhermitte-Duclos disease: report of two cases and association with Cowden's disease. AJNR Am J Neuroradiol 1992;13(1):287–90.

66. Giorgianni A, Pellegrino C, De Benedictis A, et al. Lhermitte-Duclos disease. A case report. Neurora-diol J 2013;26(6):655–60.

67. Tan TC, Ho LC. Lhermitte-Duclos disease associ-ated with Cowden syndrome. J Clin Neurosci 2007;14(8):801–5.

68. Bechtel JT, Patton JM, Takei Y. Mixed mesenchymal and neuroectodermal tumor of the cerebellum. Acta Neuropathol 1978;41(3):261–3.

69. Kleihues P, Louis DN, Scheithauer BW, et al. The WHO classification of tumors of the nervous system. J Neuropathol Exp Neurol 2002;61(3):215–25 [dis-cussion: 226–9].

70. Jackson TR, Regine WF, Wilson D, et al. Cerebellar liponeurocytoma. Case report and review of the liter-ature. J Neurosurg 2001;95(4):700–3.

71. Nishimoto T, Kaya B. Cerebellar liponeurocytoma. Arch Pathol Lab Med 2012;136(8):965–9.

72. Alkadhi H, Keller M, Brandner S, et al. Neuroimaging of cerebellar liponeurocytoma. Case report. J Neurosurg 2001;95(2):324–31.

73. Beizig N, Ziadi S, Ladib M, et al. Cerebellar liponeur-ocytoma: case report. Neurochirurgie 2013;59(1): 39–42.

74. Anghileri E, Eoli M, Paterra R, et al. FABP4 is a candidate marker of cerebellar liponeurocytomas. J Neurooncol 2012;108(3):513–9.

75. George DH, Scheithauer BW. Central liponeurocy-toma. Am J Surg Pathol 2001;25(12):1551–5.

76. Chakraborti S, Mahadevan A, Govindan A, et al. Supratentorial and cerebellar liponeurocytomas: report of four cases with review of literature. J Neurooncol 2011;103(1):121–7.

77. Wolf A, Alghefari H, Krivosheya D, et al. Cerebellar liponeurocytoma: a rare intracranial tumor with possible familial predisposition. Case report. J Neurosurg 2016;125:57–61.

78. Scoppetta TL, Brito MC, Prado JL, et al. Multifocal cerebellar liponeurocytoma. Neurology 2015; 85(21):1912.

79. Chung SB, Suh YL, Lee JI. Cerebellar liponeurocy-toma with an unusually aggressive histopathology: case report and review of the literature. J Korean Neurosurg Soc 2012;52(3):250–3.

80. Komori T, Scheithauer BW, Hirose T. A rosette-form-ing glioneuronal tumor of the fourth ventricle: infra-tentorial form of dysembryoplastic neuroepithelial tumor? Am J Surg Pathol 2002;26(5):582–91.

81. Zhang J, Babu R, McLendon RE, et al. A comprehensive analysis of 41 patients with rosette-forming glioneuronal tumors of the fourth ventricle. J Clin Neurosci 2013;20(3):335–41.

82. Medhi G, Prasad C, Saini J, et al. Imaging fea-tures of rosette-forming glioneuronal tumours (RGNTs): a series of seven cases. Eur Radiol 2016;26(1):262–70.

83. Xu J, Yang Y, Liu Y, et al. Rosette-forming glio-neuronal tumor in the pineal gland and the third ventricle: a case with radiological and clinical im-plications. Quant Imaging Med Surg 2012;2(3): 227–31.

Lymphomas–Part 1

Lara A. Brandão, MD[a,b,*], Mauricio Castillo, MD[c]

KEYWORDS

- CNS lymphoma ● Imaging findings in lymphoma ● Diffusion-weighted imaging
- Diffusion tensor imaging ● Perfusion-weighted imaging ● Dynamic contrast enhanced MR imaging
- MR spectroscopy ● Posttreatment evaluation

KEY POINTS

- Lymphoma is a highly cellular tumor with a high nuclear/cytoplasm ratio, hence typically hyperdense on CT, isointense to gray matter on T2, and with restricted diffusion.
- Elevated choline and high lipids are typical of lymphoma.
- High blood volume may not be demonstrated despite its high malignancy.
- Lymphomas may dramatically shrink or disappear after steroids.
- Restricted diffusion may not be demonstrated in lymphoma after steroid therapy.

INTRODUCTION

Primary central nervous system lymphomas (PCNSL) were previously considered rare, representing 1% of all intracranial tumors.[1,2] There is a recent increase in their incidence and it is estimated that AIDS-related PCNSL is now more common than low-grade astrocytomas and as common as meningiomas.[3]

PCNSL involves CNS without systemic disease. Lesions may be restricted to the brain, leptomeninges, spinal cord, and/or the eyes.

The origin of PCNSL remains controversial and unknown because the CNS does not have endogenous lymphoid tissues or lymphatic circulation.[4] The only established risk factor is immunodeficiency. There are three groups at risk for developing PCNSL: (1) organ transplant recipients, (2) patients with congenital immunodeficiency syndrome, and (3) those with AIDS and other systemic diseases associated with immunodeficiency.[5]

Incidence is especially high in patients with AIDS[6]; 2% to 10% of AIDS patients with AIDS develop lymphoma during their illness.[7] The frequency of PCNSL is decreasing among AIDS patients who receive highly active antiretroviral therapy.[8,9]

The common denominator present in CNS lymphoma of immunocompromised patients is a dysfunction of the suppressor T-cell system permitting proliferation and neoplastic transformation of B-cell lymphocytes.[10] Nearly all PCNSL are of the non-Hodgkin type derived from B lymphocytes.[10,11] When Hodgkin lymphoma involves the brain it is almost always in the presence of systemic disease or dural involvement.[12]

The peak age for CNS lymphoma in the non-AIDS population is during the sixth decade of life with men affected more than women.[10]

Funding Sources: None.

Conflict of Interest: None.

[a] Radiologic Department, Clínica Felippe Mattoso, Fleury Medicina Diagnóstica, Avenida das Américas 700, sala 320, Barra Da Tijuca, Rio De Janeiro, Rio De Janeiro CEP 22640-100, Brazil; [b] Radiologic Department, Clínica IRM-Ressonância Magnética, Rua Capitão Salomão, Humaitá, Rio De Janeiro, Rio De Janeiro CEP 22271-040, Brazil; [c] Division of Neuroradiology, Department of Radiology, University of North Carolina School of Medicine, Room 3326, Old Infirmary Building, Manning Drive, Chapel Hill, NC 27599-7510, USA

* Corresponding author. Clínica Felippe Mattoso, Fleury Medicina Diagnóstica, Avenida das Américas 700, sala 320, Barra Da Tijuca, Rio De Janeiro, Rio De Janeiro CEP 22640-100, Brazil.

E-mail address: larabrandao.rad@terra.com.br

1052-5149/16/© 2016 Elsevier Inc. All rights reserved.

neuroimaging.theclinics.com

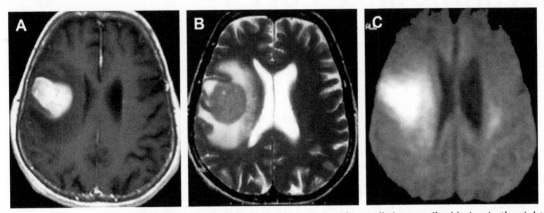

Fig. 1. Supratentorial location, solitary mass. A 71-year-old woman with a well-circumscribed lesion in the right frontal lobe with solid enhancement (*A*, axial T1 with contrast), isointense to gray matter on T2 (*B*, axial T2), and bright on diffusion-weighted imaging (DWI) (*C*) indicating restricted diffusion. Pathology was consistent with lymphoma.

IMAGING FINDINGS
Location

Approximately 70% to 85% of cases involve the supratentorial compartment (**Figs. 1** and **2**).[5,13] Focal intracerebral masses are the most common initial presentation of PCNSL,[5] whereas the subarachnoid space is a common site for recurrent disease.[2] Classic imaging findings of parenchymal lymphoma include solitary (see **Fig. 1**) or multiple (see **Fig. 2**) masses that involve the deep gray matter, periventricular regions, and corpus callosum (**Fig. 3**).[8,13] Up to 75% of lymphoma masses are in contact with

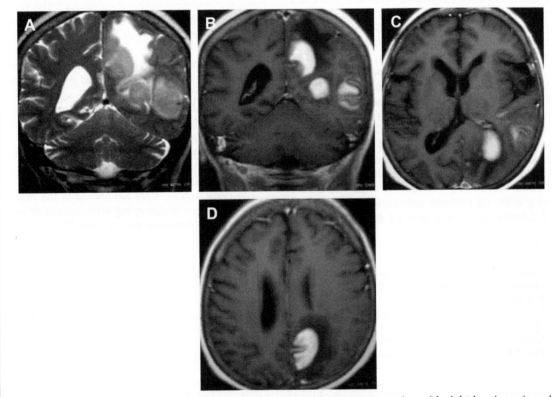

Fig. 2. Supratentorial location, multifocal lesions. A 64-year-old woman presenting with right hemiparesis and cognitive impairment. There are multifocal solid lesions in the left parietal lobe isointense to gray matter on coronal T2 (*A*) with marked enhancement (*B*, coronal; *C, D*, axial T1 with contrast).

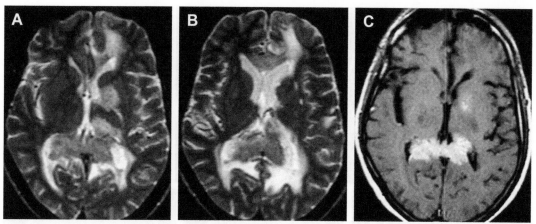

Fig. 3. Predilection for the periventricular subependymal region, deep brain nuclei, and corpus callosum. A 56-year-old man presenting with headaches and confusion. There is multifocal supratentorial lymphoma compromising the periventricular subependymal region, deep brain nuclei on the left, and corpus callosum. Lesions are isointense to gray matter on T2 (A, B). Homogeneous enhancement is demonstrated in the callosal splenium (C, axial T1 with contrast).

the ependyma, meninges, or both (Figs. 4 and 5).[13] Multiplicity is common and noted in 50% of cases. Although meningeal involvement may be demonstrated in PCNSL (Fig. 6) it is more commonly seen in secondary lymphoma (Fig. 7).[8,14] Leptomeningeal seeding in absence of parenchymal involvement commonly escapes detection by computed tomography (CT)[15] but is easily diagnosed on contrast-enhanced MR imaging. Intracranial metastasis from systemic lymphoma fall into one of two categories: leptomeningeal (see Fig. 7) (with or without parenchymal lesions) and dural-based (Fig. 8).[9] Approximately two-thirds of patients with secondary CNS lymphoma present with meningeal disease, including leptomeningeal, subependymal, dural, or cranial nerve involvement.[16]

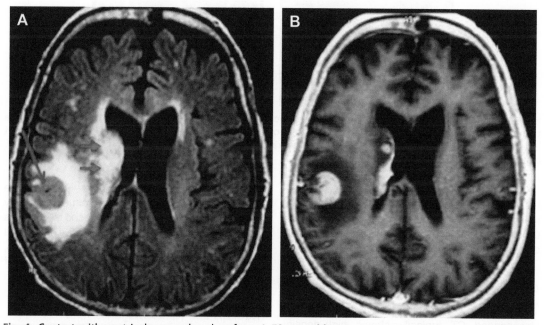

Fig. 4. Contact with ventricular ependymal surface. A 72-year-old man presenting with memory impairment, confusion, and abnormal behavior. There is a multifocal lymphoma compromising the brain parenchyma (pink arrow in A, axial fluid-attenuated inversion recovery [FLAIR]) and the right periventricular subependymal region (red arrows in A) with solid enhancement (B, axial T1 with contrast).

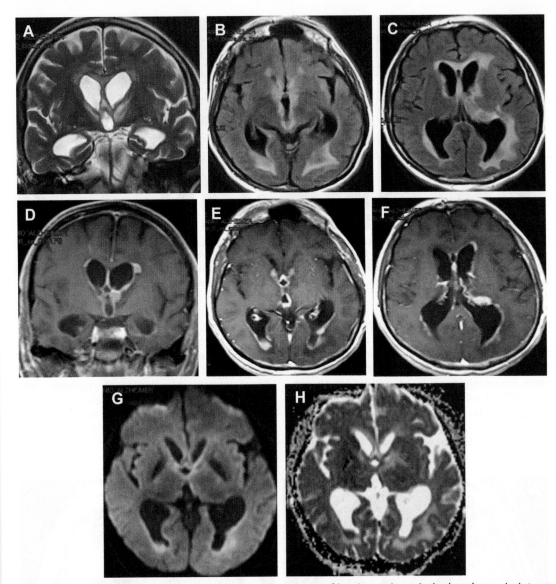

Fig. 5. Contact with ventricular ependymal surface. There is an infiltrative periventricular lymphoma, isointense to gray matter on the coronal T2 (*A*) and hyperintense on axial FLAIR images (*B, C*). Periventricular enhancement is demonstrated (*D,* coronal T1; *E, F,* axial T1 with contrast). Restricted diffusion is seen in the lesions (*G,* DWI; *H,* apparent diffusion coefficient [ADC] map).

In metastatic lymphoma to the CNS it is exceptional for parenchymal masses to occur without meningeal involvement.[11] Parenchymal masses usually represent hematogenous spread or growth of leptomeningeal neoplastic deposits.[17]

Computed Tomography and Conventional MR Imaging

Unenhanced CT typically shows high-density (70%) lesions in a central location that often reach or cross the midline (**Fig. 9**).[18] High cell density and high nuclear/citoplasmatic ratio are responsible

for their increased attenuation.[10,18] For the same reason, lymphomas tend to be isointense to gray matter on all MR imaging spin echo sequences (see **Figs. 1**B, **2**A and **3**A, B).[16,19,20] Lymphoma may be markedly hyperintense on long TR images, a finding usually demonstrated in intravascular (**Fig. 10**) and infiltrative lymphomas.[4]

Necrosis and Hemorrhage

Necrosis and hemorrhage are more common in AIDS-related lymphomas (**Fig. 11**).[18] Hemorrhage and necrosis may be demonstrated in primary

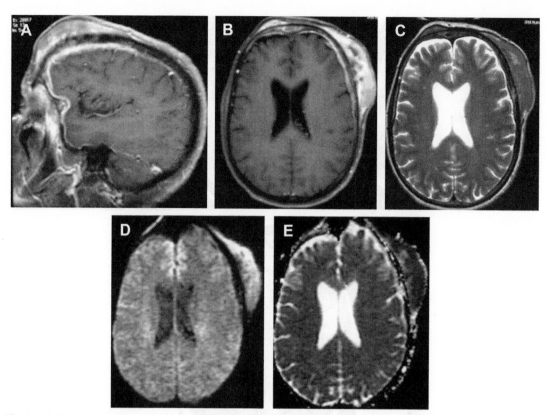

Fig. 6. PCNSL compromising the dura and adjacent bone. A 61-year-old woman presenting with frontal bulging for 6 months. There is extensive dural thickening and enhancement in the left frontal region with less involvement of the right frontal region (*A* sagittal, *B* axial T1 with contrast). The lesion extends through the bone to adjacent soft tissue where a nonhomogeneous enhancing mass (*A, B*) is demonstrated. The tumor is isointense to gray matter on T2 (*C*) and presents restricted diffusion (*D*, DWI; *E*, ADC map).

lymphomas in immunocompetent patients with Epstein-Barr virus (EBV)-positive tumors (**Fig. 12**).[21,22]

Age-related, EBV-positive, diffuse, large B-cell lymphoma is a new disease entity recognized in the 2008 World Health Organization classification as a tumor occurring in the elderly[23,24] mostly without any known immunodeficiency or prior lymphoma.

Lee and colleagues[22] compared the MR imaging features of 10 patients without AIDS with EBV-positive PCNSL with those of 45 patients without AIDS with EBV-negative PCNSL. Imaging features in the EBV-positive patients were atypical of non-AIDS PCNSL closely resembling glioblastomas (GBM) and included lesions with necrosis, hemorrhage, and irregular or peripheral contrast enhancement. In contrast, most EBV-negative cases of PCNSL presented as single or multiple relatively homogeneously enhancing lesions typical of non-AIDS PCNSL.

Calcification

Internal calcifications are unusual in CNS lymphomas[13] unless the patient has undergone prior chemotherapy or radiation therapy.[18]

Edema

The extent of edema is generally less than that seen with primary gliomas or metastasis of similar size (**Fig. 13**).[25,26] Edema and mass effect may be inconspicuous in lymphomas.[10] Prominent edema may be demonstrated in lymphomas with hemorrhage (see **Fig. 12**).[17]

Contrast Enhancement

The pattern of contrast enhancement is variable and may be as follows:

- Dense and homogeneous in most cases (see **Figs. 1–4**).[18]

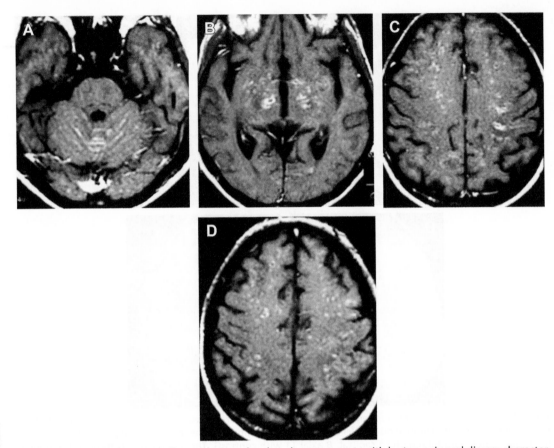

Fig. 7. Secondary lymphoma. Patient with secondary lymphoma presents with leptomeningeal disease character-ized by enhancement along the cerebellar sulci in cerebellum (*A*). Multiple enhancing nodules are also demon-strated in the perivascular spaces bilaterally (*B–D*).

- Nonhomogeneous or ring enhancement: More common in immunocompromised patients because of high prevalence of hemorrhage and necrosis (**Fig. 14**, see also **Fig. 11**). It may also be seen in EBV-positive PCNSLs.[22]
- Ependymal contrast enhancement: When enhancement is demonstrated along a ventricular surface, lymphoma should be considered (see **Figs. 4B, 5D–F,** and **14A**).
- Perivascular space contrast enhancement: Detection of enhancement in perivascular spaces suggests lymphomas (see **Fig. 7B–D**).
- Absent contrast enhancement: Infiltrative[27,28] (**Fig. 15**) and intravascular lymphomas[21] (**Fig. 16**) may not demonstrate enhancement.

Despite some characteristic conventional MR imaging findings it may be difficult or impossible to distinguish cerebral lymphomas from other aggressive brain tumors.[29,30] Accurate

preoperative differentiation between these tumors is important for appropriate treatment. Advanced MR imaging techniques, such as diffusion-weighted imaging (DWI), diffusion tensor imaging (DTI), MR spectroscopy, perfusion-weighted imaging (PWI), and dynamic contrast-enhanced (DCE)/permeability studies, may help distinguish lymphomas from other primary brain tumors.[30,31]

IMAGING CHARACTERISTICS ON ADVANCED MR IMAGING
Diffusion-Weighted Imaging

Diagnostic value
Studies have shown that apparent diffusion coefficient (ADC) can differentiate PCNSL from high-grade gliomas (HGG).[30–38] Lymphomas demonstrate low ADC values, a finding consistent with restricted water diffusion related to high tumor cell density (**Fig. 17**, see also **Figs. 6D, E, 8B,** and **10D–G**).[30–38] By contrast, HGG are relatively hyperintense to gray matter on trace DWI

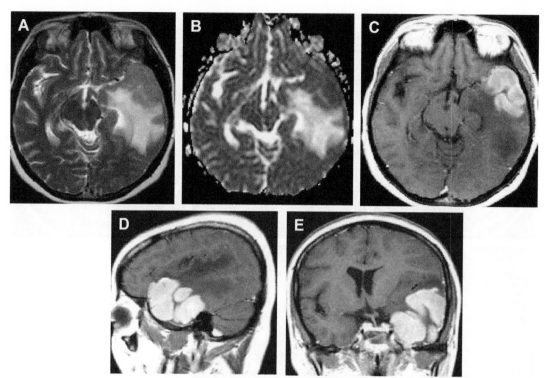

Fig. 8. Secondary lymphoma, parenchymal lesion. A 32-year-old woman with lymphoma in the left femur presenting with headaches. There is a solid mass in the left temporal region, isointense to gray matter on T2 axial (*A*) with restricted diffusion (*B*, ADC map). There is striking enhancement (*C* axial, *D* sagittal, and *E* coronal T1 with contrast). Notice the lesion is adjacent to the dura.

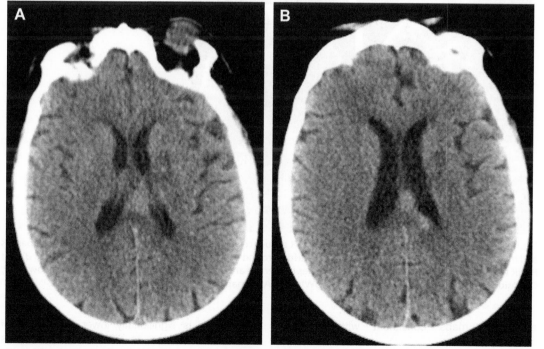

Fig. 9. Lymphoma, hyperdense on CT. A 50-year-old man presenting with headaches. Noncontrast CT shows high-density lesions (*A*, *B*) in the posterior corpus callosum adjacent to ventricular surfaces.

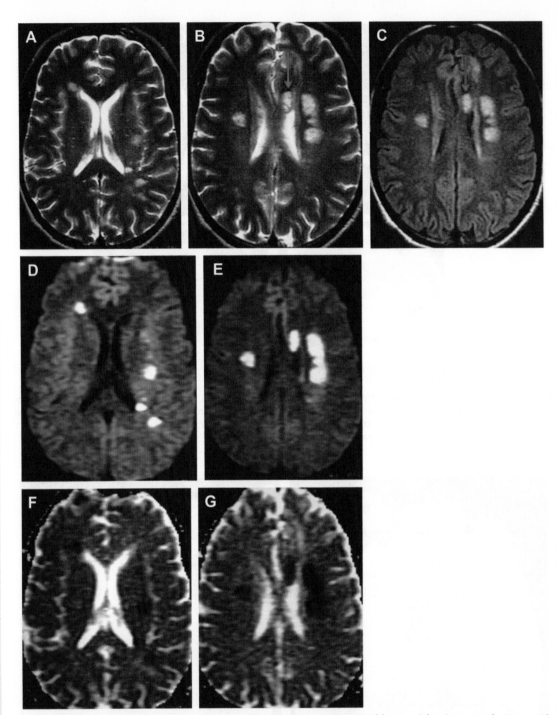

Fig. 10. Lymphoma, high signal intensity on long TR sequences. A 39-year-old man with seizures and tetraparesis and intravascular lymphoma presenting with multifocal round nodules with high signal intensity on T2 (*A*, *B*) and FLAIR (*C*) images in the region of watershed zones bilaterally and in the corpus callosum on the left (*arrows in B, C*). Lesions present restricted diffusion (*D, E*, DWI; *F, G*, ADC map).

and ADC maps consistent with elevated diffusivity.[34,36,39,40]

A study by Toh and colleagues[37] demonstrated that the fractional anisotropy (FA) and ADC of lymphomas is significantly lower than those of GBMs. Cutoff values to differentiate lymphomas from GBM were 0.192 for FA, 0.33 for FA ratio, 0.818 for ADC, and 1.06 for ADC ratio. Accuracy

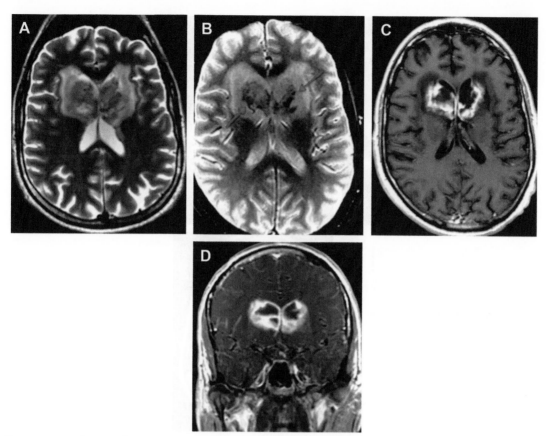

Fig. 11. Hemorrhage and necrosis in an immunocompromised patient. A 37-year-old man, human immunodeficiency virus (HIV)-positive, presenting with fever, ataxia, diplopia, and urinary incontinence. There is a mass in the deep brain nuclei adjacent to the ventricular margins. The lesion is isointense to gray matter on T2 axial (*A*) and presents with foci of low signal intensity on the gradient echo (*arrows* in *B*) consistent with hemorrhage. Enhancement is nonhomogeneous (*C* axial, *D* coronal T1 with contrast).

of 100% was reached in the distinction of lymphoma from GBM using a cutoff value of 1.06 for the ADC ratio. The specificity and accuracy of ADC were higher than of FA in differentiating the two.

ADC measurements are also useful in the distinction between lymphoma and GBM infiltrating the corpus callosum.[41] GBMs with restricted water diffusion have been reported (**Fig. 18**).[42–46] Therefore, discrimination between lymphoma and GBMs is difficult based solely on diffusion characteristics. Multimodal imaging approaches are recommended rather than ADC alone for differentiation.[47] ADC values are significantly dependent on region of interest method. According to Ahn and colleagues,[47] ADCs obtained from the whole tumor volume are the most reproducible. ADC mean from the whole tumor may aid in differentiating between lymphoma and GBM.

Prognostic biomarker

Barajas and colleagues[48] found that pretherapeutic ADC tumor measurements within contrast-enhancing regions are predictive of clinical outcome in patients with PCNSL. Specifically, ADC25% (<692) and ADCmin (<384) were predictive of shorter progression-free survival (PFS) and overall survival (OS). Additionally, an inverse correlation was found between ADC measurements and tumor cellular density. Finally, they found that patients with prolonged PFS and OS had a significant reduction in posttherapeutic ADC values. This decrease in ADC measurements is suggestive of a net reduction of extracellular water molecular motion within treated lesions. These findings were later confirmed by Valles and colleagues.[49]

DWI has been shown to complement PET in prediction of site-specific response to chemotherapy. Sites with an adequate response have a significantly lower median pretreatment ADC than those with an inadequate response.[50]

Diffusion Tensor Imaging

DTI provides diffusion anisotropy information about tissues, such as FA, linear anisotropy

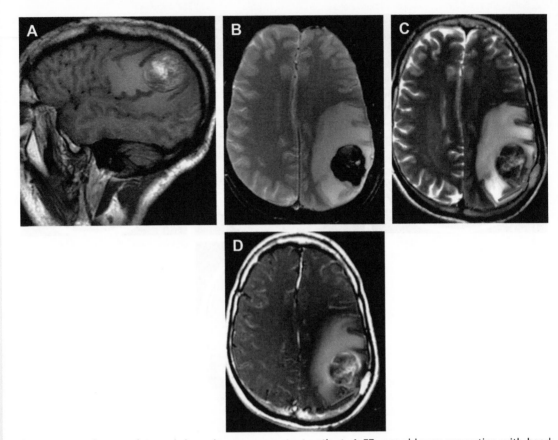

Fig. 12. Hemorrhage and necrosis in an immunocompetent patient. A 57-year-old man presenting with head-aches on the left, two seizure episodes, paresis and paresthesia on the right; HIV negative. There is a focal het-erogeneous lesion in the left parietal region presenting high signal intensity on T1 sagittal (A) and very low signal on gradient-echo axial images (B) consistent with hemorrhage. Extensive disproportional edema surrounds the lesion (B gradient recalled echo, C axial T2, D axial T1 with contrast) suggesting a neoplastic nature instead of a benign hematoma. The lesion presents with nonhomogeneous enhancement (D). Note adjacent bone compro-mise (arrows in C, D).

coefficient, planar anisotropy coefficient, and spherical anisotropy coefficient. Of these, FA has been more commonly used in the study of brain neoplasms.[51,52]

In contrast to ADC, positive[51,52] and negative correlations[37] have been reported between FA and tumor cellularity. A reason for these conflicting reports may be the heterogeneity of the tumors analyzed. Among GBMs, metastasis and PCNSL, the latter have the highest cellularity followed by GBMs and brain metastases.[31] Elevated FA from enhancing regions of GBMs in comparison with brain metastases and PCNSLs in a study by Wang and colleagues[31] indicate that diffusion anisotropy may not directly correlate with tumor cellularity. It has been reported that anisotropy in

tumors is affected by several factors including extracellular-to-intracellular space ratio, extracel-lular matrix, tortuosity, and vascularity.[53,54]

Wang and colleagues[31] demonstrated that the best model to differentiate PCNSLs from brain me-tastases comprises ADC from enhancing regions and planar anisotropy coefficient from the immedi-ate perienhancing regions with area under the curve of 0.909.

Proton MR Spectroscopy

The spectral pattern of lymphomas is similar to that of other malignant tumors and is character-ized by increased choline, reduced myoinositol, and prominent lipids (Fig. 19).[32,55,56] When lipids

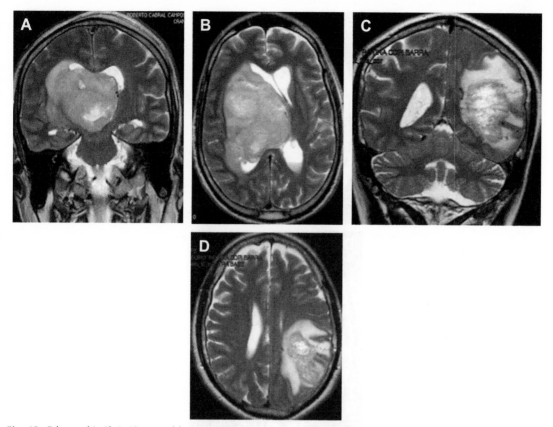

Fig. 13. Edema. (*A*, *B*) A 48-year-old man, HIV positive, presenting with confusion and seizure, diagnosed with PCNSL. A large mass is demonstrated in the right hemisphere adjacent to the ventricular margins displacing the midline. The lesion is predominantly isointense to gray matter on T2 (*A*, coronal; *B*, axial) and has no surrounding edema. (*C*, *D*) Patient for comparison, diagnosed with GBM. Despite a smaller tumor compared with the lymphoma shown in *A* and *B*, more edema is demonstrated (*C*, coronal; *D*, axial T2).

are demonstrated in solid-appearing tumors, lymphoma should be considered.[38,48–50,55–58] Lipids are also typically seen in GBMs but there they may be related to necrosis.

Dynamic Susceptibility Contrast and Dynamic Contrast-Enhanced MR Imaging

Diagnostic value

Perfusion allows discrimination of PCNSL from GBM.[59] Tumor neovascularization is absent in PCNSL and thus they have lower mean relative cerebral blood volume (rCBV) or lower rCBV max values and lower cerebral blood flow (CBF) compared with GBMs.[30,31,59–63] Because angiogenesis is not prominent in lymphomas, perfusion may not be elevated (**Figs. 20** and **21**), which helps distinguish them from HGG.[59–63] If high cell density is suggested by ADC and no elevation of rCBV is demonstrated one should consider lymphoma instead of

HGG. However, rCBV of lymphoma may be high (**Figs. 22** and **23**) overlapping with that of HGG (**Fig. 24**). In this case, ADC maps are valuable to distinguish these lesions because lymphoma shows significant restricted diffusion (compare see **Figs. 23**B and **24**C). Moreover, in patients with lymphoma, restricted diffusion tends to match areas of T2 abnormalities and contrast enhancement.

Prognostic biomarker

Besides helping to distinguish lymphoma from HGG, rCBV may be a potential prognostic biomarker in patients with PCNSL because lower values are associated with adverse prognosis.[49] Patients with low tumor rCBV values (<1.43) at pretherapy baseline have significantly shorter PFS and OS compared with patients with high tumor rCBV values. Biologic correlates of rCBV values in PCNSL remain conjectural but one

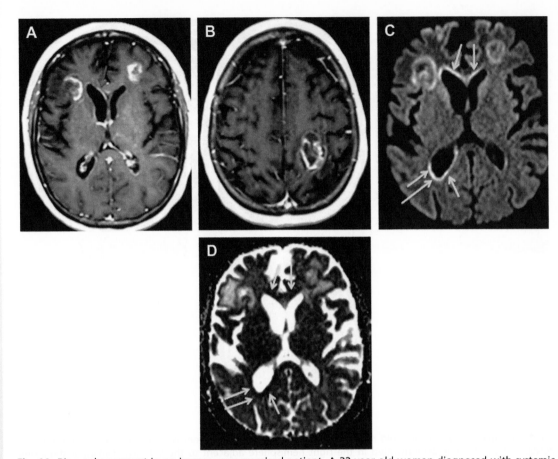

Fig. 14. Ring enhancement in an immunocompromised patient. A 32-year-old woman diagnosed with systemic lupus erythematosus presenting with headaches and disorientation. Ring-enhancing lesions are demonstrated in the frontal lobes (*A*, axial T1 with contrast) and in the left parietal lobe (*B*, axial T1 with contrast). Note ependymal enhancement (*arrow* in *A*). There is marginal restricted diffusion in the frontal lesions and along the ventricular ependyma (*arrows* in *C* DWI and *D* ADC map).

can postulate two possible explanations as to why low tumor rCBV values may be associated with adverse outcome in patients with PCNSL. First, rCBV values measure bulk vessel attenuation and thus reflect tumor angiogenesis. Second, rCBV values depend on patent vessels for delivery of intravenous gadolinium contrast agent. Therefore, low tumor rCBV values in PCNSL may signify a relative lack of tumor angiogenesis or a hypoxic microenvironment and decreased patent vessels able to deliver intravenous chemotherapy to the tumor.[49] The predictive power of adverse outcome is even greater when risk stratification is based on combined low ADC and low rCBV values suggesting the additive and complementary role of diffusion and perfusion MR imaging as prognostic biomarkers in patients with PCNSL.

Concerning permeability, in the authors' experience lymphoma usually shows no significant elevation of permeability in the maximum slope of increase map, whereas very high permeability is typical in GBM (**Fig. 25**; **Box 1**).[64,65] However, lymphomas with high permeability have been demonstrated (**Fig. 26**).

POSTTREATMENT CHANGES (RELATED TO STEROIDS)

CNS lymphoma has generated great interest because of its rising incidence in immunocompetent host and its responsiveness to systemic chemotherapy.[6,66,67] Diagnosis of PCNSL is often suggested by its imaging appearance and established by stereotactic biopsy because lesions are typically deep-seated in the brain and

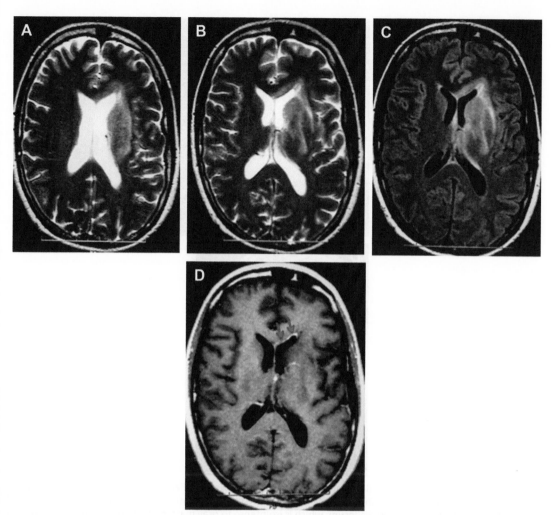

Fig. 15. No enhancement, infiltrative lymphoma. A 51-year-old woman presenting with right hemiplegia. There is an infiltrative lymphoma compromising the parenchyma adjacent to the left ventricular margin, the genu of the corpus callosum, and the deep gray nuclei (*A*, *B*, axial T2; *C*, axial FLAIR). Despite minimal ependymal enhancement (*arrows* in *D*, axial T1 with contrast) the deep infiltrative lesion shows no enhancement.

not amenable to resection. Furthermore, unlike other primary brain tumors, control of and survival from PCNSL does not improve with surgical resection.[67]

Corticosteroids are frequently administered immediately after the diagnosis of an intracranial mass is made based on imaging. In 40% to 85% of patients with PCNSL, corticosteroids cause cell lysis and tumor regression.[67] The speed of regression is variable but complete disappearance may occur in 1 to 2 days (**Fig. 27**). Some authors report complete regression at 8 hours after steroid administration.[68] Lymphoma that vanishes after steroids is known as a "ghost tumor." Even

patients with a partial response can have enough tumor lysis that nondiagnostic tissue is obtained at biopsy. Steroids may alter the findings of CNS lymphoma in the contrast-enhanced CT and MR imaging and on DWI, PWI, and in DCE studies.[69] Reduced or no contrast enhancement is seen after steroids because of normalization of the blood-brain barrier (**Fig. 28**). This finding does not indicate therapeutic response because nonenhancing tumor progression may be demonstrated on fluid-attenuated inversion recovery and T2 images (see **Fig. 28G–J**). If treatment with steroids is discontinued, contrast enhancement may reappear and new enhancing lesions develop

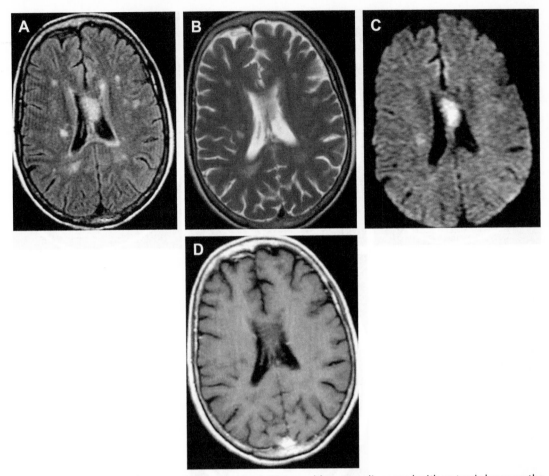

Fig. 16. No enhancement, intravascular lymphoma. A 65-year-old woman diagnosed with systemic lupus erythematosus. There are multiple high signal intensity lesions in the corona radiata (A, axial FLAIR; B, axial T2). A solid lesion is demonstrated in the corpus callosum, which is isointense to gray matter on T2 (B) and presents restricted diffusion (C, DWI). The lesion does not enhance (D, axial T1 with contrast).

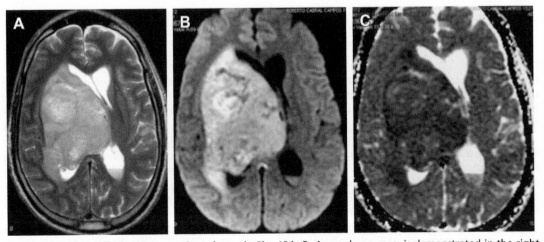

Fig. 17. Restricted diffusion. Same patient shown in Fig. 13A, B. A very large mass is demonstrated in the right hemisphere adjacent to the ventricular margins displacing the midline. The lesion is predominantly isointense to gray matter on T2 (A) and presents restricted diffusion (B, DWI; C, ADC map).

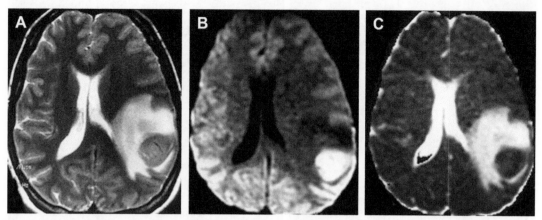

Fig. 18. Restricted diffusion in GBM. A 39-year-old woman, presenting with dysarthria. There is a solid lesion in the left parietal lobe, isointense to gray matter on T2 (A), presenting with restricted diffusion (B, DWI; C, ADC map).

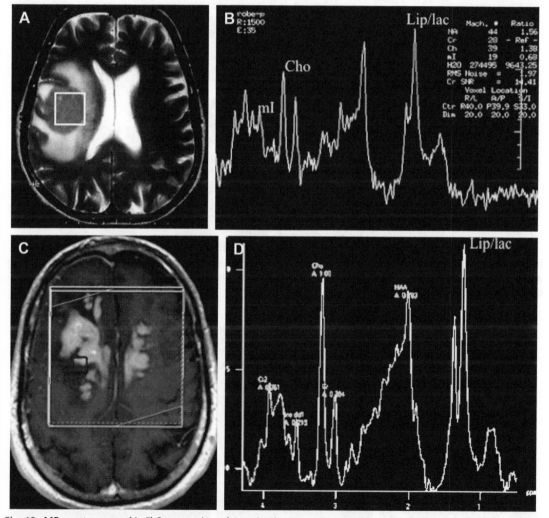

Fig. 19. MR spectroscopy. (A, B) Same patient shown in Fig. 1 presenting with lymphoma. (C, D) Different patient with multifocal lymphoma. Spectra from both tumors demonstrate low NAA, low myoinositol (mI), high choline (Cho), and a prominent lipid-lactate (lip/lac) peak consistent with lymphoma. NAA, n-acetyl-aspartate.

526

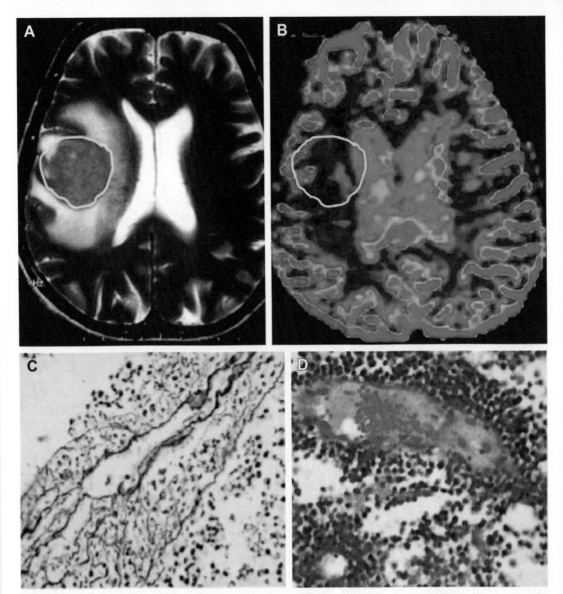

Fig. 20. Blood volume, no elevation, in an immunocompetent patient. Same patient shown in **Fig. 1** presenting with lymphoma. The lesion is isointense to gray matter on T2 (*A*) and presents hypoperfusion (*B*, rCBV map). Pathology (*C, D*) confirms the diagnosis.

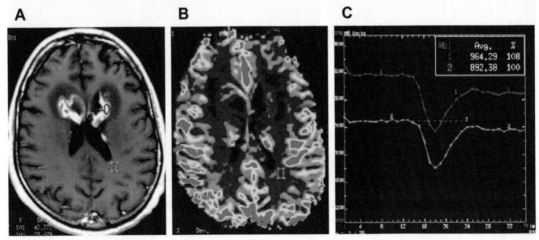

Fig. 21. Blood volume, no elevation, in an immunocompromised patient. Same patient shown in **Fig. 11**. The enhancing lesion (*A*, axial T1 with contrast) does not demonstrate elevation of blood volume (*B*, rCBV map; *C*, perfusion curve).

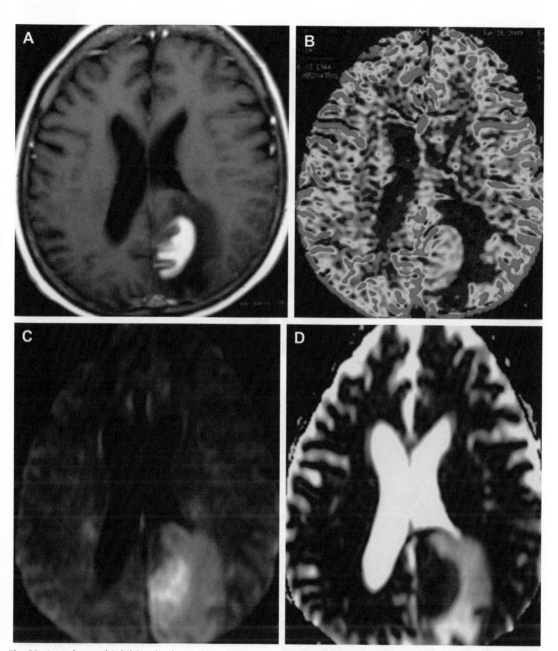

Fig. 22. Lymphoma, high blood volume, in an immunocompetent patient. Same patient shown in Fig. 2. The solid enhancing left parietal lesion (A, axial T1 with contrast) presents high blood volume (B, rCBV map) and restricted diffusion (C, DWI; D, ADC map).

(see Fig. 28K–R). Perfusion characteristics may also change after steroids.[69] Previous studies show that glucocorticoids may act by decreasing CBV or re-establishing blood-tumor barrier permeability.

Using MR imaging, ØStergaard and colleagues[69] examined the acute changes in rCBV, CBF, and blood-tumor barrier permeability with gadolinium after administration of dexamethasone in six lymphomas. Dexamethasone was found to cause a dramatic decrease in blood-tumor barrier permeability and regional CBV but no significant changes in CBF or degree of edema. No elevation of CVB may be

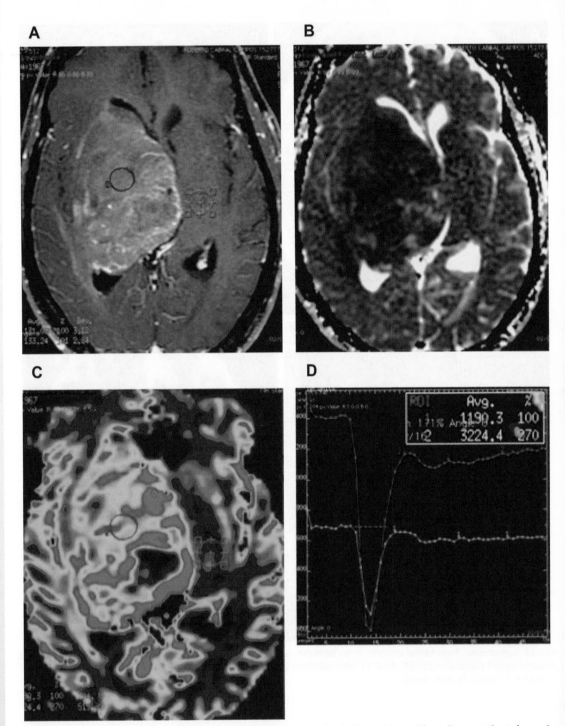

Fig. 23. Lymphoma, high blood volume, in an immunocompromised HIV-positive patient. Same patient shown in Figs. 13A, B and 17. There is a large nonhomogeneous enhancing lesion in the right frontal lobe (*A*, axial T1 with contrast) with restricted diffusion (*B*, ADC map) and high blood volume (*C*, rCBV map; *D*, curve from the perfusion study).

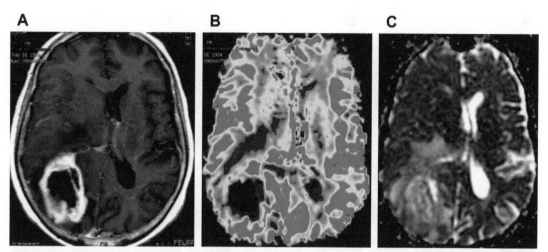

Fig. 24. GBM for comparison. A 76-year-old woman presenting with left hemiparesis. There is a nonhomogeneous ring-enhancing lesion in the right parietal lobe (*A*, axial T1 with contrast) with high blood volume (*B*, rCBV map). However, as opposed to the restricted diffusion typically seen in lymphomas (see **Fig. 23**B), high diffusivity is demonstrated in this GBM (*C*, ADC map).

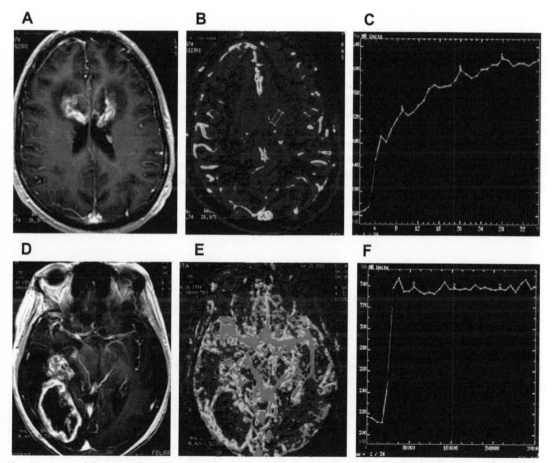

Fig. 25. Permeability, lymphoma and GBM. (*A–C*) Lymphoma, same patient shown in **Figs. 11** and **21**. The enhancing lesion (*A*, axial T1 with contrast) shows no significant elevation of permeability (*B*, maximum slope of increase map). There is slow progressive elevation of the permeability curve (*C*). (*D–F*) GBM, same patient shown in **Fig. 24**. The enhancing temporal nodule (*D*, axial T1 with contrast) presents high permeability (*E*, maximum slope of increase map; *F*, permeability curve).

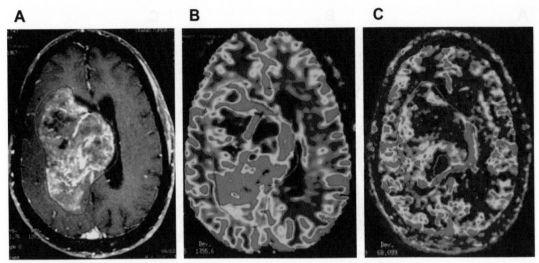

A   **B**   **C**

Fig. 26. Lymphoma with high permeability. Same patient shown in **Figs. 13, 17** and **23**. There is a large nonhomogeneous enhancing lesion in the right frontal lobe (*A*, axial T1 with contrast) with high blood volume (*B*, rCBV map) and areas of high permeability (*C*, maximum slope of increase map).

demonstrated in a previously highly perfused lymphoma after steroid therapy (**Fig. 29**).

ADC of lymphoma may also change after steroid therapy and restricted ADC may resolve (**Fig. 30**) making a diagnosis more difficult based solely on ADC values.

Resection of lymphoma does not increase survival and, in some cases, causes neurologic deterioration because of the deep location of most lesions.[70] Furthermore, there is a theoretic concern that craniotomy may cause spillage of tumor cells into the subarachnoid space possibly seeding the leptomeninges.[71]

Steroid Therapy, Take Home Messages

- Lymphomas may diminish in size or completely disappear after steroids.
- No contrast enhancement in a previously enhancing lesion may be demonstrated in lymphoma after steroids; this does not necessarily mean therapeutic response.
- No elevation of CVB may be demonstrated in a previously highly perfused lymphomatous mass if the patient is under steroid therapy.
- Restricted ADC may resolve after steroids.

Box 1
Key points to remember

- Restricted diffusion is typical of lymphoma but may also be demonstrated in HGG. In lymphoma, restricted diffusion matches the T2 abnormality, whereas in HGG, low ADC is usually restricted to small areas within the tumor.
- Although high lipids are typical of necrotic brain tumors, such as GBM, lipids are demonstrated in solid-appearing lymphomas.
- Despite its aggressiveness, lymphoma may not present elevated blood volumes on perfusion studies.
- Significant elevation of permeability (DCE) is usually not demonstrated in lymphoma.

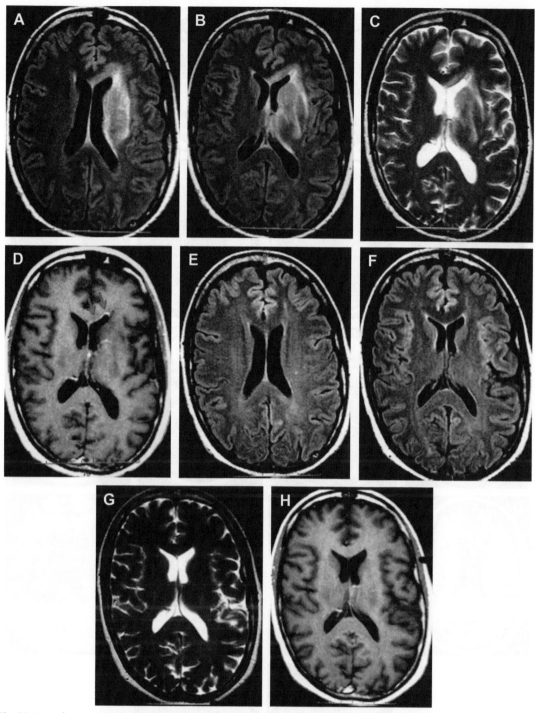

Fig. 27. Lymphoma, complete regression after steroids. Same patient shown in Fig. 15. There is an ill-defined infiltrative lesion adjacent to the left ventricle compromising the genu of the corpus callosum on the left and the deep gray nuclei (*A, B*, axial FLAIR; *C*, axial T2) with subtle subependymal enhancement (*arrows* in *D*, axial T1 with contrast). Four months after steroids (*E, F*, axial FLAIR; *G*, axial T2) no tumor infiltration or enhancement is demonstrated (*H*, axial T1 with contrast).

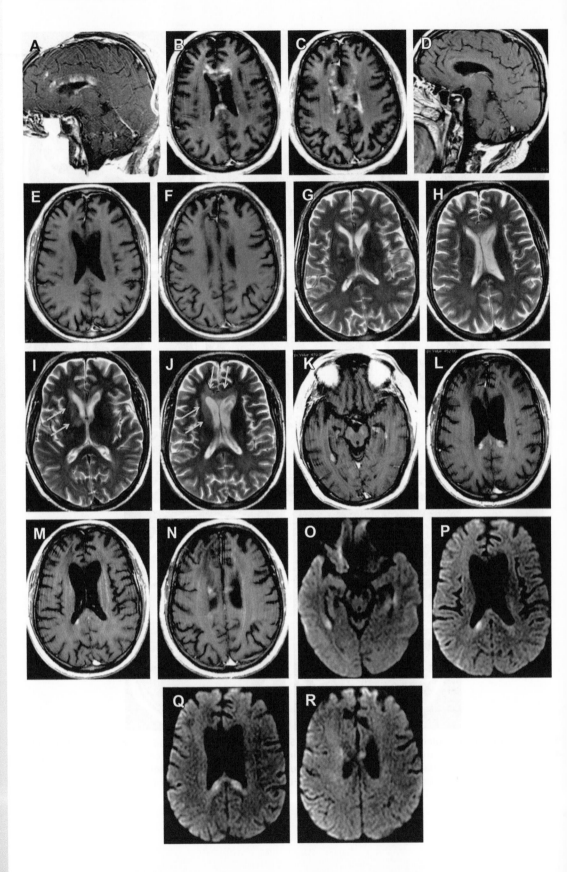

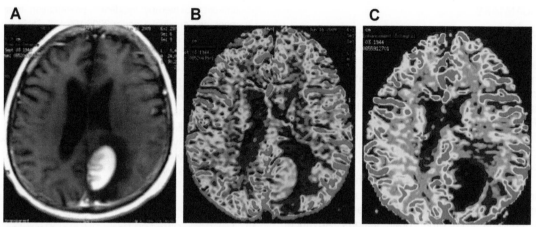

Fig. 29. Lymphoma, no elevation of the blood volume after steroids. Same patient shown in **Fig. 2**. There is a solid enhancing lesion in the left parietal lobe (*A*, axial T1 with contrast) with high perfusion (*B*, rCBV map). Reduced perfusion is demonstrated after steroid therapy (*C*, rCBV map).

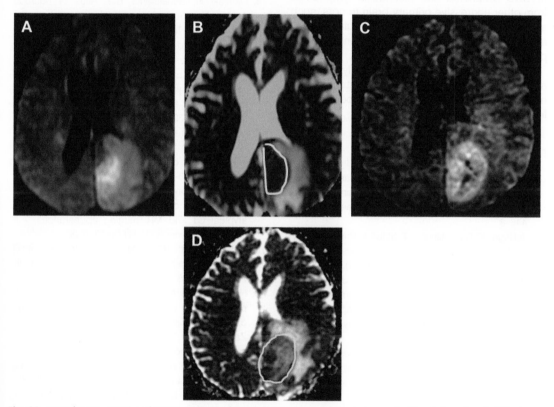

Fig. 30. Lymphoma, restricted ADC resolves after steroids. Same patient shown in **Fig. 2**. Restricted diffusion is demonstrated before treatment (*A*, DWI; *B*, ADC map). Less restriction is seen after steroids (*C*, DWI; *D*, ADC map).

Fig. 28. Lymphoma, no enhancement after steroids. A 56-year-old man diagnosed with primary CNS lymphoma presents an infiltrative enhancing lesion in the corpus callosum and ventricular ependyma. (*A* sagittal and *B, C* axial T1 with contrast). After steroids (*D*, sagittal T1; *E, F*, axial T1 with contrast) no enhancement is demonstrated. Despite no enhancement, areas of tumor infiltration have progressed with more extensive lesions in the periventricular parenchyma as demonstrated on T2 axial images (*G, H* before steroids vs *I, J* after steroids *arrows*). Steroid administration was discontinued and follow-up MR imaging 3 months later demonstrates new enhancing lesions adjacent to the ventricular margins (*K–N*, axial T1 with contrast) with restricted diffusion (*O–R*, DWI).

SUMMARY

When PCNSL is suspected, contrast-enhanced MR imaging is the technique of choice. Secondary CNS lymphomas present as meningeal metastases in two-thirds of patients and as parenchymal metastases in one-third. In PCNSL, almost all patients have parenchymal lesions. Parenchymal lymphomas have a predilection for the periventricular and superficial regions, often abutting the ventricular or meningeal surfaces.

Although CNS lymphomas may have characteristic imaging findings on traditional MR imaging, no technique unequivocally differentiates CNS lymphoma from other brain lesions. Advanced MR imaging techniques, such as DWI, DTI, MRS, PWI, and DCE studies, help establish a diagnosis of CNS lymphoma and distinguish lymphomas from other aggressive primary brain tumors, such as GBM. If ADC suggests high cellular density and no elevation of rCBV is seen, consider lymphoma as the main diagnosis.

Following administration of steroids, lymphomas may partially or completely regress, restricted ADC may resolve, and a previously hyperperfused lesion may demonstrate low rCBV.

REFERENCES

1. Atlas SW. Extra-axial brain tumors. In: Atlas SW, editor. Magnetic resonance imaging of the brain and spine. 2nd edition. Philadelphia: Lippincott Raven; 1996. p. 446–8.

2. Jellinger K, Radszkiewicz T, Slowk F. Primary malignant lymphoma of the central nervous system in man. Acta Neuropathol 1975;(Suppl VI):95.

3. Baumgartner J, Rachin J, Beckstead J, et al. Primary central nervous system lymphomas: natural history and response to radiation therapy in 55 patients with acquired immunodeficiency syndrome. J Neurosurg 1990;73:206–11.

4. Atlas SW. Intra-axial brain tumors. In: Atlas SW, editor. Magnetic resonance imaging of the brain and spine. 2nd edition. Philadelphia: Lippincott Raven; 1996. p. 404–7.

5. Hochberg FH, Miller DC. Primary central nervous system lymphoma. J Neurosurg 1988;68:835–53.

6. Nasir S, Deangelis LM. Update on the management of primary CNS lymphoma. Oncology 2000;14(2): 228–37.

7. Forsyth PA, DeAngelis LM. Biology and management of AIDS-associated primary CNS lymphomas. Hematol Oncol Clin North Am 1996;10:1125–34.

8. Diamond C, Taylor TH, Aboumrad T, et al. Changes in acquired immuno- deficiency syndrome-related non-Hodgkin lymphoma in the era of highly active antiretroviral therapy: incidence, presentation, treatment, and survival. Cancer 2006;106:128–35.

9. Besson C, Goubar A, Gabarre J, et al. Changes in AIDS-related lymphoma since the era of highly active antiretroviral therapy. Blood 2001;98:2339–44.

10. Greenberg JO, Polachini I. Intracranial neoplasms. In: Greenberg JO, editor. Neuroimaging. A companion to Adams and Victor's principles of neurology. Mc-Graw-Hill, Inc; 1995. p. 340–2.

11. Russel DS, Rubinstein LJ. Pathology of tumors of the central nervous system. 5th edition. Baltimore (MD): Williams & Wilkins; 1989.

12. Clark W, Callihan T, Schwartzberg L, et al. Primary intracranial Hodgkin's lymphoma without dural attachment. J Neurosurg 1992;76:692–5.

13. Jack CR Jr, O'Neill BP, Banks PM, et al. Central nervous system lymphoma: histologic types and CT appearance. Radiology 1988;167:211–5.

14. Okazaki H, Scheithauer BW. Atlas of neuropathology. New York: Gower; 1988.

15. Enzmann DR, Tokye KC, Hayward R. CT in leptomeningeal spread of tumor. J Comput Assist Tomogr 1978;2:448–55.

16. Haldorsen IS, Espeland A, Larsson AM. Central nervous system lymphoma: characteristic findings on traditional and advanced imaging. AJNR Am J Neuroradiol 2011;32(6):984–92.

17. Nacif MS, Jauregui GF, Mello RAF, et al. Linfoma adrenal primário bilateral com envolvimento do sistema nervoso central: relato de caso. Radiol Bras 2005;38(3):235–8.

18. Erdag N, Bhorade RM, Alberico RA. Primary lymphoma of the central nervous system. Typical and atypical CT and MR imaging appearances. AJR Am J Roentgenol 2001;176(5):1319–26.

19. Tang YZ, Booth TC, Bhogal P, et al. Imaging of primary central nervous system lymphoma. Clin Radiol 2011;66(8):768–77.

20. Haque S, Law M, Abrey LE, et al. Imaging of lymphoma of the central nervous system, spine, and orbit. Radiol Clin North Am 2008;46(2):339–61.

21. Zambrano AD, Berkowitz F. Primary central nervous system lymphoma: what the radiologist needs to know. Presented at the ASNR Annual Meeting. Quebec (Canada), May 17–22, 2014. p. eEdE18.

22. Lee HY, Kim HS, Park JW, et al. Atypical imaging features of Epstein-Barr virus–positive primary central nervous system lymphomas in patients without AIDS. AJNR Am J Neuroradiol 2013;34:1562–7.

23. Oyama T, Ichimura K, Suzuki R, et al. Senile EBV+ B-cell lymphoproliferative disorders: a clinicopathologic study of 22 patients. Am J Surg Pathol 2003; 27:16–26.

24. Nakamura S, Jaffe ES, Swerdlow SH. EBV positive diffuse large B-cell lymphoma of the elderly. In: Swerdlow SH, Campo E, Harris NL, et al, editors. WHO classification of tumours of haematopoietic

and lymphoid tissues. Lyon (France): IARS Press; 2008. p. 243–4.

25. Eichler AF, Batchelor TT. Primary central nervous system lymphoma: presentation, diagnosis and staging. Neurosurg Focus 2006;21:E15.

26. Go JL, Lee SC, Kim PE. Imaging of primary central nervous system lymphoma. Neurosurg Focus 2006; 21:E4.

27. Choi CY, Lee CH, Joo M. Lymphomatosis cerebri. J Korean Neurosurg Soc 2013;54(5):420–2.

28. Keswani A, Bigio E, Grimm S. Lymphomatosis cerebri presenting with orthostatic hypotension, anorexia, and paraparesis. J Neurooncol 2012;109:581–6.

29. Poon T, Matoso I, Tchertkoff V, et al. CT features of primary cerebral lymphoma in AIDS and non-AIDS patients. J Comput Assist Tomogr 1989;13:6–9.

30. Stadnick TW, Demaerel P, Luypaert RR, et al. Imaging tutorial: differential diagnosis of bright lesions on diffusion-weighted MR images. Radiographics 2003;23:e7.

31. Wang S, Kim S, Chawla S, et al. Differentiation between glioblastomas, solitary brain metastases, and primary cerebral lymphomas using diffusion tensor and dynamic susceptibility contrast-enhanced MR imaging. AJNR Am J Neuroradiol 2011;32:507–14.

32. Calli C, Kitis O, Yunten N, et al. Perfusion and diffusion MR imaging in enhancing malignant cerebral tumors. Eur J Radiol 2006;58(3):394–403.

33. Cha S. Neuroimaging in neuro-oncology. Neurotherapeutics 2009;6(3):465–77.

34. Brandão LA, Shiroishi MS, Law M. Brain tumors: a multimodality approach with diffusion-weighted imaging, diffusion tensor imaging, magnetic resonance spectroscopy, dynamic susceptibility contrast and dynamic contrast-enhanced magnetic resonance imaging. In modern imaging evaluation of the brain, body and spine. Magn Reson Imaging Clin N Am 2013;21(2):203–7.

35. Guo AC, Cummings TJ, Dash RC, et al. Lymphomas and high-grade astrocytomas: comparison of water diffusibility and histologic characteristics. Radiology 2002;224(1):177–83.

36. Yamasaki F, Kurisu K, Satoh K, et al. Apparent diffusion coefficient of human brain tumors at MR imaging. Radiology 2005;235:985–91.

37. Toh CH, Castillo M, Wong AC, et al. Primary cerebral lymphoma and glioblastoma multiforme: differences in diffusion characteristics evaluated with diffusion tensor imaging. AJNR Am J Neuroradiol 2008;29:471–5.

38. Stadnik TW, Chaskis C, Michotte A, et al. Diffusion-weighted MR images of intracerebral masses: comparison with conventional MR imaging and histologic findings. AJNR Am J Neuroradiol 2001;22:969–76.

39. Sugahara T, Korogi Y, Kochi M, et al. Usefulness of diffusion-weighted MRI with echo-planar techniques in the evaluation of cellularity in gliomas. J Magn Reson Imaging 1999;9:53–60.

40. Kono K, Inoue Y, Nakayama K, et al. The role of diffusion-weighted imaging in patients with brain tumors. AJNR Am J Neuroradiol 2001;22:1081–8.

41. Horger M, Fenchel M, Nägele T, et al. Water diffusivity: comparison of primary CNS lymphoma and astrocytic tumor infiltrating the corpus callosum. AJR Am J Roentgenol 2009;193:1384–7.

42. Batra A, Tripathi RP. Atypical diffusion-weighted magnetic resonance findings in glioblastoma multiforme. Australas Radiol 2004;48:388–91.

43. Hakyemez B, Erdogan C, Yildirim N, et al. Glioblastoma multiforme with atypical diffusion-weighted MR findings. Br J Radiol 2005;78:989–92.

44. Toh CH, Chen YL, Hsieh TC, et al. Glioblastoma multiforme with diffusion-weighted magnetic resonance imaging characteristics mimicking primary brain lymphoma. Case report. J Neurosurg 2006;105:132–5.

45. Baehring JM, Bi WL, Bannykh S, et al. Diffusion MRI in the early diagnosis of malignant glioma. J Neurooncol 2007;82:221–5.

46. Chang YW, Yoon HK, Shih HJ, et al. MR imaging of glioblastoma in children: usefulness of diffusion/perfusion-weighted MRI and MR spectroscopy. Pediatr Radiol 2003;33:836–42.

47. Ahn SJ, Shin HJ, Chang JH, et al. Differentiation between primary cerebral lymphoma and glioblastoma using the apparent diffusion coefficient: comparison of three different ROI methods. PLoS One 2014; 9(11):e112948.

48. Barajas RF, Rubenstein JL, Chang JS, et al. Diffusion-weighted MR imaging derived apparent diffusion coefficient is predictive of clinical outcome in primary central nervous system lymphoma. AJNR Am J Neuroradiol 2010;31:60–6.

49. Valles FE, Perez-Valles CL, Regalado S, et al. Combined diffusion and perfusion MR imaging as biomarkers of prognosis in immunocompetent patients with primary central nervous system lymphoma. AJNR Am J Neuroradiol 2013;34:35–40.

50. Punwani S, Taylor SA, Saad ZZ, et al. Diffusion-weighted MRI of lymphoma: prognostic utility and implications for PET/MRI? Eur J Nucl Med Mol Imaging 2013;40(3):373–85.

51. Beppu T, Inoue T, Shibata Y, et al. Measurement of fractional anisotropy using diffusion tensor MRI in supratentorial astrocytic tumors. J Neurooncol 2003;63:109–16.

52. Kinoshita M, Hashimoto N, Goto T, et al. Fractional anisotropy and tumor cell density of the tumor core show positive correlation in diffusion tensor magnetic resonance imaging of malignant brain tumors. Neuroimage 2008;43:29–35.

53. Vargova L, Homola A, Zamecnik J, et al. Diffusion parameters of the extracellular space in human gliomas. Glia 2003;42:77–88.

54. Zamecnik J. The extracellular space and matrix of gliomas. Acta Neuropathol 2005;110:435–42.

55. Brandão L, Domingues R. Intracranial neoplasms. In: McAllister L, Lazar T, Cook RE, editors. MR spectroscopy of the brain. Philadelphia: Lippincott Williams & Wilkins; 2004. p. 130–67.

56. Brandão LA, Castillo M. Adult brain tumors: clinical applications of magnetic resonance spectroscopy. Neuroimag Clin N Am 2013;23(3):527–55.

57. Knopp EA. Advanced MR imaging of tumors using spectroscopy and perfusion. Presented at the 39th Annual Meeting of the American Society of Neuroradiology. Boston, April 23–27, 2001.

58. Castillo M. Proton MR spectroscopy of common brain tumors. Neuroimaging Clin N Am 1998;8(4):733–52.

59. Toh CH, Wei KC, Chang CN, et al. Differentiation of primary central nervous system lymphomas and glioblastomas: comparisons of diagnostic performance of dynamic susceptibility contrast-enhanced perfusion MR imaging without and with contrast-leakage correction. AJNR Am J Neuroradiol 2013;34:1145–9.

60. Liao W, Liu Y, Wang X, et al. Differentiation of primary central nervous system lymphoma and high-grade glioma with dynamic susceptibility contrast-enhanced perfusion magnetic resonance imaging. Acta Radiol 2009;50(2):217–25.

61. Cha S, Knop EA, Jhonson G, et al. Intracranial mass lesions: dynamic contrast enhanced susceptibility-weighted echo-planar perfusion MR imaging. Radiology 2002;223:11–29.

62. Rowland LA, Pedley TA, Merritt HH. Distinguishing of primary cerebral lymphoma from high grade glioma with perfusion-weighted magnetic resonance imaging. Neurosci Lett 2003;338:119–22.

63. Weber MA, Zoubaa S, Schileter M, et al. Diagnostic performance of spectroscopic and perfusion MRI for distinction of brain tumors. Neurology 2006;66:1899–906.

64. Patankar TF, Haroon HA, Mills SJ, et al. Is volume transfer coefficient (Ktrans) related to histologic grade in human gliomas? AJNR Am J Neuroradiol 2005;26:2455–65.

65. Cha S, Yang L, Johnson G, et al. Comparison of microvascular permeability measurements, K trans, determined with conventional steady-state T1-weighted and first pass T2*-weighted MR imaging methods in gliomas and meningiomas. AJNR Am J Neuroradiol 2006;27:409–17.

66. Eby NL, Grufferman S, Flanelly CM, et al. Increasing incidence of primary brain lymphoma in the US. Cancer 1998;62:2461–5.

67. DeAngelis LM. Current management of primary central nervous system lymphoma. Oncology (Williston Park) 1995;9:63–71.

68. Samani A, Davagnanam I, Cockerell OC, et al. Lymphomatosis cerebri: a treatable cause of rapidly progressive dementia. J Neurol Neurosurg Psychiatry 2015;86(2):238–40.

69. ØStergaard L, Hochberg FH, Rabinov J, et al. Early changes measured by magnetic resonance imaging in cerebral blood flow, blood volume, and blood-brain barrier permeability following dexamethasone treatment in patients with brain tumors. J Neurosurg 1999;90(2):300–5.

70. DeAngelis LM, Yahalom J, Heinemann M-H, et al. Primary CNS lymphoma: combined treatment with chemotherapy and radiotherapy. Neurology 1990;40:80–6.

71. Henry JM, Heffner RR Jr, Dillard SH. Primary malignant lymphomas of the nervous system. Cancer 1974;34:1293–302.

Lymphomas–Part 2

Lara A. Brandão, MD[a,b,*], Mauricio Castillo, MD[c]

KEYWORDS

- Lymphomatosis cerebri • Intravascular lymphoma • Lymphomatoid granulomatosis

KEY POINTS

- Lymphomatosis cerebri (LC) is a rare type of infiltrative lymphoma that usually does not enhance.
- In LC, restricted diffusion is minimal or absent.
- Magnetic resonance spectroscopy (MRS) may distinguish LC from gliomatosis cerebri (GC).
- Intravascular lymphoma (IVL) may mimic ischemic lesions.

SPECIAL LYMPHOMA TYPES

Lymphomatosis Cerebri

LC is a rare variant of primary central nervous system (CNS) lymphoma (PCNSL) pathologically characterized by diffuse cerebral infiltration of a noncohesive mass of malignant lymphoid cells.[1–6] The clinical picture is variable and includes abnormal behavior, personality changes, gait disturbance, seizures, memory deficits, and rapidly progressive dementia and weight loss.[4–8]

White matter abnormalities in LC affect all of the brain. MR imaging findings are extensive, diffuse T2 and FLAIR-weighted hyperintense lesions without formation of a cohesive mass and no contrast enhancement in both cerebral hemispheres and brainstem (Fig. 1).[6–11] Subtle or patchy enhancement may be seen.[8,10] There may be a transition from nonenhancing to enhancing lesions suggesting that progression and evolution is associated with disruption of the blood-brain barrier.[4] Restricted diffusion may be minimal or absent (see Figs. 1F, G).[10] Many cases respond to steroids alone, at least initially. To achieve complete remission, steroids are usually followed by radiotherapy, cisplatin, or methotrexate.[12]

Pearls

- LC is a diagnostic challenge.
- In patients presenting with diffuse, bilateral, asymmetric signal abnormalities in white matter, infiltrative lymphoma should be considered, especially if there is callosal involvement.
- Consider brain biopsy in rapidly progressive cognitive decline to allow earlier therapy for a potentially curable disease.[4]
- Awareness of this rare disease and early biopsy are required for preventing a poor clinical outcome.[6]

Intravascular Lymphoma

IVL was originally described in 1959[13] and designated as "angioendotheliomatosis proliferans systemisata." Since then, it has been referred to as neoplastic angioendotheliosis, malignant angioendotheliomatosis, and angiotropic large-cell lymphoma.[14–17]

IVL is a rare subtype of extranodal diffuse large B-cell lymphoma with a distinct presentation. Anatomically, it is characterized by proliferation of clonal lymphocytes within small vessels with

Funding Sources: None.

Conflict of Interest: None.

[a] Radiologic Department, Clínica Felippe Mattoso, Fleury Medicina Diagnóstica, Avenida das Américas 700, sala 320, Barra Da Tijuca, Rio De Janeiro, Rio De Janeiro CEP 22640-100, Brazil; [b] Radiologic Department, Clínica IRM- Ressonância Magnética, Rua Capitão Salomão, Humaitá, Rio De Janeiro, Rio De Janeiro CEP 22271-040, Brazil; [c] Division of Neuroradiology, Department of Radiology, University of North Carolina, School of Medicine, Room 3326, Old Infirmary Building, Manning Drive, Chapel Hill, NC 27599-7510, USA

* Corresponding author. Clínica Felippe Mattoso, Fleury Medicina Diagnóstica, Avenida das Américas 700, sala 320, Barra Da Tijuca, Rio De Janeiro, Rio De Janeiro CEP 22640-100, Brazil.

E-mail address: larabrandao.rad@terra.com.br

1052-5149/16/© 2016 Elsevier Inc. All rights reserved.

neuroimaging.theclinics.com

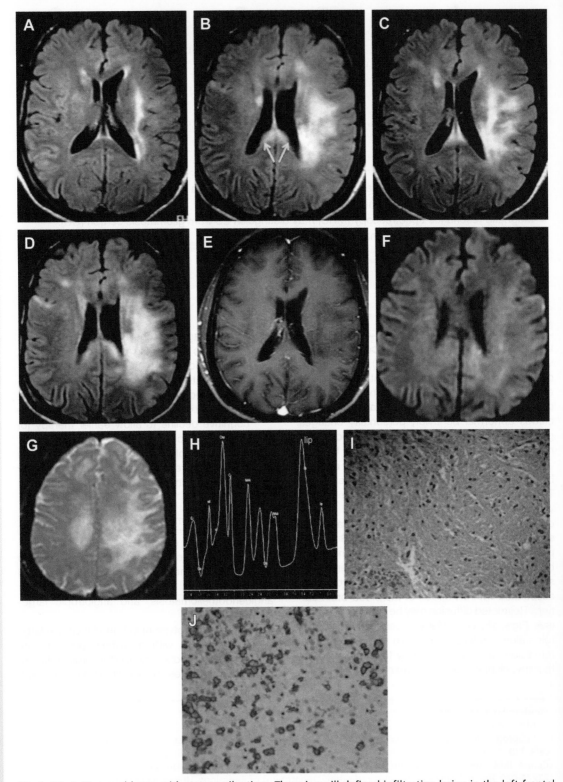

Fig. 1. LC. A 40-year-old man with status epilepticus. There is an ill-defined infiltrating lesion in the left frontal and parietal lobes ([*A, B*] axial FLAIR), extending to the splenium of the corpus callosum ([*B*] *arrows*). MR imaging 1 month later ([*C, D*] axial FLAIR) shows progression. No enhancement is demonstrated ([*E*] axial T1 with contrast) and there is no restricted diffusion ([*F*] DWI, [*G*] ADC map). (*H*) MRS shows low NAA and mI, high Cho, and lipid peaks, characteristic of LC ([*I, J*] confirmed at pathology). ADC, apparent diffusion coefficient. (*Courtesy of* Dr Leonardo Avanza, Vitória, Rio De Janeiro, Brazil; and Leila Chimelli, MD, Rio De Janeiro, Brazil.)

relative sparing of surrounding tissues.[18] The degree of sparing of surrounding tissues and absence of lymphoma cells in lymph nodes and reticuloendothelial system is a hallmark of the disease.[18]

Epidemiology and risk factors

IVL is a rare disease with an incidence of less than 1 person per million. It has been described in patients ranging from 34 to 90 years of age with a

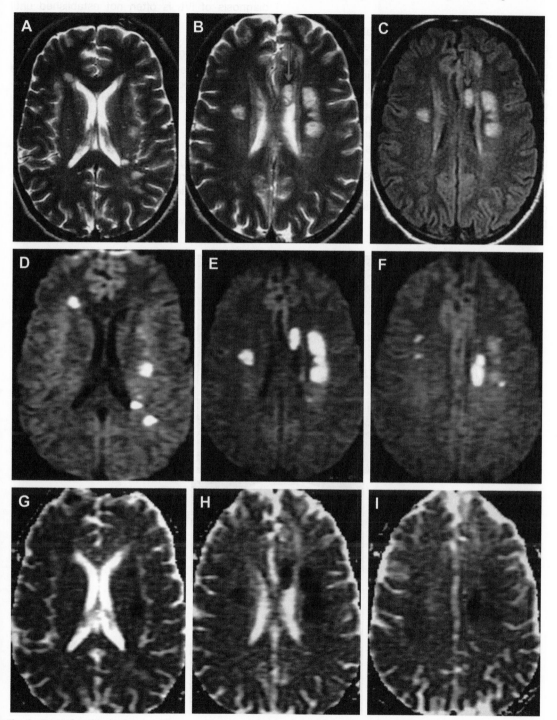

Fig. 2. IVL–infarctlike lesions. A 39-year-old man with seizures and tetraparesis. IVL shows multifocal round nodules hyperintense on (*A, B*) T2 and (*C*) FLAIR in the watershed zones bilateraly mimicking infarcts. A lesion is seen in the corpus callosum ([*B, C*] *arrows*), which suggests IVL. The restricted diffusion ([*D–F*] DWI and [*G–I*] ADC map) is also very characteristic of IVL.

median age of 70 years and occurs equally in women and men.[19] There are no known risk factors for IVL.

Clinical features

IVL is heterogeneous in its clinical presentation and affects the small vessels in nearly every organ. Although IVL is a clonal proliferation of lymphocytes, it is uncommon to find significant adenopathy, hepatosplenomegaly, or malignant cells in the peripheral blood. Absence of IVL in the traditional sites of presentation of lymphoma makes accurate and timely diagnosis difficult. Clinical symptoms depend on specific organ involvement, which most often includes the CNS and skin. Patients with CNS compromise present with focal sensory or motor deficits, generalized weakness, altered sensorium, rapidly progressive dementia, seizures, hemiparesis, dysarthria, ataxia, vertigo, and transient visual loss.[20–23] Initial diagnoses of stroke, encephalomyelitis, Guillain-Barré syndrome, vasculitis, and multiple sclerosis (MS) are often made and a diagnosis of IVL is often not established until autopsy.[21,24–26]

Laboratory findings

Anemia, elevated lactate dehydrogenase, and elevated erythrocyte sedimentation rate are common laboratory abnormalities in IVL.[19] A majority of studies have shown IVL absent in peripheral blood smears.

Imaging findings

The diffuse nature of brain involvement, with multifocal abnormalities, is reflected by its MR imaging appearance.[27–30] MR imaging findings of IVL include the following.[28]

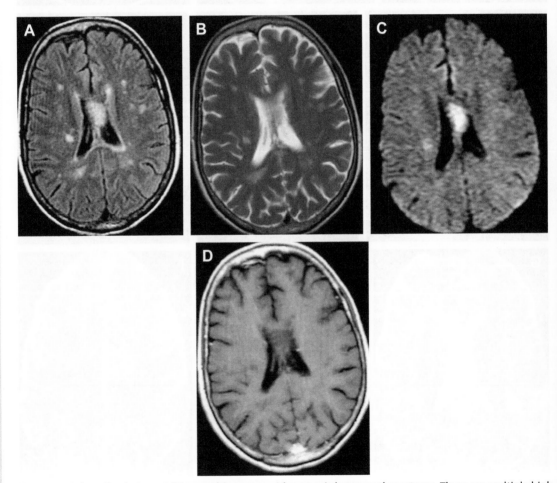

Fig. 3. IVL–infarct-like lesions. A 65-year-old woman with systemic lupus erythematosus. There are multiple high signal intensity lesions in the corona radiata bilaterally ([A] axial FLAIR and [B] axial T2). A solid lesion is demonstrated in the corpus callosum, hyperintense on (A) FLAIR, isointense to gray matter on (B) T2, and (C) having restricted diffusion (DWI). (D) No enhancement is seen.

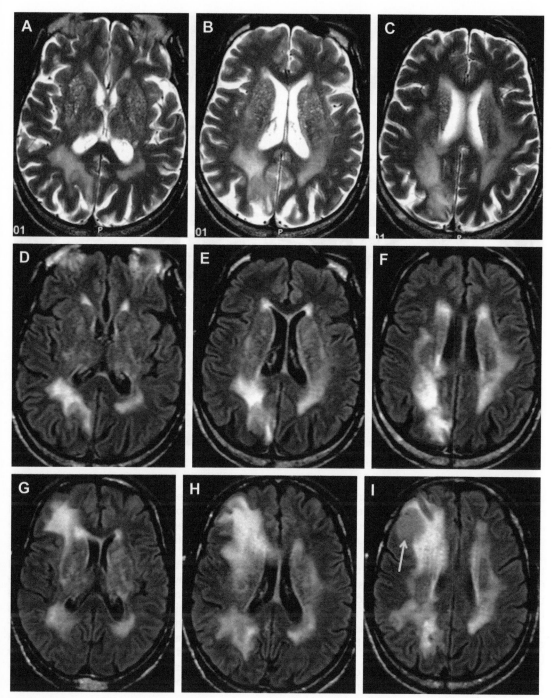

Fig. 4. IVL–nonspecific white matter lesions and masslike lesions. Extensive high signal intensity lesions are demonstrated in the (*A–C*) axial T2 and (*D–F*) FLAIR mainly in the white matter as well as in the deep gray nuclei resembling vascular lesions. (*G–I*) Two months later the lesions progressed and are diffuse. (*I*) A solid mass is demonstrated in the right frontal lobe (*arrow*). (*J–O*) Axial T1 with contrast shows enhancing lesions adjacent to the (*J*) right ventricular atrium, (*K*) in the right parietal region, and (*L*) in the left frontal lobe. Again, 2 months later the right occipital enhancing nodule (demonstrated in [*J*]) disappeared and (*M–O*) a new lesion in the right frontal area is demonstrated. (*K*) The enhancing lesion in the right parietal region seen in the first MR imaging resolved and (*N*) new enhancing foci are noted anteriorly. (*L*) The left frontal enhancing nodules (*O*) almost disappeared.

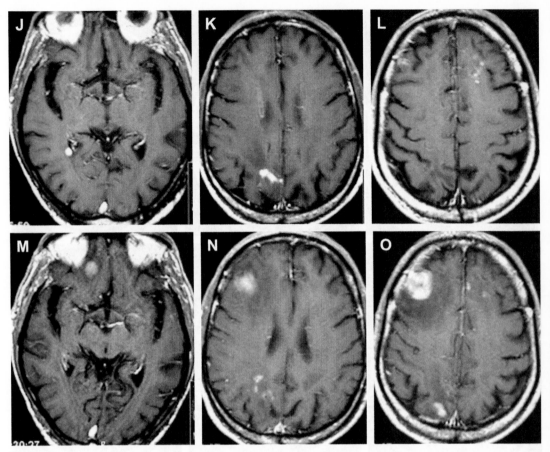

Fig. 4.

Infarct-like lesions Multiple, round or oval metachronous cortical or subcortical lesions that are hyperintense on T2-weighted and fluid-attenuated inversion recovery (FLAIR) images, some presenting with restricted diffusion suggestive of small vessel ischemia or demyelination (**Figs. 2** and **3**).[22,27] Although classically IVL is thought to remain strictly confined to vascular lumina in the CNS, parenchymal[14] and callosal involvement may represent extravascular spread of tumor and may help suggest the diagnosis (see **Figs. 2** and **3**).[23]

Infarct-like lesions correlate with commonly reported findings of multiple recent or resolving infarctions.[17] The lesions may not enhance (see **Fig. 3**D). Infarct-like lesions suggest that the tumor predominantly involves small arteries.[31] This pattern was reported in 36% of patients with IVL who had brain MR imaging.[27]

Nonspecific white matter lesions Poorly defined nonspecific white matter lesions have been reported, especially in the periventricular areas, mimicking leukoaraiosis (**Fig. 4**).[27] Some

investigators speculate that severe vascular infiltration by tumor cells leads to small vessel occlusion, ischemia, and infarction, which are responsible for these imaging findings.[32]

Masslike lesions Williams and colleagues[27] noticed that intraparenchymal mass lesions have extensive vasogenic edema and mass effect contrary to the characteristic features of tumor cell infiltration predominantly in the vascular lumen. Nodular-enhancing lesions may disappear in follow-up MR imaging studies and be replaced by other enhancing lesions in other locations reflecting a dynamic behavior of IVL (see **Fig. 4**J–O).

Meningeal enhancement Meningeal enhancement is sometimes present in patients with IVL, although the nature of this finding is unclear.[27] Severe meningeal inflammatory reaction with tumor cells has been demonstrated in post mortem examinations.[28]

Hyperintense T2 lesions in the pons T2 hyperintense lesions in the central pons without contrast enhancement or diffusion restriction have been

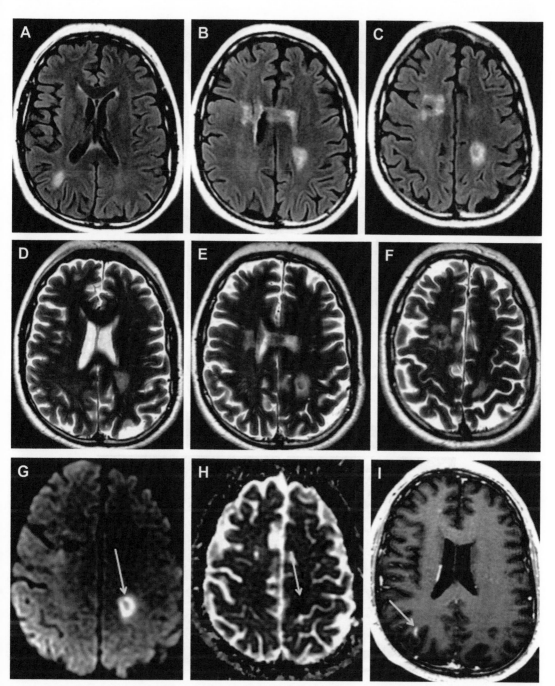

Fig. 5. LG. A 59-year-old man presents with memory impairment, left facial palsy, and headaches. Multiple high signal intensity lesions are demonstrated in the white matter and corpus callosum ([*A–C*] axial FLAIR and [*D–F*] axial T2). Restricted diffusion is demonstrated in the lesion located in the left parietal white matter ([*G*] *arrows*, DWI, and [*H*] ADC map). (*I–K*) Axial T1 with contrast: (*I*) linear, (*J*) nodular, and (*K*) ring enhancement are demonstrated (*arrows*). Perfusion is variable, with some lesions presenting with high blood volume ([*L*] axial FLAIR and [*M*] rCBV map) and some with no elevation of the blood volume ([*N*] axial FLAIR and [*O*] rCBV map). Permeability is not significantly elevated ([*P*] axial T1 with contrast and [*Q*] maximum slope of increase map).

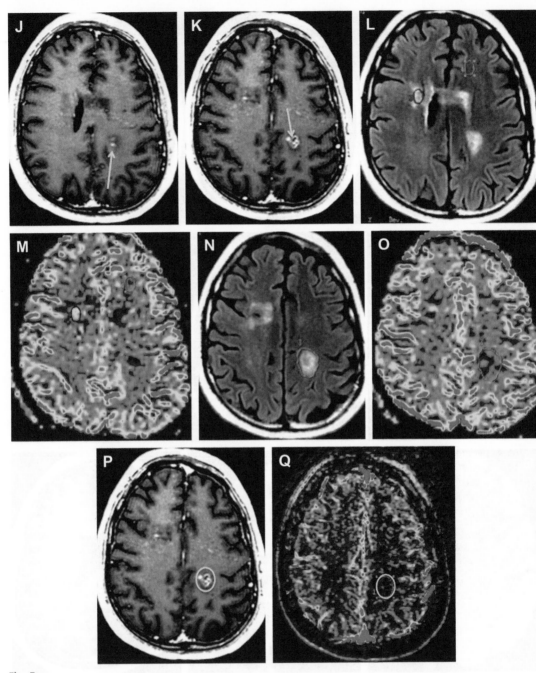

Fig. 5.

reported. These lesions in the central pons exclude the pontine tegmentum and ventrolateral region and are similar to those of pontine osmolytic demyelination and posterior reversible encephalopathy syndrome or those from intracranial dural arteriovenous fistula with venous congestion.[33–38]

Occlusion of capillaries causes diffuse white matter abnormal intensities. Some investigators[38] speculate that the hyperintense pons lesions result from occlusion of capillaries.

A majority of cases of IVL present as CNS abnormalities, particularly with diffuse encephalopathy, and/or subacute progressive multifocal neurologic deficits and MR imaging findings that resemble vasculitis.[39]

Lymphomatoid Granulomatosis

Lymphomatoid granulomatosis (LG) is a rare angiocentric, destructive lymphoproliferative disorder. It mainly involves the lungs followed by the skin and brain.[40,41] Isolated CNS involvement is rare.[42–48] When it affects the CNS, it is more commonly due to spread of systemic LG to the CNS. Although it may develop in the immunocompetent, LG is more common in the immune suppressed, including AIDS patients.[48]

Clinical picture
Clinical features of CNS involvement are highly variable, including headache, seizure, blindness, cranial nerve palsies, hemiparesis, ataxia, spastic gait, dementia, and altered consciousness.[42,43]

Imaging findings
LG presents diverse neuroimaging features, such as multiple punctuate or linear enhancement, ring-like enhancement, large mass lesions, and lepto-meningeal and choroid plexus involvement.[49–51] Multifocal T2 hyperintensities with linear or punctuate contrast enhancement are common (**Fig. 5**)[49] and thought to be due to the angiocentric and angiodestructive nature of the disease. The lesions typically involve the white matter and deep gray nuclei. Leptomeningeal and cranial nerve enhancement are also common.

MR imaging is more sensitive than cerebrospinal fluid (CSF) analysis or flow cytometry for detecting CNS involvement from LG.[49]

DIFFERENTIAL DIAGNOSIS
Focal and Multifocal Brain Lesions

When CNS lymphoma presents with focal or multifocal brain lesions, the main differential diagnoses are the following.

Glioblastoma
It may be difficult or even impossible to distinguish lymphoma from glioblastoma (GBM).[52,53] Both tumors may present with isointense to hypointense signal to gray matter on T2 (**Fig. 6**).

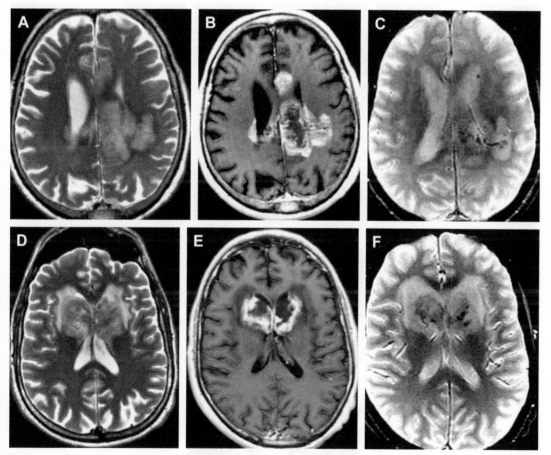

Fig. 6. Lymphoma versus GBM. (*A–C*) A 79-year-old man, presenting with progressive right hemiparesis diagnosed with GBM. (*D–F*) A 37-year-old man HIV+ presenting with fever and memory impairment diagnosed with lymphoma. Both patients present infiltrative lesions surrounding the lateral ventricles, isointense to gray matter on T2 ([*A, D*] axial T2), with nonhomogeneous enhancement, due to necrosis and hemorrhage, ([*B, E*] axial T1 with contrast and [*C, F*] axial gradient-echo).

Necrosis and hemorrhage, although more common in GBM, also may be demonstrated in lymphoma, even in immunocompetent patients. Advanced MR imaging techniques, such as diffusion-weighted imaging (DWI) (**Fig. 7**), MRS (**Fig. 8**), perfusion-weighted imaging (**Fig. 9**), and dynamic contrast-enhanced studies (**Fig. 10**) may help distinguish these lesions.[53] (For a complete description of imaging findings on advanced MR Imaging techniques in lymphomas and GBM, see Lara A. Brandão and Mauricio Castillo's article, "Lymphomas- Part 1," in this issue.)

Multifocal glioma

High-grade gliomas (HGGs) may present as multifocal brain lesions, mimicking multifocal lymphoma (**Fig. 11**). Hypoperfusion and no significant elevation of permeability suggest lymphoma. Lymphomas with high blood volumes and high permeability, however, have been documented. Diffusion plays a significant role in the distinction between these lesions. In lymphoma, restricted diffusion usually matches the T2 abnormality, whereas in HGGs small foci of restricted diffusion may be demonstrated within the lesion.

Multiple sclerosis

PCNSL can be misdiagnosed as MS in patients who present with nonenhancing periventricular lesions and CSF pleocytosis.[54] Administration of corticosteroids causes clinical improvement and regression of PCNSL in some patients, which may be interpreted as a steroid-induced remission of MS. Sustained clinical dependence on corticosteroids is unusual in MS and should lead to consideration of PCNSL. Repeat CNS examination

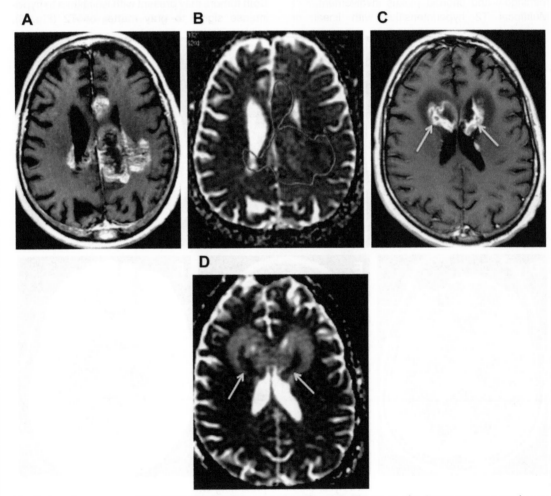

Fig. 7. Lymphoma versus GBM-DWI/ADC. (*A, B*) Same patient shown in **Fig.** 6A–C. The GBM presents a nonhomogeneous enhancement ([*A*] axial T1 with contrast) and high ADC ([*B*] ADC map). (*C, D*) Same patient as shown in **Fig.** 6D–F. The lymphoma ([*C*] *arrows*, axial T1 with contrast) demonstrates low ADC ([*D*] *arrows*, ADC map) consistent with restricted water diffusion due to high cell density.

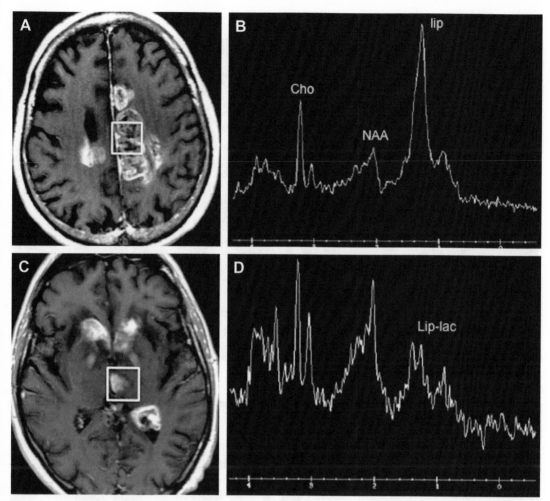

Fig. 8. Lymphoma versus GBM-MRS. (*A, B*) Same patient shown in Fig. 6A–C. The GBM demonstrates high Cho, low NAA, and a large lipid peak. (*C, D*) Same patient shown in Fig. 6D–F. MRS from the left thalamic lesion demonstrates high lipids and lactate. When lipids are demonstrated in a solid-appearing tumor, lymphoma should be considered.

and gadolinium-enhanced MR imaging obtained off corticosteroids help differentiate between the two (Fig. 12).

Contrast enhancement Despite enhancement may be demonstrated in acute MS plaques, if all lesions enhance lymphoma should be considered (Fig. 13).

Diffusion-weighted imaging/apparent diffusion coefficient Restricted diffusion may be demonstrated in some MS plaques whereas restricted diffusion is typically seen in all lymphoma brain masses usually matching the T2 abnormalities.

Perfusion and permeability High blood volumes and permeability, although not common, may be seen in lymphoma, but are not typically demonstrated in MS.

Tumefactive demyelinating lesions
Tumefactive demyelinating lesions (TDLs) are frequently encountered in clinical practice and when they appear as solitary masses greater than 2 cm in diameter they can cause symptoms mimicking brain neoplasms.[55] Differentiating between PCNSLs and TDLs by conventional MR imaging can be challenging, especially when there are atypical features in PCNSLs. Considering the rapid progression of PCNSLs, early differentiation is important because both treatment effectiveness and patient survival substantially decrease if there is delayed radiation therapy and/or chemotherapy.[56] Accurate differentiation is important to avoid unnecessary biopsies of TDLs.

Valuable clues to the diagnosis
- Vessels crossing the lesion: Linear vascular structures may be demonstrated within a

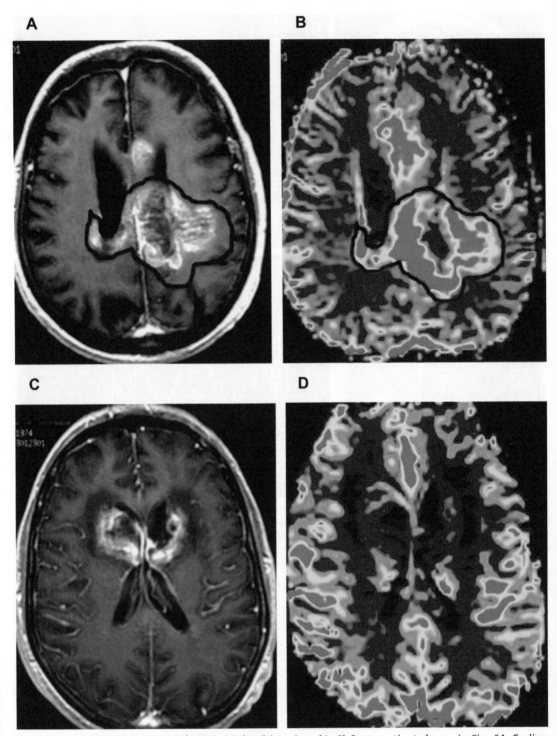

Fig. 9. Lymphoma versus GBM-perfusion weighted imaging. (*A, B*) Same patient shown in Fig. 6A–C, diagnosed with GBM. The nonhomogeneous enhancing lesion (region of interest in [*A*] axial T1 with contrast) demonstrates high perfusion ([*B*] rCBV map) consistent with high vascular density and high count of microvascular tumor vessels. (*C, D*) Same patient shown in Fig. 6D–F. The nonhomogeneous enhancing lymphoma ([*C*] axial T1 with contrast) presents hypoperfusion ([*D*] rCBV map), a finding different than that seen in GBM.

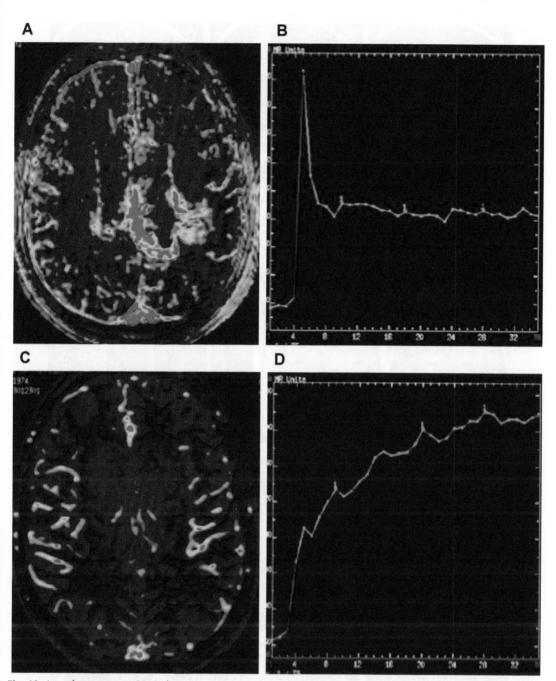

Fig. 10. Lymphoma versus GBM–dynamic contrast-enhanced study. (*A, B*) Same patient shown in **Fig.** 6A–C, diagnosed with GBM. There is very high permeability in the lesion ([*A*] map of maximum slope of increase and [*B*] curve). (*C, D*) Same patient shown in **Fig.** 6D–F. There is no significant permeability in this lymphoma ([*C*] map of maximum slope of increase and [*D*] curve), a finding that helps distinguish lymphoma from GBM.

TDL, indicating perivascular demyelination (**Fig. 14**).

- Pattern of enhancement: A peripheral open ring of enhancement suggests a TDL,[55,57]

whereas solid enhancement suggests lymphoma (**Fig. 15**).

- Diffusion-weighted imaging/apparent diffusion coefficient measurements: A peripheral rim of

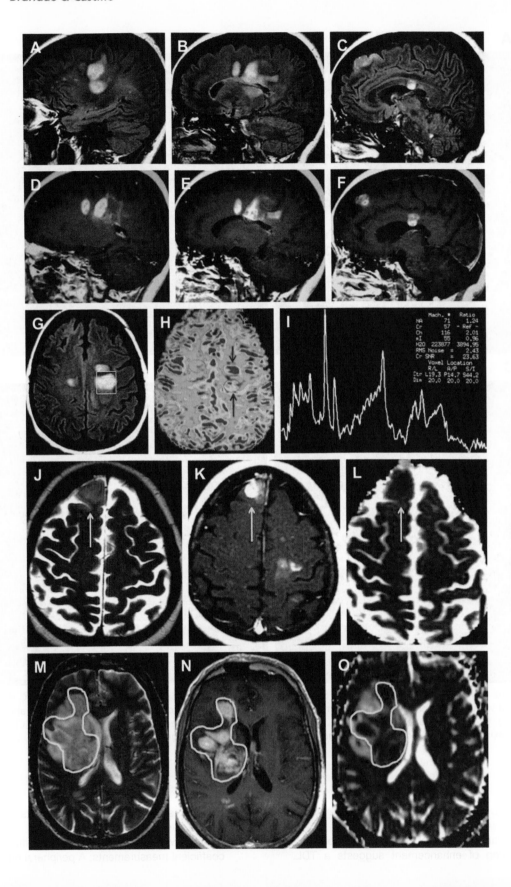

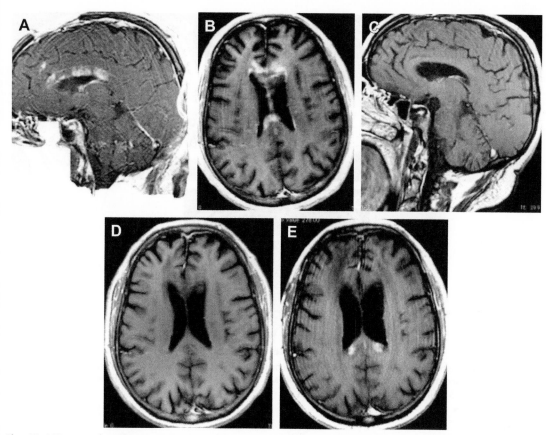

Fig. 12. MS versus lymphoma. A 56-year-old man presenting with enhancing lesions in the corpus callosum and periventricular white matter ([A] sagittal and [B] axial T1 with contrast). After steroid therapy ([C] sagittal and [D] axial T1 with contrast) no enhancement is demonstrated. Steroid administration was discontinued and a follow-up MR imaging 3 months later ([E] axial T1 with contrast) demonstrates new enhancing lesions adjacent to the ventricular margins, in the splenium of the corpus callosum bilaterally. Final diagnosis: PCNSL.

restricted diffusion suggests a TDL (see **Fig. 15**C) instead of lymphoma (see **Fig. 15**F).[58]

- Magnetic resonance spectroscopy: Differentiation between aggressive brain tumors and acute demyelinating lesions based on MRS alone is difficult because of histopathologic similarities, which include hypercellularity, reactive astrocytes, mitotic figures, and areas of necrosis.[59–61]

Aggressive brain tumors and demyelinating plaques present elevated choline (Cho), reduced N-acetyl aspartate (NAA), and increased lipids and lactate.[61–63] Elevation of glutamine and glutamate helps differentiate TDL from neoplastic masses (**Fig. 16**).[63] Lu and colleagues[64] demonstrated that lymphoma can be suggested when Cho/creatine (Cr) ratio is greater than 2.58, Cho/NAA ratio is greater than

Fig. 11. Multifocal HGG versus lymphoma. A 78-year-old woman presenting with hemiparesis on the right, dizziness, dysartria, dysphagia, blurred speech, and hyperreflexia due to grade III glioma. (A–C) Multiple round and oval lesions with high signal intensity on FLAIR are demonstrated in (A, B) deep white matter, corpus callosum, and (C) cortex. All lesions enhance ([D–F] sagittal T1 with contrast), which makes the diagnosis of MS unlikely. The hyperintense lesions on FLAIR ([G] axial FLAIR) have hyperperfusion (arrows in [H] rCBV map), more consistent with the diagnosis of HGG. (I) Spectroscopy shows low NAA, high Cho, and presence of lipids/lac. Only 1 solid lesion ([J] arrow, axial T2, and [K] axial T1 with contrast) presents restricted diffusion ([L] ADC map), different from what is expected in lymphomas (M–O) where restricted diffusion matches the T2 abnormalities as well the areas of enhancement ([M] axial T2, [N] axial T1 with contrast, and [O] ADC map).

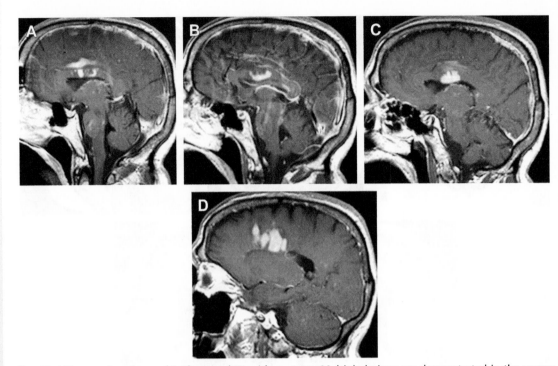

Fig. 13. MS versus lymphoma. (*A–D*) sagittal T1 with contrast. Multiple lesions are demonstrated in the corpus callosum and adjacent white matter, which resemble MS lesions. All lesions enhance, however, which makes the diagnosis of MS unlikely. Final diagnosis: PCNSL.

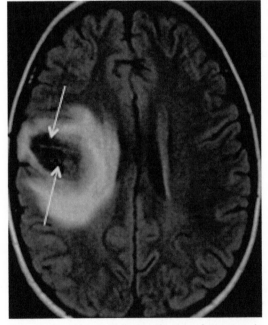

Fig. 14. TDL versus lymphoma. There is a large mass in the right frontal lobe, surrounded by extensive edema with high signal intensity on FLAIR (axial T1). Linear structures can be demonstrated crossing the lesion, suggesting vascular structures, indicating perivascular demyelination (*arrows*).

1.73, and high lipid and/or lactate peaks are seen. Very high Cho, Cho/Cr, and Cho/NAA ratios, however, as well as high lipid and lactate peaks may also be seen in TDL (see Fig. 16).

Perfusion and permeability: If high blood volume and high permeability are present, lymphoma should be considered. Low relative cerebral blood volume (rCBV) along with no significant elevation of permeability may be demonstrated, however, in lymphoma and TDL.

Toxoplasmosis

Accurate differentiation of focal brain masses in AIDS patients is critical for timely initiation of therapy.[65,66] The 2 most common masses in this population are toxoplasmosis and lymphoma and frequently have similar characteristics on both CT and MR imaging.[65–68]

Diffusion-weighted imaging/apparent diffusion coefficient Apparent diffusion coefficient (ADC) values can play a role in the neurologically impaired AIDS patients whose brain lesions show a nonspecific appearance.

Camacho and colleagues[66] demonstrated that ADC values in toxoplasmosis are significantly greater than those in lymphoma. According to

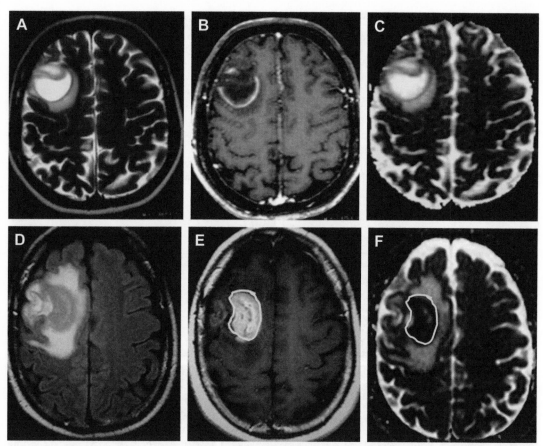

Fig. 15. TDL versus lymphoma. (*A–C*) TDL. Patient presenting with a right frontal lesion, hyperintense on T2 ([*A*] axial T2), with an open ring of enhancement ([*B*] axial T1 with contrast) and a peripheral rim of restricted diffusion ([*C*] ADC map). (*D–F*) Lymphoma. There is a right frontal lesion isointense to gray matter on (*D*) FLAIR, with solid enhancement ([*E*] axial T1 with contrast) and restricted diffusion that matches the enhancing area ([*F*] region of interest, ADC map).

their study, if a focal brain mass is identified on brain MR imaging and if the ADC ratio in that lesion is greater than 1.6, the patient should be given a trial of antitoxoplasma therapy. If the ADC ratio is less than 1.6, in particular less than 1.0, additional imaging or early biopsy may be needed.

Magnetic resonance spectroscopy An overlap in metabolic profiles of lymphoma and toxoplasmosis is often demonstrated.[69–71] Elevation of Cho and presence of lipids and low NAA are often demonstrated in both lesions.[71]

Perfusion and permeability Distinction between lymphoma and toxoplasmosis is easy when blood volumes are elevated in lymphomas.[72] Some lymphomas, however, do not demonstrate elevation of blood volumes or permeability, making the distinction between lymphoma and toxoplasmosis difficult.

Infiltrative Diffuse Lesion with No Discernible Mass

Lymphomatois cerebri versus gliomatosis cerebri

Imaging findings in LC are similar with those of GC. Discrete or no enhancement is demonstrated in both tumors. MRS may help differentiate LC from GC grades II and III. A high myo-inositol (mI) peak is characteristic of GC grade II, even if Cho is not elevated.[73–76]

On the other hand, LC is characterized by reduced NAA and mI peaks along with elevation of Cho and lipid (**Fig. 17**).[73] In GC grade III, the Cho peak is high due to a high cell density similar to what is demonstrated in LC. No elevation of lipids, however, is demonstrated in GC grade III (**Fig. 18**).

Lymphomatosis cerebri versus microangiopathy (Binswanger disease)

Rarely, PCNSL presents as a diffuse, infiltrating condition without formation of a mass and is called

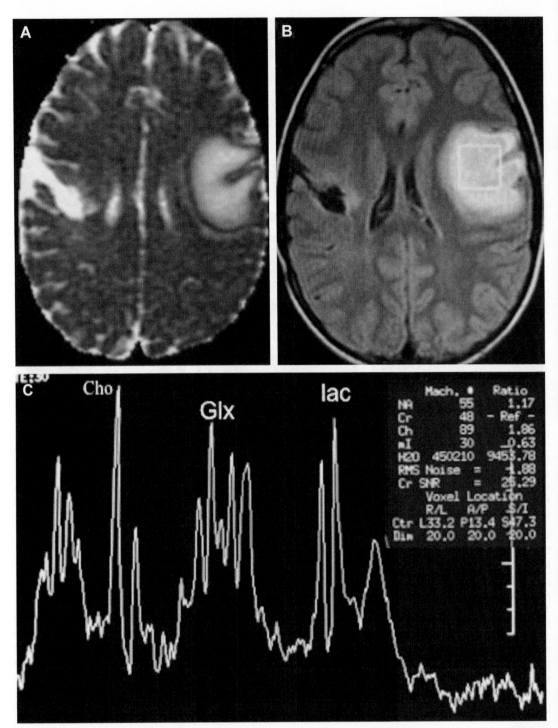

Fig. 16. TDL versus lymphoma. There is a left frontal lesion presenting with a peripheral rim of restricted diffusion ([A] ADC map) typical of TDL. Spectroscopy ([B] voxel location and [C] curve) shows high Cho and high lactate, along with a very high glutamate and glutamine peak also typical of demyelination.

LC and may be mistaken for diffuse leukoencephalopathy.[4,6] In cases of presumed vascular dementia based on MR imaging and an unusually rapidly progressive cognitive decline and a presumed chronic encephalomyelitis, LC should be considered, especially when marked additional signal changes in basal ganglia and thalamus are present.[11]

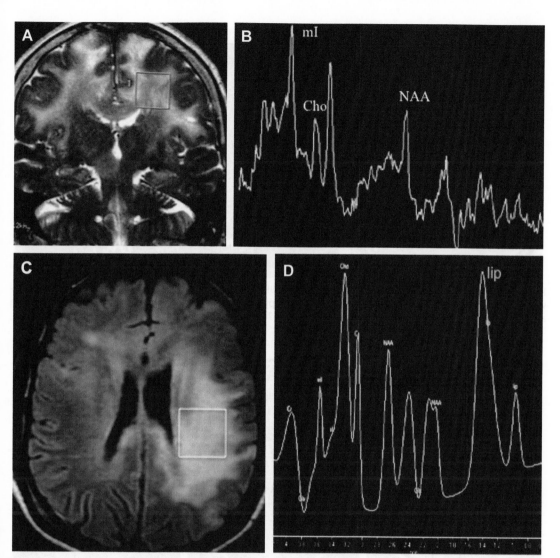

Fig. 17. LC versus GC grade II. (*A, B*) GC grade II. There is an infiltrating lesion in both cerebral hemispheres ([*A*] coronal T2). (*B*) Spectroscopy demonstrates high mI peak, along with reduced NAA. There is no elevation of the Cho peak. (*B, C*) LC. There is an infiltrating lesion in the frontal and parietal lobes, mainly on the left (*C*). (*D*) Spectroscopy shows high Cho, reduced NAA and mI, and a huge lipid peak, not present in GC grade II.

Rapid progression of structural changes combined with new foci of enhancement should prompt a brain biopsy.[77] Detection of subcortical hypermetabolism by FDG-PET may indicate LC.[78]

Lymphomatosis cerebri versus progressive multifocal leukoencephalopathy

Progressive multifocal leukoencephalopathy (PML) in immunocompromised patients may present as diffuse infiltrative white matter lesions even compromising the brainstem and cerebellum. Infiltration of the brain by PML may be misdiagnosed as LC. No enhancement is typically demonstrated in both PML and LC. PML has a peculiar presentation on DWI that may be of help in the differential

diagnosis.[79] In PML, the appearance on DWI varies according to the disease stage.[80] In new active lesions, there is a rim of diffusion restriction and a central core of facilitated diffusion (**Fig. 19**).[80–83] The rim is usually incomplete and signifies active infection.[81] Beyond the rim of restricted diffusion, multiple small lesions with restricted diffusion, consistent with active inflammation are demonstrated.[82] Follow-up imaging may demonstrate the multiple punctuate lesions that evolve into a confluent hemispheric lesion and atrophy.

Intravascular Lymphoma

Intravascular lymphoma versus embolic infarcts
IVL may present as infarct-like lesions.

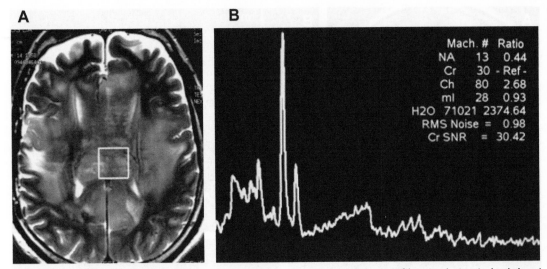

Fig. 18. GC grade III. Patient diagnosed with GC grade III, presenting with an infiltrative lesion in both hemi-spheres crossing the midline ([A] axial T2). (B) Spectroscopy shows high Cho, along with low NAA and mI. There are no lipids as opposed to what is seen in LC (see Fig. 17D).

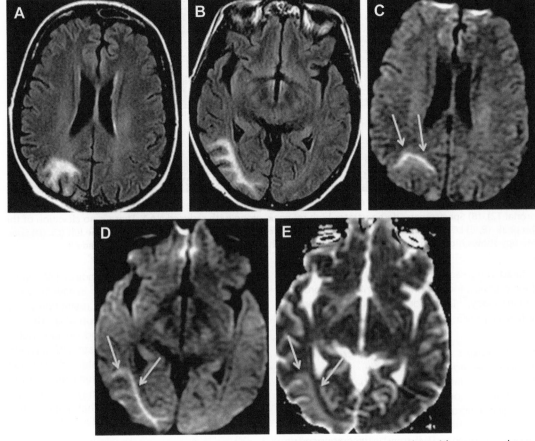

Fig. 19. PML versus lymphomatosis. A 55-year-old man diagnosed with PML, presenting with tremor and pares-thesia in the left hand. There is an infiltrative subcortical parietal and occipital lesion on the right, hyperintense on FLAIR ([A, B] axial FLAIR), presenting with a rim of high signal on DWI ([C, D] arrows) and restricted ADC ([E] arrows) typical of PML.

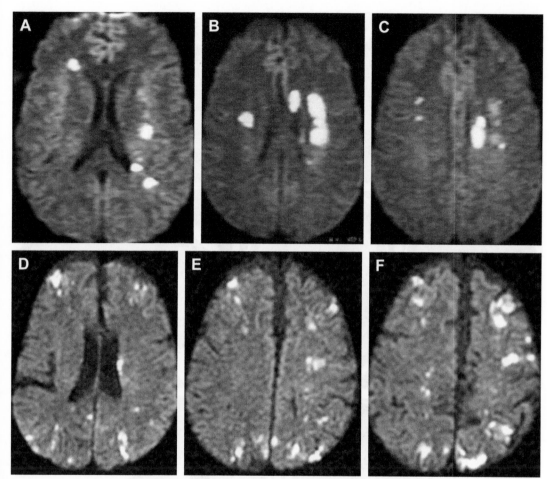

Fig. 20. IVL versus ischemic infarcts. Multiple round and oval lesions are demonstrated in both cerebral hemispheres in the topography of watershed zones in a patient diagnosed with IVL ([A–C] axial DWI). This imaging aspect overlaps with that of a patient presenting with infarcts secondary to hypereosinophilic sybdrome ([D–F] axial DWI). Note lesion in the corpus callosum of patient diagnosed with IVL (B). (*Courtesy of* Dr Leonardo Macedo, Cedimagem, MG-Brazil.)

Multiple cerebral emboli may result in dementia. The clinical history, however, usually discloses abrupt episodes of neurologic deterioration as opposed to the more insidious compromise of IVL.[19] Differentiation of IVL from embolic infarcts may be difficult on conventional MR imaging because scattered foci of high signal intensity on T2 FLAIR are demonstrated in both in the topography of the vascular watershed zones. Restricted diffusion may also be seen in both (**Fig. 20**). If a lesion involves the corpus callosum, IVL should be considered.

Intravascular lymphoma versus vasculitis

There are no pathognomonic neuroradiological findings for IVL. The most common alternative diagnosis is CNS vasculitis.[21,25] Small foci of enhancement may be demonstrated in

vasculitis, such as in Behçet disease (**Fig. 21**), as well as in chronic lymphocytic inflammation with pontine perivascular enhancement responsive to steroids (CLIPPERS). In patients with CLIPPERS, lesions predominantly occur in the pons and middle cerebelar peduncle (**Fig. 22**).

In cases of vasculitis, the clinical history may suggest the diagnosis. Vasculitis may be a cause of small vessel occlusions with resulting gray or white matter abnormalities on MR imaging. The extensive dural/arachnoid enhancement found in some cases of IVL, however, is atypical for vasculitis.

Ependymal Enhancement

When periventricular, subependymal enhancement is demonstrated, the main diagnostic

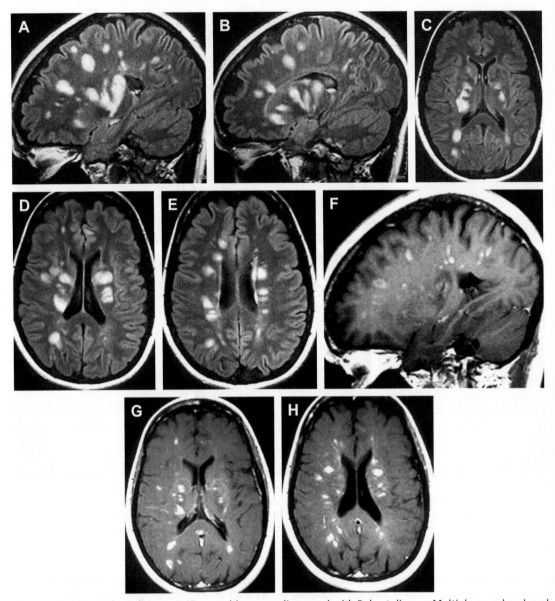

Fig. 21. IVL versus Behçet disease. A 45-year-old woman diagnosed with Behçet disease. Multiple round and oval lesions deeply located, adjacent to the ventricular margins as well as in the deep brain nuclei are seen in the (*A, B*) sagittal and (*C–E*) axial FLAIR images. Contrast enhancement is demonstrated in all lesions ([*F*] sagittal and [*G, H*] axial T1 with contrast), which is atypical for MS. Clinical history may help distinguish these lesions from those associated with IVL.

considerations are (**Fig. 23**) lymphoma, HGG, metastasis, cytomegalovirus infection, and neuromyelitis optica (NMO). NMO is a severe demyelinating disease with a propensity to selectively affect the optic nerves and spinal cord causing recurrent attacks of blindness and paralysis.[84]

NMO has a worldwide distribution and a poor prognosis and, although thought to be a variant of MS, its clinical, laboratory, immunologic, and pathologic characteristics are different. Presence of a highly specific serum autoantibody marker (NMO-IgG) differentiates NMO from MS. NMO-IgG binds selectively to aquaporin 4, which is highly concentrated in astrocytic foot processes and is not restricted to the optic nerves and spinal cord. Aquaporin 4 is found throughout the brain.[85–88]

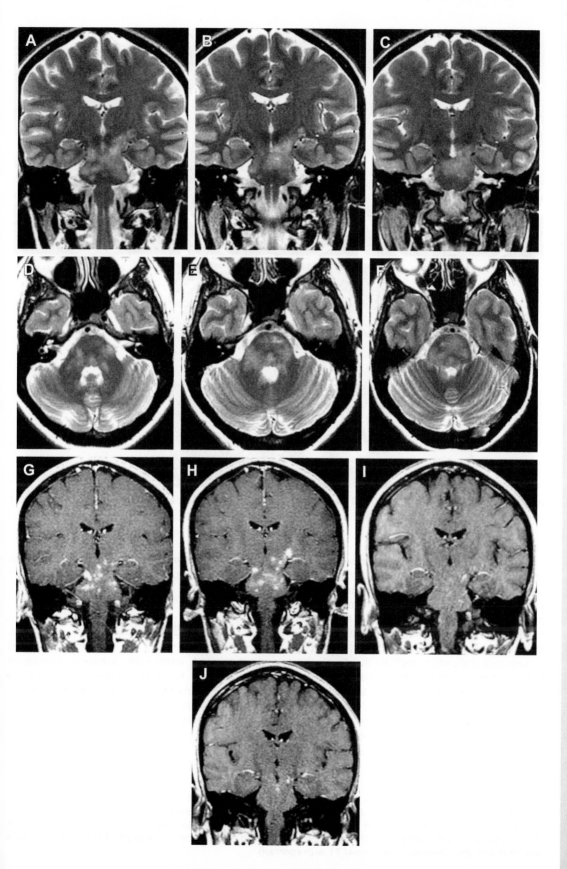

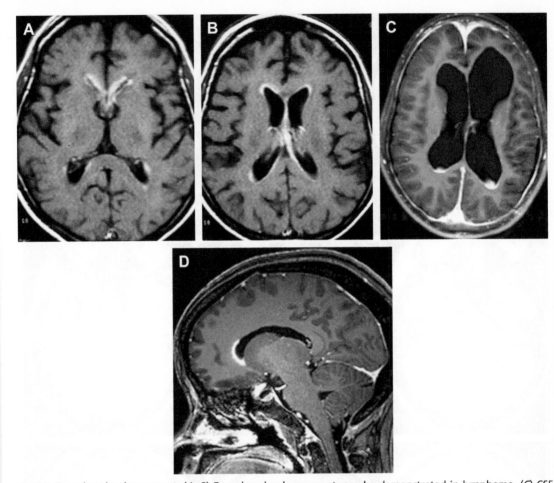

Fig. 23. Ependymal enhancement. (*A, B*) Ependymal enhancement may be demonstrated in lymphoma, (*C*) CSF spread of primary intracranial tumors and (*D*) NMO, among other diseases.

MR imaging demonstrates evidence of myelitis and optic neuritis and brain lesions in a distribution not consistent with MS.[89] Despite traditional views that the lesions of NMO are restricted to optic nerves and spinal cord, recent MR imaging studies have revealed evidence of brain lesions in 60% of patients who also fulfill the 1999 criteria of Wingerchuk and colleagues[84] for the diagnosis of NMO. Lesions in the hypothalamus or brainstem (floor of the fourth ventricle) are typical of NMO[90–93] (Fig. 24). Because of infiltration of the brain parenchyma, adjacent to the lateral, third and fourth ventricles, callosal involvement, and ependymal enhancement are seen in some (see Fig. 23D) NMO patients, it may be mistaken for lymphoma.

Meningeal Enhancement

Lymphomas represent an important differential diagnosis of extra-axial lesions.[2] Meningeal enhancement is demonstrated in lymphoma, meningioma, metastasis, tuberculosis, sarcoidosis, and cerebral spinal fluid (CSF) hypotension. Clinical history may help distinguish these lesions.

Fig. 22. IVL versus CLIPPERS. A 31-year-old woman diagnosed with Clippers. Multiple high signal intensity lesions are seen on the (*A–C*) coronal and (*D–F*) axial T2 images in the brainstem and middle cerebellar peduncles. Punctate and linear-nodular enhancement within the areas of T2 hyperintensities are seen along perivascular spaces ([*G, H*] coronal T1 with contrast). Significant improvement with disappearance of almost all enhancing lesions is demonstrated after steroids ([*I, J*] coronal T1 with contrast).

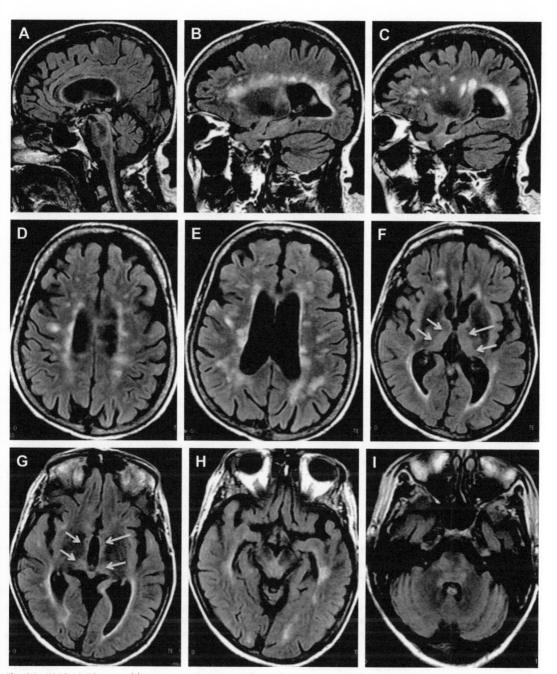

Fig. 24. NMO. A 58-year-old woman presenting with weakness and paresthesia in all limbs. High signal intensity round and oval lesions in the corpus callosum and adjacent to the margins of the lateral ventricles are demonstrated ([A–C] sagittal and [D, E] axial FLAIR), resembling MS. Lesions adjacent to the (F, G) third ventricle (arrows), however, as well as the (H) periaqueductal region and close to the (I) anterior portion of the fourth ventricle suggest NMO.

SUMMARY

Special types of lymphoma with particular imaging findings include diffuse infiltrating tumor, known as LC, IVL, and LG. Awareness of these uncommon lymphoma types is essential for prompt diagnosis.

Lymphomas that present with focal or multifocal masses should be distinguished from gliomas, MS, TDLs and infection. In patients with LC, distinction from GC, Biswanger disease, and PML is essential. Patients with IVL may be misdiagnosed as having vascular ischemic disease and vasculitis. Meningeal enhancement is a well-known presentation of lymphoma. Other diagnostic considerations are sarcoidosis, tuberculosis, and CSF hypotension.

REFERENCES

1. Broadbent M, Supakul N, Mehta P, et al. The faces of CNS lymphoma. Indiana University. Department of Radiology. School of Medicine. Presented at the 50th Annual meeting of the American Society of Neurorradiology. Montreal, May 17–22, 2014.

2. Atlas SW. Extra-axial brain tumors. In: Atlas SW, editor. Magnetic resonance imaging of the brain and spine. 2nd edition. Philadelphia: Lippincot Raven; 1996. p. 446–8.

3. Atlas SW. Intra-axial brain tumors. In: Atlas SW, editor. Magnetic resonance imaging of the brain and spine. 2nd edition. Philadelphia: Lippincot Raven; 1996. p. 404–7.

4. Samani A, Davagnanam I, Cockerell OC, et al. Lymphomatosis cerebri: a treatable cause of rapidly progressive dementia. J Neurol Neurosurg Psychiatr 2015;86(2):238–40.

5. Bakshi R, Mazziotta JC, Mischel PS, et al. Lymphomatosis cerebri presenting as a rapidly progressive dementia: clinical, neuroimaging and pathologic findings. Dement Geriatr Cogn Disord 1999;10: 152–7.

6. Choi CY, Lee CH, Joo M. Lymphomatosis cerebri. J Korean Neurosurg Soc 2013;54(5):420–2.

7. Keswani A, Bigio E, Grimm S. Lymphomatosis cerebri presenting with orthostatic hypotension, anorexia, and paraparesis. J Neurooncol 2012;109: 581–6.

8. Kitai R, Hashimoto N, Yamate K, et al. Lymphomatosis cerebri : clinical characteristics, neuroimaging, and pathological findings. Brain Tumor Pathol 2012; 29:47–53.

9. Lewerenz J, Ding X, Matschke J, et al. Dementia and leukoencephalopathy due to lymphomatosis cerebri. J Neurol Neurosurg Psychiatr 2007;78(7):777–8.

10. Raz E, Tinelli E, Antonelli M, et al. MRI findings in lymphomatosis cerebri : description of a case and revision of the literature. J Neuroimaging 2011;21: e183–6.

11. Rollins KE, Kleinschmidt-DeMasters BK, Corboy JR, et al. Lymphomatosis cerebri as a cause of white matter dementia. Hum Pathol 2005;36:282–90.

12. Leschziner G, Rudge P, Lucas S, et al. Lymphomatosis cerebri presenting as a rapidly progressive dementia with a high methylmalonic acid. J Neurol 2011;258:1489–93.

13. Pfleger V, Tappeiner J. Zur Kenntnis der Systemisierten Endothe- liomatose der Cutanen Blutgefasse (reticuloendotheliose?). Hautarzt 1959;10:359–63.

14. Wick M, Mills S. Intravascular lymphomatosis: clinicopathologic features and differential diagnosis. Semin Diagn Pathol 1991;8:91–101.

15. Wick M, Mills S, Scheithauer B, et al. Reassessment of malignant "angioendotheliomatosis": evidence in favor of its reclassification as "intravascular lymphomatosis". Am J Surg Pathol 1986;10:112–23.

16. DiGiuseppe J, Nelson W, Seifter E, et al. Intravascular lymphomatosis: a clinicopathologic study of 10 cases and assessment of responses to chemotherapy. J Clin Oncol 1994;12:2573–9.

17. Clark W, Dohan F, Moss T, et al. Immunocytochemical evidence of lymphocytic derivation of neoplastic cells in malignant anigoendotheliomatosis. J Neurosurg 1991;74:757–62.

18. Zuckerman D, Seliem R, Hochberg E. Intravascular lymphoma: the oncologist's "great imitator". Oncologist 2006;11(5):496–502.

19. Ferreri AJ, Campo E, Seymour JF, et al. Intravascular lymphoma: clinical presentation, natural history, management and prognostic factors in a series of 38 cases, with special emphasis on the 'cutaneous variant'. Br J Haematol 2004;127:173–83.

20. Nakahara T, Saito T, Muroi A, et al. Intravascular lymphomatosis presenting as an ascending cauda equina: conus medullaris syndrome: remission after biweekly CHOP therapy. J Neurol Neurosurg Psychiatr 1999;67:403–6.

21. Calamia KT, Miller A, Shuster EA, et al. Intravascular lymphomatosis. A report of ten patients with central nervous system involvement and a review of the disease process. Adv Exp Med Biol 1999;455:249–65.

22. Vieren M, Sciot R, Robberecht W. Intravascular lymphomatosis of the brain: a diagnostic problem. Clin Neurol Neurosurg 1999;101:33–6.

23. Glass J, Hochberg FH, Miller DC. Intravascular lymphomatosis. A systemic disease with neurologic manifestations. Cancer 1993;71:3156–64.

24. Hsu YH, Tseng BY, Shyu WC, et al. Intravascular lymphomatosis mimicking acute disseminated encephalomyelitis: a case report. Kaohsiung J Med Sci 2005;21:93–7.

25. Legerton CW 3rd, Sergent JS. Intravascular malignant lymphoma mimicking central nervous system lupus. Arthritis Rheum 1993;36:135.

26. Fredericks RK, Walker FO, Elster A, et al. Angiotropic intravascular large-cell lymphoma (malignant angioendotheliomatosis): report of a case and review of the literature. Surg Neurol 1991;35:218–23.

27. Williams RL, Meltzer CC, Smirniotopoulos JG, et al. Cerebral MR imaging in intravascular lymphomatosis. AJNR Am J Neuroradiol 1998;19:427–31.

28. Yamamoto A, Kikuchi Y, Homma K, et al. Characteristics of intravascular large B-cell lymphoma on cerebral MR imaging. AJNR Am J Neuroradiol 2012; 33:292–6.

29. Bahering JM, Henchclife C, Ledezma CJ, et al. Intravascular lymphoma: magnetic resonance imaging correlates of disease dynamics within the central nervous system. J Neurol Neurosurg Psychiatr 2005;76:540–4.

30. Jitpratoom P, Yuckpan P, Sitthinamsuwan P, et al. Pregressive multifocal cerebral infarction from intravascular large B cell lymphoma presenting in a man: a case report. J Med Case Rep 2011;5:24.

31. Ganguly S. Acute intracerebral hemorrhage inintravascular lymphoma: a serious infusion related adverse event of rituximab. Am J Clin Oncol 2007; 30:211–2.

32. Otrakji C, Voigt W, Amador A, et al. Malignant angioendotheliomatosis—a true lymphoma: a case of intravascular malignant lymphomatosis studied by Southern blot hybridization analysis. Hum Pathol 1988;19:475–8.

33. Endo Y, Oda M, Hara M. Central pontine myelinolysis:a study of 37cases in 1,000 consecutive autopsies. Acta Neuropathol 1981;53:145–53.

34. Crosley CJ, Rorke LB, Evans A, et al. Central nervous system lesions in childhood leukemia. Neurology 1978;28:678–85.

35. Marchioli CC, Graziano SL. Paraneoplastic syndromes associated with small cell lung cancer. Chest Surg Clin N Am 1997;7:65–80.

36. Miller GM, Baker HL Jr, Okazaki H, et al. Central pontine myelinolysis and its imitators: MR findings. Radiology 1988;168:795–802.

37. Iwasaki M, Murakami K, Tomita T, et al. Cavernous sinus dural arteriovenous fistula complicated by pontine venous congestion: a case report. Surg Neurol 2006;65:516–8.

38. Domizio P, Hall PA, Cotter F, et al. Angiotropic large cell lymphoma (ALCL): morphological, immunohistochemical and genotypic studies with analysis of previous reports. Hematol Oncol 1989;7: 195–206.

39. Song DK, Boulis NM, McKeever PE, et al. Angiotropic large cell lymphoma with imaging characteristics of CNS vasculitis. AJNR Am J Neuroradiol 2002; 23:239–42.

40. Sohn EH, Song CJ, Lee HJ, et al. Central nervous system lymphomatoid granulomatosis presenting with parkinsonism. J Clin Neurol 2007;3(2):108–11.

41. Liebow A, Carrington C, Friedman P. Lymphomatoid granulomatosis. Hum Pathol 1972;3:457–558.

42. Bae WK, Lee KS, Kim PN, et al. Lymphomatoid granulomatosis with isolated involvement of the brain. J Korean Med Sci 1991;6:255–9.

43. Paspala AB, Sundaram C, Purohit AK, et al. Exclusive CNS involvement by lymphomatoid granolomatosis in a 12-year-old boy: a case report. Surg Neurol 1999;51:258–60.

44. Agarwal V, Agarwal A, Pal L, et al. Arthritis in lymphomatoid granulomatosis: report of a case and review of literature. Indian J Med Sci 2004; 58(2):67–71.

45. Gitelson E, Al-Saleem T, Smith MR. Review: lymphomatoid granulomatosis: challenges in diagnosis and treatment. Clin Adv Hematol Oncol 2009;7(1):68–70.

46. Lucantoni C, De Bonis P, Doglietto F, et al. Primary cerebral lymphomatoid granulomatosis: report of four cases and literature review. J Neurooncol 2009;94(2):235–42.

47. Nishihara H, Tateishi U, Itoh T, et al. Immunohistochemical and gene rearrangement studies of central nervous system lymphomatoid granulomatosis. Neuropathology 2007;27(5):413–8.

48. Wyen C, Stenzel W, Hoffmann C, et al. Fatal cerebral lymphomatoid granulomatosis in an HIV-1-infected patient. J Infect 2007;54(3):e175–8.

49. Patsalides AD, Atac G, Hedge U, et al. Lymphomatoid granulomatosis: abnormalities of the brain at MR imaging. Radiology 2005;237:265–73.

50. Tateishi U, Terae S, Ogata A, et al. MR imaging of the brain in lymphomatoid granulomatosis. AJNR Am J Neuroradiol 2001;22:1284–90.

51. Jaffe ES, Wilson WH. Lymphomatoid granulomatosis: pathogenesis, pathology and clinical implications. Cancer Surv 1997;30:233–48.

52. Stadnick TW, Demaerel P, Luypaert RR, et al. Imaging tutorial: differential diagnosis of bright lesions on diffusion-weighted MR images. Radiographics 2003;23:e7.

53. Brandão LA, Shiroishi MS, Law M. Brain tumors: a multimodality approach with diffusion-weighted imaging, diffusion tensor imaging, magnetic resonance spectroscopy, dynamic susceptibility contrast and dynamic contrast-enhanced magnetic resonance imaging. Magn Reson Imaging Clin N Am 2013;21(2):203–7.

54. DeAngelis LM. Primary central nervous system lymphoma imitates multiple sclerosis. J Neurooncol 1990;9:177–81.

55. Given CA 2nd, Stevens BS, Lee C. The MRI appearance of tumefactive demyelinating lesions. AJR Am J Roentgenol 2004;182:195–9.

56. Erdag N, Bhorade RM, Alberico RA, et al. Primary lymphoma of the central nervous system: typical and atypical CT and MR imaging appearances. AJR Am J Roentgenol 2001;176:1319–26.

57. Masdeu JC, Quinto C, Oliveira C, et al. Open-ring imaging sign Highly specific for atypical brain demyelination. Neurology 2000;54(7):1427–33.

58. Cohen B, Valles FE, Rubenstein JL, et al. Differentiating tumefactive demyelinating lesions and primary CNS lymphoma using quantitative apparent diffusion coeficiente analysis. Presented at the ASNR. Seattle, June 4–9, 2011, EP 058.

59. Cha S. Update on brain tumor imaging: from anatomy to physiology. AJNR Am J Neuroradiol 2006; 27:475–87.

60. Rand SD, Prost R, Haughton V, et al. Accuracy of single voxel proton MR specotrocopy in distinguishing neoplastic from non neoplastic brain lesions. AJNR Am J Neuroradiol 1997;18:1695.

61. Saindane AM, Cha S, Law M, et al. Proton MR spectroscopy of tumefactive demyelinating lesions. AJNR Am J Neuroradiol 2002;23:1378–86.

62. De Stefano N, Caramanos Z, Preil MC, et al. In vivo differentiation of astrocytic brain tumors and isolated demyelinating lesions of the type seen in multiple sclerosis using ^{1}H magnetic resonance sptectroscopic imaging. Ann Neurol 1998; 44:273–8.

63. Cianfoni A, Niku S, Imbesi SG, et al. Metabolite findings in tumefactive demyelinating lesions using short echo time proton magnetic resonance spectroscopy. AJNR Am J Neuroradiol 2007;28: 272–7.

64. Lu S-S, Kim SJ, Kim HS, et al. Utility of proton MR spectroscopy for differentiating typical and atypical primary central nervous system lymphomas from tumefactive demyelinating lesions. AJNR Am J Neuroradiol 2014;35:270–7.

65. Circillo SF, Rosenblum ML. Use of CT and MR imaging to distinguish intracranial lesions and to define the need for biopsy in AIDS patients. J Neurosurg 1990;73(5):720–4.

66. Camacho DLA, Smith JK, Castillo M. Differentiation of Toxoplasmosis and lymphoma in AIDS patients by using apparent diffusion coefficients. AJNR Am J Neuroradiol 2003;24:633–7.

67. Dina TS. Primary central nervous system lymphoma versus toxo- plasmosis in AIDS. Radiology 1991; 179:823–8.

68. Smirniotopoulos JG, Koeller KK, Nelson AM, et al. Neuroimaging-autopsy correlations in AIDS. Neuroimaging Clin N Am 1997;7:615–37.

69. Pomper MG, Constantinides CD, Barker PB, et al. Quantitative MR spectroscopic imaging of brain lesions in patients with AIDS. Acad Radiol 2002;9: 398–409.

70. Chinn RJS, Wilkinson ID, Hall-Craggs MA, et al. Toxoplasmosis and primary central nervous system lymphoma in HIV infection: diagnosis with MR spectroscopy. Radiology 1995;197:649–54.

71. Brandão L, Domingues R. Intracranial neoplasms. In: MR spectroscopy of the brain. Philadelphia: Lippincott Williams & Wilkins; 2003. p. 130–67.

72. Ernst TM, Chang L, Witt MD, et al. Cerebral toxoplasmosis and lymphoma in AIDS: perfusion MR imaging experience in 13 patients. Radiology 1998; 208:663–9.

73. Brandão LA, Castillo M. Adult brain tumors: clinical applications of magnetic resonance spectroscopy. Neuroimag Clin N Am 2013;23(3):527–55.

74. Mohana Borges AV, Imbesi SG, Dietrich R, et al. Role of magnetic resonance spectroscopy in the diagnosis of gliomatosis cerebri. J Comput Assist Tomogr 2004;28(1):103–5.

75. Sarafi Lavi E, Bowen BC, Pattany PM, et al. Proton MR spectroscopy of gliomatosis cerebri: case report of elevated myoinositol with normal choline levels. AJNR Am J Neuroradiol 2003;24:946–51.

76. Guzman-de-Villoria JA, Sánchez Gonzalez J, Muñoz L, et al. [1]H MR spectroscopy in the assessment of gliomatosis cerebri. AJR Am J Roentgenol 2007;188:710–4.

77. Kanai R, Shibuya M, Hata T, et al. A case of 'lymphomatosis cerebri' diagnosed in an early phase and treated by whole brain radiation: case report and literature review. J Neurooncol 2008;86:83–8.

78. Mielke R, Kessler J, Szelies B, et al. Vascular dementia: perfusional and metabolic disturbances and effects of therapy. J Neural Transm Suppl 1996;47:183–91.

79. Bag AK, Curé JK, Chapman PR, et al. JC virus infection of the brain. AJNR Am J Neuroradiol 2010;31: 1564–76.

80. Bergui M, Bradac GB, Oguz KK, et al. Progressive multifocal leukoencephalopathy: diffusion-weighted imaging and pathological correlations. Neuroradiology 2004;46:22–5.

81. Henderson RD, Smith MG, Mowat P, et al. Progressive multifocal leukoencephalopathy. Neurology 2002;58:1825.

82. Usiskin SI, Bainbridge A, Miller RF, et al. Progressive multifocal leukoencephalopathy: serial high-b-value diffusion-weighted MR imaging and apparent diffusion coefficient measurements to assess response to highly active antiretroviral therapy. AJNR Am J Neuroradiol 2007;28:285–6.

83. Huisman TA, Boltshauser E, Martin E, et al. Diffusion tensor imaging in progressive multifocal leukoencephalopathy: early predictor for demyelination? AJNR Am J Neuroradiol 2005;26:2153–6.

84. Wingerchuk DM, Hogancamp WF, O' Brien PC, et al. The clinical course of neuromyelitis optica (Devic's syndrome). Neurology 1999;53:1107–14.

85. Amiry-Moghaddam M, Ottersen OP. The molecular basis of water transport in the brain. Nat Rev Neurosci 2003;4:991–1001.

86. Nielsen S, Nagelhus EA, Amiry-Moghaddam M, et al. Specialized membrane domains for water transport in glial cells: high-resolution immunogold cytochemistry of aquaporin-4 in rat brain. J Neurosci 1997;17:171–80.

87. Jung JS, Bhat RV, Preston GM, et al. Molecular characterization of an aquaporin cDNA from brain: candidate osmoreceptor and regulator of water balance. Proc Natl Acad Sci U S A 1994;91(26): 13052–6.

88. Frigeri A, Gropper MA Turck CW, Verkman AS. Immunolocalization of the mercurial-insensitive water channel and glycerol intrinsic protein in epithelial

cell plasma membranes. Proc Natl Acad Sci U S A 1995;924:328–31.

89. Pittock SJ, Weinshenker BG, Lucchinetti CF, et al. Neuromyelitis optica brain lesions localized at sites of high aquaporin 4 expression. Arch Neurol 2006; 63(7):964–8.

90. Nicchia GP, Nico B, Camassa LMA, et al. The role of aquaporin-4 in the blood-brain barrier development and integrity: studies in animal and cell culture models. Neuroscience 2004;129:935–45.

91. Pittock SJ, Lennon VA, Krecke K, et al. Brain abnormalities in patients with neuromyelitis optica (NMO). Arch Neurol 2006;633:90–396.

92. Poppe AY, Lapierre Y, Melancon D, et al. Neuromyelitis optica with hypothalamic involvement. Mult Scler 2005;11:617–21.

93. Nakashima I, Fujihara K, Miyazawa I, et al. Clinical and MRI features of 14 Japanese MS patients with NMO-IgG. J Neurol Neurosurg Psychiatry 2006; 77(9):1073–5.

Pretreatment Evaluation of Glioma

Ali Mohammadzadeh, MD[a], Vahid Mohammadzadeh, MD[b],
Soheil Kooraki, MD[c], Houman Sotoudeh, MD[d], Sakineh Kadivar, MD[e],
Madjid Shakiba, MD[f], Bahman Rasuli, MD[f], Ali Borhani, MD[f],
Maryam Mohammadzadeh, MD[g],*

KEYWORDS

- Glioma • CNS tumor • Grading • MR imaging • PET • Perfusion imaging • DTI • SWI

KEY POINTS

- Despite their limited role, conventional computed tomography and magnetic resonance (MR) imaging are traditionally considered the primary techniques for characterization of central nervous system (CNS) glioma; however, advanced imaging methods have evolved the imaging of glioma.
- Various modern imaging techniques, such as diffusion-weighted imaging, perfusion imaging, MR spectroscopy, and susceptibility-weighted imaging, might be used to assess presurgical grading, prognosis, and biopsy planning of CNS gliomas.
- The use of functional MR imaging and diffusion tensor imaging to delineate the relation of the tumor to important anatomic and functional areas has been promising. These techniques are shown to be useful in decreasing postoperative disability and allowing maximum tumor resection. Both techniques are subject to various limitations and need further technical improvements.
- PET is valuable for evaluation of the various aspects of the cellular metabolism of gliomas, which can potentially aid in surgical planning of gliomas and predicting their prognosis.

INTRODUCTION

Glioma, the most common primary brain tumor, refers to all the tumors originating from glial cells.[1] Gliomas constitute approximately 27% of all primary central nervous system (CNS) tumors and 80% of malignant tumors.[2] Glioma includes all the neoplasms arising from astrocytic, ependymal, and oligodendroglial cells or choroid plexus. Astrocytomas (originating from astrocytes) can be either circumscribed or diffuse. Circumscribed astrocytomas include pilocytic astrocytoma, pleomorphic xanthoastrocytoma, and subependymal giant cell astrocytoma. Diffuse astrocytomas consist of low-grade fibrillary astrocytoma, anaplastic astrocytoma, gliomatosis cerebri, and glioblastoma multiforme (GBM).[1,3] Based on the World Health Organization (WHO) guidelines, gliomas are classified into 4 grades[3,4] (Table 1). Mortality increases in higher-grade tumors but, depending on the anatomic location, and the tendency for local infiltration and later malignant transformation, even grade I tumors can be fatal.[5]

Disclosure: The authors have nothing to disclose.
[a] Department of Radiology, Rajaie Hospital, Iran University of Medical Sciences, Tehran, Iran; [b] Department of Ophthalmology, Farabi Hospital, Tehran University of Medical Sciences, Tehran, Iran; [c] Department of Radiology, Shariati Hospital, Tehran University of Medical Sciences, Tehran, Iran; [d] St Louis Children's Hospital, Mallinckrodt Institute of Radiology, Washington University in St Louis, St Louis, MO, USA; [e] Department of Ophthalmology, Amiralmomenin Hospital, Guilan University of Medical Sciences, Rasht, Iran; [f] Advanced Diagnostic and Interventional Radiology Research Center, Tehran University of Medical Science, Tehran, Iran; [g] Division of Neuroradiology, Department of Radiology, Amiralam Hospital, Tehran University of Medical Sciences, Tehran, Iran
* Corresponding author. 28451 Shrike Drive, Laguna Niguel, CA 92677.
E-mail addresses: m-mohammadzadeh@sina.tums.ac.ir; mm1361@yahoo.com

1052-5149/16/© 2016 Elsevier Inc. All rights reserved.

neuroimaging.theclinics.com

Table 1
CNS glioma WHO grading

Tumor Origin	Grade 1	Grade 2	Grade 3	Grade 4
Astrocytic	• Pilocytic astrocytoma • Subependymal giant cell astrocytoma	• Pleomorphic xanthoastrocytoma • Pilomyxoid astrocytoma • Diffuse astrocytoma (fibrillary, gemistocytic)	Anaplastic astrocytoma	• GBM • Gliosarcoma • Gliomatosis cerebri
Oligodendroglial	—	• Oligodendroglioma • Oligoastrocytoma	Anaplastic oligodendroglioma/ oligoastrocytoma	—
Ependymal	Subependymoma	Ependymoma	Anaplastic ependymoma	—
Choroid plexus	Choroid plexus papilloma	Atypical choroid plexus papilloma	Choroid plexus carcinoma	—
Others	Angiocentric glioma	Chordoid glioma	—	

Imaging plays an important role in the diagnosis and management of gliomas. In the past, computed tomography (CT) scan and conventional magnetic resonance (MR) imaging techniques were used for detection and characterization of gliomas. With recent advances in brain tumor imaging, preoperative assessment of glioma has progressed. Modern imaging techniques evaluate all aspects of initial diagnosis, including the extent of disease, grading, surgical planning, and prognosis. The gold standard in the diagnosis and grading of gliomas remains histopathology. However, in daily practice, because the sampling is difficult and subject to possible morbidities, the therapeutic plan of many individuals with CNS glioma is performed based on the imaging features. The use of preoperative functional and anatomic imaging methods has evolved the therapeutic plans, resulting in safer surgical approach, increased survival, and decreased postoperative functional disability.

This article discusses the role of preoperative routine conventional imaging in individuals with CNS gliomas, along with more detailed description of specific modern imaging methods.

CONVENTIONAL IMAGING TECHNIQUES

CT might be used as the primary modality for identification of the brain mass, but its role in the characterization of primary CNS neoplasms and differentiation from nonneoplastic conditions is limited. The appearance of astrocytomas on CT scan varies from usually homogeneous in low-grade gliomas to heterogeneous in higher grades. CT scan is usually considered superior to conventional MR imaging for demonstration of intratumoral calcification, most frequently seen in oligodendrogliomas. Conventional MR imaging is the mainstay of CNS glioma imaging. However, it is not accurate enough for differentiation of tumor subtypes and estimation of tumor grade.[6] Exceptions are juvenile pilocytic astrocytoma,[7] subependymal giant cell astrocytoma,[8] and pleomorphic xanthoastrocytoma,[9] which show characteristic features on conventional MR imaging.

Overall, low-grade gliomas are hypointense on T1 and hyperintense on T2 with absent or minimal mass effect. As the tumor progresses to higher grades, it becomes more heterogeneous with ill-defined and irregular borders, apparent peripheral edema, and mass effect (**Fig. 1**A, B) Hemorrhage may contribute to the heterogeneity of these tumors. Central coagulative necrosis is the hallmark of grade 4 glioma. Intravenous gadolinium-based agents increase the accuracy of MR imaging. In general, the presence of contrast enhancement is associated with higher-grade gliomas (**Fig. 1**C). The peripheral, irregular, and nodular enhancement is characteristic for GBM, whereas anaplastic astrocytoma shows patchy or no enhancement. It is notable that several subtypes of low-grade gliomas show contrast enhancement; the most important is the mural nodule of juvenile pilocytic astrocytoma[7] and pleomorphic xanthoastrocytoma.[10] In addition, nonenhancing gliomas are reported to be high grade in about one-third of cases.[11] In high-grade gliomas, infiltration of tumoral cells into surrounding edema beyond the margin of enhanced area is described as infiltrative edema. Conventional MR imaging techniques are unable to show the

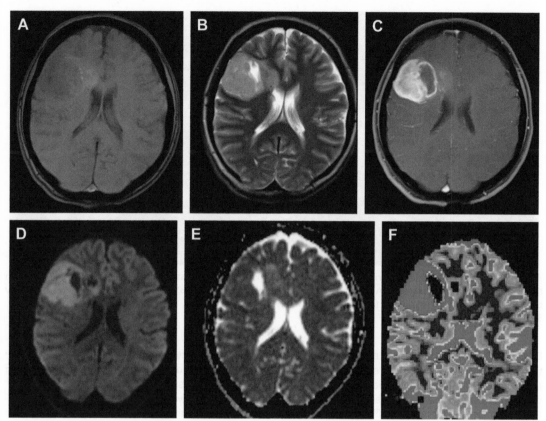

Fig. 1. Brain MR imaging of a 23-year-old woman with high-grade glioma, showing a solid enhancing mass in the right frontoparietal area. The enhancing part shows restricted diffusion on diffusion-weighted imaging (DWI) and apparent diffusion coefficient (ADC) and increased rCBV. T1-weighted (*A*), T2-weighted (*B*), contrast-enhanced T1-weighted (*C*), DWI (*D*), ADC (*E*), and rCBV (*F*).

areas of infiltrative edema. Altogether, conventional CT and MR imaging are not accurate modalities to characterize low-grade and high-grade gliomas.

MODERN IMAGING TECHNIQUES
Magnetic Resonance Perfusion Imaging

Neoangiogenesis is vital for glial tumor growth. Traditionally, the tumor vascularity is evaluated with contrast-enhanced CT or MR imaging, although the pattern of enhancement in gliomas does not allow accurate estimation of tumor vascular density, because it depends on the integrity of the blood-brain barrier, the amount of the contrast in the intra-arterial compartment, diffusion of the extravasated contrast to the adjacent tissues, and reabsorption of the contrast.[12] Dynamic CT and MR perfusion imaging are more accurate noninvasive methods for assessment of tumor vascularity. MR perfusion can be performed either with or without intravenous contrast. The favored techniques of contrast-enhanced MR perfusion include T2*-weighted dynamic susceptibility contrast-enhanced (DSC) and T1-weighted dynamic

contrast-enhanced (DCE). These techniques allow calculation of the cerebral blood volume (CBV) and endothelial transfer coefficient (K^{trans}) respectively. DSC is the most common perfusion technique used in preoperative glioma imaging for a range of applications, including pretherapeutic glioma grading, differentiating high-grade glioma from CNS lymphoma or solitary brain metastases, and predicting prognosis.[13] The most common perfusion parameter to assess glioma angiogenesis is the relative CBV (rCBV). rCBV has reportedly shown the ability to differentiate low-grade from high-grade glioma, but it can be misleading in oligodendrogliomas (because of the so-called chicken-wire capillary architecture) and pilocytic astrocytomas.[14–17] Overall, low-grade gliomas show normal/minimally increased rCBV. As the tumor transforms to higher grades, rCBV value increases, with GBMs showing markedly increased rCBV[17–19] (**Figs. 1F, 2,** and **4D**). Moreover, by showing the most malignant part of a CNS tumor, rCBV maps can be used to guide biopsy.[12]

The second MR perfusion technique with intravenous contrast agent is DCE. The advantage of

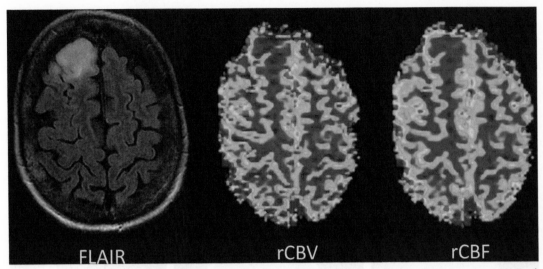

FLAIR   rCBV   rCBF

Fig. 2. A 70-year-old female with right frontal low grade glioma (diffuse astrocytoma, IDH mutant, WHO Grade II). This mass is hyperintense on FLAIR and demonstrates slightly reduced rCBV and rCBF on dynamic susceptibility contrast perfusion imaging. (*Courtesy of* Michael Iv and Max Wintermark, Stanford University Medical Center, Stanford, CA).

DCE is the superior spatial resolution, less susceptibility artifact, and three-dimensional acquisitions.[16] K^{trans} is the main indicator of capillary permeability and neoangiogenesis in DCE. Similar to rCBV, there is evidence that K^{trans} is an effective way to distinguish high-grade from low-grade glioma.[16,20,21] DCE is limited because institutions use different sorts of postprocessing algorithms to calculate K^{trans}; this needs to be standardized for future studies.

The third MR perfusion technique, arterial spin labeling (ASL) requires no intravenous contrast. In ASL, the brain signal is measured in the presence and absence of magnetic labeling of arterial water proton. The differences in these signals correlates with the inflow of labeled blood to the tissue (the cerebral blood flow).[22] The ASL technique is still evolving and so far there are no definite data regarding its application for pretreatment glioma planning, although the primary reports are promising.[23]

Diffusion-weighted Imaging

Diffusion-weighted imaging (DWI) reflects a measure of the random brownian motion of the water molecules. The role of DWI and its quantitative counterpart, apparent diffusion coefficient (ADC), in diagnosis and grading of CNS gliomas has been widely investigated. At present, DWI is used as a routine sequence in most of the preoperative imaging studies of gliomas.

The degree of restricted diffusion in gliomas is variable. Tumors with higher proliferation rate

(higher Ki-67 level index) have increased cellular density and reduced extracellular spaces, yielding restricted diffusion of the water molecules[24,25] (**Fig. 1**D, E). Several studies have detected an inverse relationship between ADC value and glioma grade.[26–28] Lower pretreatment minimum ADC value is related to dismal prognosis of supratentorial gliomas.[26] Higano and colleagues[27] observed a significant negative association between minimum ADC and Ki-67 index in malignant gliomas. Also, they reported that an ADC cutoff value of 0.90×10^{-3} mm^2/s had the highest accuracy for predicting prognosis. Other studies have not found ADC map to be valuable in preoperative characterization of gliomas.[29–31] In a study of a small group of high-grade gliomas, substantial overlap was found between ADC values of tumor, surrounding edema, and normal brain tissue.[30] According to Kono and colleagues,[32] ADC was not capable of detecting tumor infiltration in peripheral edema surrounding brain gliomas. An important drawback of many of these studies is that the evolution of ADC values with time is not well established for determining how it changes as the tumor progresses from low grade to high grade.

Whether ADC can discriminate glioma from metastasis is unclear. Some clinicians have shown ADC not to be powerful for differentiation between glioblastoma and metastasis.[28,33] Lee and colleagues[34] showed minimum ADC values of infiltrative edema in GBM to be significantly lower than those of metastasis.

These controversies might be partly explained by the differences in selecting the regions of interest (ROIs). Different grades of gliomas might exist in a single tumor. In addition, the presence of cystic, necrotic, and hemorrhagic areas within tumor confound the interpretation of DWI. Most glial tumors show heterogeneous mixed ADC pattern and manual selection of ROIs may lead to sampling bias. Several recent studies have advocated using a mean of minimum ADC values instead of a total mean ADC value. Kang and colleagues[35] used histogram analysis of whole-tumor ADC and showed that both minimum ADC and lowest fifth percentile at b values of 1000 and 3000 were valuable to discriminate high-grade from low-grade gliomas, whereas only higher-end values (75th percentile) were powerful in differentiation of grade 3 and 4 gliomas. Moreover, the number of high-ADC voxels was significantly higher in grade 4 compared with grade 3 glioma. The investigators justified this finding as being related to the presence of necrosis in glioblastoma. It is important to exclude areas of gross necrosis while selecting ROIs for measuring ADC value.

Lower ADC value can represent higher metabolic activity in tumor. In a pixel-by-pixel analysis, Holodny and colleagues[36] identified a strong overlap between data from ADC maps and 2-deoxy-2-[18F] fluoro-D-glucose (FDG)-PET. They reported a greater association between FDG-PET and ADC than between FDG-PET and gadolinium-enhanced MR imaging. Hilario and colleagues[37] proposed a preoperative prognostic model for diffuse gliomas depending only on minimum ADC and maximum rCBV. They showed ADC to be a stronger prognostic marker than rCBV, with a median survival of 8 months in tumors with ADC value less than 0.799×10^{-3} mm^2/s.

By locating areas with higher-grade tumor, DWI can aid in biopsy planning far better than conventional MR imaging.

Susceptibility-weighted Imaging

Recently, susceptibility-weighted imaging (SWI) has emerged as a complementary sequence in various CNS imaging studies. SWI is a T2* gradient echo sequence that measures the magnetic susceptibility signals of various tissues based on blood oxygen level–dependent (BOLD) technique. SWI is very sensitive for visualization of small veins, blood products, and calcification. Both unenhanced[38,39] and contrast-enhanced SWI (CE-SWI)[40–43] have been examined for characterization of CNS gliomas.

SWI is more accurate than conventional MR imaging techniques for detection of intratumoral microhemorrhages.[39] CE-SWI is superior to contrast-enhanced T1 in showing microvascularity and microbleeding within the tumor.[42] The presence of small vessels and microbleeding within a tumor is suggested to be a sign of neoangiogenesis. Neoangiogenesis is directly associated with tumor grade. Several studies have proposed SWI features to be useful for glioma grading. A study on a small group of patients with glioma by Hori and colleagues[43] showed that the ratio of susceptibility effects within tumor is significantly higher in high-grade compared with low-grade gliomas. Moreover, they showed that the presence of surrounding bright enhancement on CE-SWI is only seen in high-grade gliomas. Intratumoral susceptibility signals are identified more frequently on CE-SWI compared with unenhanced SWI.[40] Pinker and colleagues[44] examined the potential of CE-SWI at 3 T for differentiation of gliomas and showed a strong association between the frequency of intratumoral susceptibility signal intensity (ITSS) and tumor grade determined by PET and histopathology. In the study by Park and colleagues,[38] a powerful correlation was found between the grade of ITSS (on unenhanced SWI) and maximum rCBV in the same tumor segment. These studies suggest ITSS to be a helpful marker for showing tumor vascularity and for grading gliomas.

Furthermore, SWI provides reliable identification of intratumoral calcification, precluding complementary CT scan for identifying calcification.[45]

Using SWI in 1.5-T MR units was limited by long acquisition time and low signal/noise ratio; however, with advances in 3-T MR imaging, acquisition of SWI has become more practical and feasible in imaging of brain tumors. A study using 7-T MR imaging proposed fractal dimension (FD) as a quantitative index of SWI pattern in brain glioma. Higher FD (higher geometric complexity) was related to tumoral necrosis and microhemorrhage, whereas lower FD was a correlate of microvascularity.[46]

Magnetic Resonance Spectroscopy

Magnetic resonance spectroscopy (MRS) offers insight into metabolites of tissue in vivo. The potentials of various metabolite have been evaluated in the diagnosis and grading of CNS gliomas, such as N-acetylaspartate (NAA), creatine (Cr), choline (Cho), myoinositol (Mi), lactate, and lipid. MRS can be performed at different echo times (TEs). It is desirable to use both short time of echo (TE) (30 milliseconds) and long TE (144 milliseconds); however, if only a single TE is chosen, short TE is preferred.[47] Rather than diagnostic value, MRS can influence target boundary for radiotherapy. In a study on 34 high-grade gliomas, MRS detected evidence of active tumor outside the T2 tumor region in 88% of patients.[48] Furthermore, MRS can assist in biopsy guiding by identifying the most active tumor regions.

As a marker of neuronal density, NAA level decreases in all types of gliomas with an inverse correlation between NAA level and tumor grade. Decrease in NAA level is associated with infiltration and destruction of neurons by tumoral tissue. Investigated by numerous studies, increased Cho (a marker of cell membrane turnover) concentration occurs in all grades of gliomas. The relative signal intensity of Cho and Cho/Cr ratio increases significantly from low-grade toward high-grade gliomas[49] (**Figs. 3** and **4**). A strong correlation is described between rCBV with ADC and choline level in glioblastomas.[31] Increased choline concentration (>45%) on serial MRS is described as an indicator of malignant transformation in low-grade gliomas.[50] However, characterization of gliomas based on choline index should be made with caution. Shimizu and colleagues[51] reported a powerful correlation of choline level and Ki-67 index in gliomas with homogeneous MR imaging pattern, but not in heterogeneous gliomas. They suggested that choline is not reliable for predicting malignancy in heterogeneous gliomas. In glioblastomas with extensive necrosis and less viable cells, Cho/Cr and Cho/NAA ratios are diminished,[52] but areas with high cellular density show Cho/Cr ratios greater than 2 in these high-grade

tumors.[53] In contrast, absence of choline peak does not exclude CNS glioma.[54]

It is important to know that MRS choline peak consists of several choline products, but only phosphocholine (Pcho) indicates malignant cell overgrowth.[52] Increased Cho/Cr ratio is seen in pediatric pilocytic astrocytoma (WHO grade 1).[55] This choline peak consists mainly of glycerophosphocholine and low levels of Pcho.[56]

Peritumoral Cho/Cr and Cho/NAA ratios are significantly different between low-grade and high-grade gliomas, making MRS superior to DWI in assessing peritumoral changes. The combination of mean and maximum tumor ADC values with peritumoral metabolites ratio yields a sensitivity of 91.5% and specificity of 100% for differentiation of low-grade from high-grade gliomas.[57]

Cr, a marker of cellular hemostasis, usually has constant levels. Hence, it is used as a reference for calculation of metabolite ratios for in vivo MRS. Total Cr level might be used as a prognostic marker, as shown in the study of Hattingen and colleagues[58] in which low-grade gliomas with relative total Cr less than 1 had more stable course and later malignant transformation than those with normal or increased relative total Cr level. Myoinositol is an indicator of brain osmolarity. Higher Mi/Cr level is detected in low-grade gliomas compared with grade 3 and 4 gliomas.[59]

Increased levels of lactate and lipid are frequently seen in high-grade gliomas. Increased lactate peaks are found in pediatric pilocytic astrocytoma without distinct lipid peaks.[55] Although

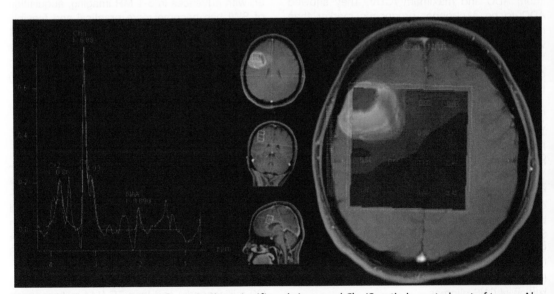

Fig. 3. MRS of the same patient shown in **Fig. 1** significantly increased Cho/Cr ratio in central part of tumor. Also, an MRS color map reveals significantly increased Cho/NAA ratio in central (9.56) and peripheral parts of the tumor (2.12–2.35) compared with normal brain tissue.

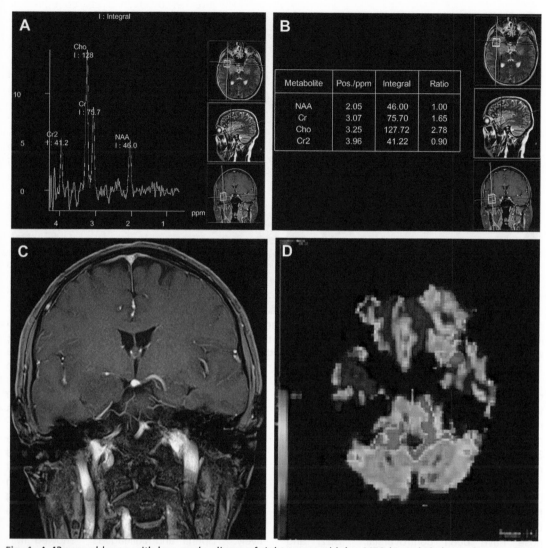

Fig. 4. A 43-year-old man with low-grade glioma of right temporal lobe; MRS (*A* and *B*) shows decreased NAA within the mass associated with increased choline. However, less than 3-fold increase in choline/NAA ratio is compatible with low-grade glioma. Note the lack of enhancement on coronal contrast-enhanced T1-weighted image (*C*) decreased rCBV is also noted on perfusion imaging (*D*).

both lipid and lactate peaks are associated with worse prognosis, higher lipid level is a stronger indicator of high-grade glioma. Lactate is a marker of relative hypoxia and anaerobic glycolysis, whereas high levels of lipid exist in glioblastoma as a result of cell death and necrosis.

Functional MR imaging

Evaluation of the relationship between brain tumors and eloquent functional cortex is of great importance in allowing maximum tumor resection with minimal postoperative disability. Intraoperative electrocortical mapping (ECM) is considered the gold standard for this purpose. However, it is invasive and necessitates intraoperative active cooperation of the patient. Preoperative task-based functional MR (fMR) imaging is now increasingly being used for such assessment (**Fig. 5**). BOLD fMR imaging is performed either at rest, called resting state fMR imaging (RS-fMR imaging) or while performing a task, named task-based fMR imaging. The probable role of RS-fMR imaging in glioma imaging needs further investigation and is currently limited to noncooperative patients such as children and individuals with existing motor deficits.[16] Numerous studies have assessed the potentials of preoperative task-based fMR imaging compared with ECM, but discrepancies in fMR imaging protocols have resulted in controversial

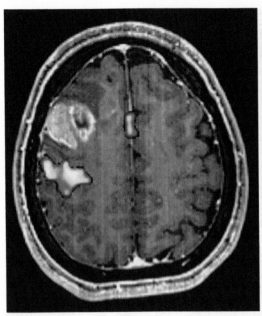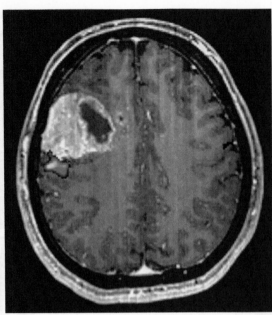

Fig. 5. fMR imaging of the same patient in Fig. 1 shows BOLD signal of the left-hand motor function and tongue motor, respectively. Left-hand motor area is activated in the normal area and is not in the vicinity of the tumor, whereas the tongue motor area is in close proximity to the tumor.

results. fMR imaging can significantly alter the therapeutic plan in individuals with potentially resectable CNS tumors.[60] fMR imaging allowed a more aggressive surgical approach in 18 out of 39 patients with brain tumors as described by Petrella and colleagues.[61]

Task-based fMR imaging is being increasingly used for preoperative lateralization of language function. The results of various studies on sensitivity and specificity of fMR imaging for this purpose have been controversial.[62] Bizzi and colleagues[63] found a sensitivity and specificity of 80% and 78%, respectively, for identification of language laterality on fMR imaging compared with intraoperative ECM. In the study by Stippich and colleagues,[64] fMR imaging with sentence generation and word generation paradigms had 98% accuracy for recognizing language areas in individuals with brain tumors. Giussani and colleagues[65] reviewed the findings of 9 studies that had compared the accuracy of language fMR imaging versus direct cortical mapping and found wide controversy between several studies, with sensitivities and specificities ranging from 59% to 100% and 0% to 97% respectively. They suggest that fMR imaging should be used as a complementary tool to direct mapping and not as an alternative. Lesion-to-activation distance (LAD) and lateralization index (LI) have frequently been addressed as promising language fMR imaging parameters. LI is a quantitative index, and shows the differences between activated areas of the right and left hemispheres. LAD less than 1 cm is associated with poorer postoperative outcome.[66] In contrast with the language function, motor cortex function assessment with fMR imaging has shown higher validation and higher agreement with ECM.[67] In a study on 87 individuals with brain gliomas, fMR imaging accuracy for localizing visual cortex, sensorimotor cortex, and language cortex was 100%, 91.9%, and 85.4%, respectively.[68] Spena and colleagues[69] showed fMR imaging accuracy of 92.3% for outlining sensorimotor area, but only 42.8% for language area.

Functional MR imaging is reported to be more accurate in low-grade than high-grade gliomas.[68] As neovascularization occurs in high-grade glioma, there is loss of autoregulation within tumor vasculature. This phenomenon confounds interpretation of BOLD fMR imaging by preventing blood flow augmentation in the activated area. Furthermore, the presence of arteriovenous shunting, and mechanical vasoconstriction caused by tumoral mass effect, alter the diagnostic power of the BOLD signal, which largely depends on changes of hemoglobin oxygenation state.[70] Likewise, the presence of intratumoral hemorrhage may decrease the accuracy of fMR imaging. In summary, preoperative fMR imaging is widely used to increase the accuracy of direct cortical mapping and aid in more delicate surgical planning.

Diffusion Tensor Imaging

Diffusion tensor imaging (DTI) measures multidimensional gaussian distribution of water diffusion with characterization of the magnitude and direction of diffusion anisotropy. DTI provides valuable preoperative anatomic information for neurosurgeons. Various DTI-driven algorithms have been investigated in presurgical brain tumor imaging. Details of these indices are beyond the scope of this article. The most widely investigated, fractional anisotropy (FA), assesses microstructural white matter integrity of brain tissue, whereas mean diffusivity (MD) is an index of diffusion magnitude.[16] FA values are between 0 and 1, which are consistent with isotropic voxel (free water) and highly anisotropic voxel respectively. Glial tumors may displace, infiltrate, or disrupt white matter fibers, leading to decreased anisotropy.[71] Decreased FA of the adjacent white matter might be an indicator of occult tumoral invasion.[72]

At present, diffusion tensor (DT) tractography is the most practical technique used in CNS tumor imaging for delineating a three-dimensional view of the white matter tracts and their relationship with the tumor. Tractography can be used for navigation purposes to reduce the risk of injury to critical tracts. A high correlation between presurgical DT tractography of pyramidal tracts (PT) and direct intraoperative subcortical stimulation is reported.[73] DTI-based neuronavigation of both low-grade and high-grade gliomas with involvement of PT allows maximum resection of the tumor along with better postoperative functional outcome and increased survival.[74] An integrated fMR imaging–DT tractography protocol, used by Smits and colleagues,[75] showed that direct tracking of PT from BOLD-activated area allows discrimination of various components of the tract. Rather than the PT, various studies have found beneficial effects of DTI for mapping optic tracts, superior longitudinal fasciculus, and arcuate fasciculus in individuals with brain tumors.[76]

DTI might be used for characterization of the tumoral tissue. Neuronal integrity decreases continuously from the periphery toward the center of the glioma. Increased cellular density in high-grade gliomas leads to reduced MD and increased FA.[77] However, several studies have not found significant differences between the FA of low-grade and high-grade gliomas,[78,79] and the correlation between FA and tumor grade is low according to Zou and colleagues.[80]

It is essential to be familiar with the potential drawbacks of DTI, including image noise, diffusion artifacts, and crossing fibers. Wide anisotropic variations exist within regional crossing fibers, which cofound DTI measures.[81] Variations in tractography software and other user-dependent factors can also influence DTI results. In addition, intraoperative brain shift can alter the reliability of DTI guidance.[76] The technical aspects of DTI need further improvement and validation.

Diffusion kurtosis imaging (DKI) has emerged as an alternative technique for more accurate estimation of diffusion. Unlike DTI, diffusion kurtosis shows variations from nongaussian distribution, which can be used as an indicator of tissue organization and heterogeneity.[82] DKI is helpful in showing the microstructural pattern of CNS gliomas.[83] Van Cauter and colleagues[84] showed that mean kurtosis is more accurate than FA and MD for discrimination between low-grade and high-grade gliomas, with higher-grade gliomas showing higher mean kurtosis. Further studies are required to assess the potential of DKI in glioma imaging.

PET

Despite the extensive anatomic and functional information provided by CT scan and MR imaging techniques, they cannot access tumor metabolism. PET imaging is now the only clinically available technique to evaluate the metabolism of CNS gliomas. PET can evaluate various aspects of cell metabolism, including glucose metabolism, cell proliferation rate, cell membrane biosynthesis, tissue hypoxia, and expression of amino acid transporters.

Glucose Metabolism

FDG is the most common PET tracer used in oncology. In general, the higher the glioma grade, the more the FDG uptake, which is helpful in pretreatment grading, selection of biopsy target, and following the tumor to detect transformation to higher grades. The most recent data showed the accuracy of glioma grading by FDG-PET and fluoroethyltyrosine (FET)-PET to be almost equal to that of FDG-PET, with a sensitivity of 0.38 and specificity of 0.86 for diagnosis of glioma.[85] It is notable that FDG is a marker of glucose metabolism rather than cell proliferation. High FDG uptake in normal brain cortex, basal ganglia, and thalamus, and nonspecific uptake in other disorders, such as inflammation/infection, is a major limiting factor.

Amino Acid Transport and Protein Synthesis

The more cellular proliferation and the higher the cellular grade, the more use of amino acids. So far, [^{11}C]-methionine ([^{11}C]-MET), [^{18}F]-fluorotyrosine, [^{18}F]-FET, [^{18}F]-fluoromethyltyrosine, and [^{18}F]-fluorodopa ([^{18}F]-DOPA) have been used to evaluate brain neoplasms.[86] In general, the amino acid uptake is higher in glioma compared with normal tissue, regardless of the glioma grading. L-Methyl-[^{11}C]-MET was one of the first tracers that was developed for glioma evaluation. There is some evidence that methionine uptake correlates with the glioma grade and Ki-67 index.[87] Nonspecific uptake in inflammation/infection and short half-life of the tracer (20 minutes) are the limitations. Based on the meta-analysis data, FET-PET has a sensitivity of 94% and pooled specificity of 88% for diagnosing glioma.[88] Dynamic imaging with [^{18}F]-FET is 97% accurate to differentiate between low-grade and high-grade gliomas.[88] Higher [^{18}F]-DOPA uptake is reported in high-grade gliomas (sensitivity of 85% and specificity of 89%).[89]

Proliferation Rate

Application of 3-deoxy-3-[18F] fluorothymidine (FLT), a tumor-proliferating tracer, has been promising in glioma detection and grading. FLT uptake is very low in normal brain parenchyma, providing a low-background image. There is evidence that the maximum and mean values of [18F]-FLT uptake are more accurate than the conventional and advanced MR imaging techniques for glioma grading.[90]

Membrane Biosynthesis

In general, the higher the cell proliferation rate, the higher the cell membrane biosynthesis. [18F]-fluorocholine and [11C]-choline uptake have been reported to correlate with glioma grading. Data about the primary evaluation of glioma by [18F]/[11C]-choline are controversial and most of the suggestions are based on studies with small patient numbers; overall, [18F]/[11C]-choline PET grading of glioma is feasible and tumor/normal tissue uptake ratio is high.

Oxygen Metabolism

Rapid cell proliferation in high-grade tumor leads to relative hypoxia of tumoral mass. Tumoral hypoxia is a high-grade marker and is associated with poor treatment response. [18F]-fluoromisonidazole (FMISO) and [18F]-fluoroazomycin-arabinoside (FAZA) have been used as markers for hypoxia. Increased [18F]-FMISO uptake is seen in high-grade but not low-grade gliomas.[91]

Perfusion

Increased tumor perfusion is helpful to predict glioma grade. The most common PET tracer for this purpose is [15O]-labeled water; however, in the clinical setting MR perfusion is more often used.[86]

Biopsy Targeting

High uptake of choline PET in the high-grade component of tumor may play a role in biopsy planning.[92] Amino acid tracers (FET-PET) are preferred to FDG-PET and postcontrast MR imaging for biopsy targeting with a sensitivity of 93% and specificity of 94%.[93]

Radiation Therapy Planning with PET

Although the gross tumor volume (GTV), clinical tumor volume, and planning target volume are usually determined by conventional imaging, preradiation planning by PET may correlate more accurately with biological target volume (BTV). It is assumed that, in high-grade glioma, BTV would be more accurate than GTV, although the application of radiation planning with amino acid tracer PET is not completely understood.[94,95] In addition, preradiation use of hypoxia-specific tracers may change the plan and the dose of radiation.[91,96]

PET/Magnetic Resonance

Although FDG-PET–CT is now standard of care for many neoplasms and provides both diagnostic and prognostic information, hybrid PET/MR scanners are being approved for clinical applications. The main advantages of PET/MR are lack of ionizing radiation for anatomic imaging and attenuation correction, the ability to acquire functional data (eg, MRS, DWI, SWI, fMR imaging), less misregistration artifact, and improved soft tissue resolution. As with PET/CT, PET/MR technology is compatible with all aforementioned tracers. Using simultaneous methionine PET/MR, Bisadas and colleagues[97] showed the feasibility of PET/MR before histopathologic sampling in glioma, although the regions of high methionine uptake did not always match the regions of increased Cr/NAA. The PET/MR technology is still in its infancy and more studies are needed of its application in pretreatment planning in gliomas.

SUMMARY

Histopathology remains the gold standard for diagnosis and classification of gliomas. Advanced neuroimaging techniques have an important role in diagnosis, prognosis, biopsy planning, and pretreatment planning. The effect of advanced imaging on the patients' survival rate and posttreatment recurrence is not well understood but preliminary results are promising. Further studies are needed to establish the standard of care using the new imaging multimodalities.

REFERENCES

1. Schwartzbaum JA, Fisher JL, Aldape KD, et al. Epidemiology and molecular pathology of glioma. Nat Clin Pract Neurol 2006;2(9):494–503 [quiz 1 p following 16].
2. Ostrom QT, Gittleman H, Fulop J, et al. CBTRUS Statistical report: primary brain and central nervous system tumors diagnosed in the United States in 2008-2012. Neuro Oncol 2015;17(Suppl 4):iv1–62.
3. Louis DN, Perry A, Reifenberger G, et al. The 2016 World Health Organization Classification of Tumors of the Central Nervous System: a summary. Acta Neuropathol 2016;131(6):803–20.
4. Louis DN, Ohgaki H, Wiestler OD, et al. The 2007 WHO classification of tumours of the central nervous system. Acta Neuropathol 2007;114(2):97–109.
5. McKinney PA. Brain tumours: incidence, survival, and aetiology. J Neurol Neurosurg Psychiatr 2004; 75(Suppl 2):ii12–7.
6. Upadhyay N, Waldman AD. Conventional MRI evaluation of gliomas. Br J Radiol 2011;84(Spec No 2): S107–11.
7. Koeller KK, Rushing EJ. From the archives of the AFIP: pilocytic astrocytoma: radiologic-pathologic correlation. Radiographics 2004;24(6):1693–708.
8. Clarke MJ, Foy AB, Wetjen N, et al. Imaging characteristics and growth of suibependymal giant cell astrocytomas. Neurosurg Focus 2006;20(1):E5.
9. Yu S, He L, Zhuang X, et al. Pleomorphic xanthoastrocytoma: MR imaging findings in 19 patients. Acta Radiol 2011;52(2):223–8.
10. Lipper MH, Eberhard DA, Phillips CD, et al. Pleomorphic xanthoastrocytoma, a distinctive astroglial tumor: neuroradiologic and pathologic features. AJNR Am J Neuroradiol 1993;14(6):1397–404.
11. Scott JN, Brasher PM, Sevick RJ, et al. How often are nonenhancing supratentorial gliomas malignant? A population study. Neurology 2002;59(6):947–9.
12. Jain R. Measurements of tumor vascular leakiness using DCE in brain tumors: clinical applications. NMR Biomed 2013;26(8):1042–9.
13. Barajas RF Jr, Cha S. Benefits of dynamic susceptibility-weighted contrast-enhanced perfusion MRI for glioma diagnosis and therapy. CNS Oncol 2014;3(6):407–19.
14. Cha S, Tihan T, Crawford F, et al. Differentiation of low-grade oligodendrogliomas from low-grade astrocytomas by using quantitative blood-volume measurements derived from dynamic susceptibility contrast-enhanced MR imaging. AJNR Am J Neuroradiol 2005;26(2):266–73.
15. Lev MH, Ozsunar Y, Henson JW, et al. Glial tumor grading and outcome prediction using dynamic spin-echo MR susceptibility mapping compared with conventional contrast-enhanced MR: confounding effect of elevated rCBV of oligodendrogliomas [corrected]. AJNR Am J Neuroradiol 2004;25(2): 214–21.
16. Mabray MC, Barajas RF Jr, Cha S. Modern brain tumor imaging. Brain Tumor Res Treat 2015;3(1):8–23.
17. Svolos P, Kousi E, Kapsalaki E, et al. The role of diffusion and perfusion weighted imaging in the differential diagnosis of cerebral tumors: a review and future perspectives. Cancer Imaging 2014;14:20.
18. Di Costanzo A, Pollice S, Trojsi F, et al. Role of perfusion-weighted imaging at 3 Tesla in the assessment of malignancy of cerebral gliomas. Radiol Med 2008;113(1):134–43.
19. Senturk S, Oguz KK, Cila A. Dynamic contrast-enhanced susceptibility-weighted perfusion imaging of intracranial tumors: a study using a 3T MR scanner. Diagn Interv Radiol 2009;15(1): 3–12.
20. Roberts HC, Roberts TP, Bollen AW, et al. Correlation of microvascular permeability derived from dynamic contrast-enhanced MR imaging with histologic grade and tumor labeling index: a study in human brain tumors. Acad Radiol 2001;8(5):384–91.
21. Roberts HC, Roberts TP, Ley S, et al. Quantitative estimation of microvascular permeability in human brain tumors: correlation of dynamic Gd-DTPA-enhanced MR imaging with histopathologic grading. Acad Radiol 2002;9(Suppl 1):S151–5.
22. Watts JM, Whitlow CT, Maldjian JA. Clinical applications of arterial spin labeling. NMR Biomed 2013; 26(8):892–900.
23. Telischak NA, Detre JA, Zaharchuk G. Arterial spin labeling MRI: clinical applications in the brain. J Magn Reson Imaging 2015;41(5):1165–80.
24. Kiss R, Dewitte O, Decaestecker C, et al. The combined determination of proliferative activity and cell density in the prognosis of adult patients with supratentorial high-grade astrocytic tumors. Am J Clin Pathol 1997;107(3):321–31.
25. Calvar JA, Meli FJ, Romero C, et al. Characterization of brain tumors by MRS, DWI and Ki-67 labeling index. J Neurooncol 2005;72(3):273–80.
26. Murakami R, Sugahara T, Nakamura H, et al. Malignant supratentorial astrocytoma treated with postoperative radiation therapy: prognostic value of pretreatment quantitative diffusion-weighted MR imaging. Radiology 2007;243(2):493–9.
27. Higano S, Yun X, Kumabe T, et al. Malignant astrocytic tumors: clinical importance of apparent diffusion coefficient in prediction of grade and prognosis. Radiology 2006;241(3):839–46.
28. Yamasaki F, Kurisu K, Satoh K, et al. Apparent diffusion coefficient of human brain tumors at MR imaging. Radiology 2005;235(3):985–91.
29. Lam WW, Poon WS, Metreweli C. Diffusion MR imaging in glioma: does it have any role in the preoperation determination of grading of glioma? Clin Radiol 2002;57(3):219–25.

30. Castillo M, Smith JK, Kwock L, et al. Apparent diffusion coefficients in the evaluation of high-grade cerebral gliomas. AJNR Am J Neuroradiol 2001; 22(1):60–4.

31. Catalaa I, Henry R, Dillon WP, et al. Perfusion, diffusion and spectroscopy values in newly diagnosed cerebral gliomas. NMR Biomed 2006;19(4):463–75.

32. Kono K, Inoue Y, Nakayama K, et al. The role of diffusion-weighted imaging in patients with brain tumors. AJNR Am J Neuroradiol 2001;22(6):1081–8.

33. Oh J, Cha S, Aiken AH, et al. Quantitative apparent diffusion coefficients and T2 relaxation times in characterizing contrast enhancing brain tumors and regions of peritumoral edema. J Magn Reson Imaging 2005;21(6):701–8.

34. Lee EJ, terBrugge K, Mikulis D, et al. Diagnostic value of peritumoral minimum apparent diffusion coefficient for differentiation of glioblastoma multiforme from solitary metastatic lesions. AJR Am J Roentgenol 2011;196(1):71–6.

35. Kang Y, Choi SH, Kim YJ, et al. Gliomas: histogram analysis of apparent diffusion coefficient maps with standard- or high-b-value diffusion-weighted MR imaging–correlation with tumor grade. Radiology 2011; 261(3):882–90.

36. Holodny AI, Makeyev S, Beattie BJ, et al. Apparent diffusion coefficient of glial neoplasms: correlation with fluorodeoxyglucose-positron-emission tomography and gadolinium-enhanced MR imaging. AJNR Am J Neuroradiol 2010;31(6):1042–8.

37. Hilario A, Sepulveda JM, Perez-Nunez A, et al. A prognostic model based on preoperative MRI predicts overall survival in patients with diffuse gliomas. AJNR Am J Neuroradiol 2014;35(6):1096–102.

38. Park MJ, Kim HS, Jahng GH, et al. Semiquantitative assessment of intratumoral susceptibility signals using non-contrast-enhanced high-field high-resolution susceptibility-weighted imaging in patients with gliomas: comparison with MR perfusion imaging. AJNR Am J Neuroradiol 2009;30(7): 1402–8.

39. Li C, Ai B, Li Y, et al. Susceptibility-weighted imaging in grading brain astrocytomas. Eur J Radiol 2010; 75(1):e81–5.

40. Fahrendorf D, Schwindt W, Wolfer J, et al. Benefits of contrast-enhanced SWI in patients with glioblastoma multiforme. Eur Radiol 2013;23(10):2868–79.

41. Pinker K, Noebauer-Huhmann IM, Stavrou I, et al. High-field, high-resolution, susceptibility-weighted magnetic resonance imaging: improved image quality by addition of contrast agent and higher field strength in patients with brain tumors. Neuroradiology 2008;50(1):9–16.

42. Zhang H, Tan Y, Wang XC, et al. Susceptibility-weighted imaging: the value in cerebral astrocytomas grading. Neurol India 2013;61(4):389–95.

43. Hori M, Mori H, Aoki S, et al. Three-dimensional susceptibility-weighted imaging at 3 T using various image analysis methods in the estimation of grading intracranial gliomas. Magn Reson Imaging 2010; 28(4):594–8.

44. Pinker K, Noebauer-Huhmann IM, Stavrou I, et al. High-resolution contrast-enhanced, susceptibility-weighted MR imaging at 3T in patients with brain tumors: correlation with positron-emission tomography and histopathologic findings. AJNR Am J Neuroradiol 2007;28(7):1280–6.

45. Mohammed W, Xunning H, Haibin S, et al. Clinical applications of susceptibility-weighted imaging in detecting and grading intracranial gliomas: a review. Cancer Imaging 2013;13:186–95.

46. Di Ieva A, God S, Grabner G, et al. Three-dimensional susceptibility-weighted imaging at 7 T using fractal-based quantitative analysis to grade gliomas. Neuroradiology 2013;55(1):35–40.

47. Majos C, Julia-Sape M, Alonso J, et al. Brain tumor classification by proton MR spectroscopy: comparison of diagnostic accuracy at short and long TE. AJNR Am J Neuroradiol 2004;25(10):1696–704.

48. Pirzkall A, McKnight TR, Graves EE, et al. MR-spectroscopy guided target delineation for high-grade gliomas. Int J Radiat Oncol Biol Phys 2001;50(4): 915–28.

49. Moller-Hartmann W, Herminghaus S, Krings T, et al. Clinical application of proton magnetic resonance spectroscopy in the diagnosis of intracranial mass lesions. Neuroradiology 2002;44(5):371–81.

50. Tedeschi G, Lundbom N, Raman R, et al. Increased choline signal coinciding with malignant degeneration of cerebral gliomas: a serial proton magnetic resonance spectroscopy imaging study. J Neurosurg 1997;87(4):516–24.

51. Shimizu H, Kumabe T, Shirane R, et al. Correlation between choline level measured by proton MR spectroscopy and Ki-67 labeling index in gliomas. AJNR Am J Neuroradiol 2000;21(4):659–65.

52. Bulik M, Jancalek R, Vanicek J, et al. Potential of MR spectroscopy for assessment of glioma grading. Clin Neurol Neurosurg 2013;115(2):146–53.

53. Saraswathy S, Crawford FW, Lamborn KR, et al. Evaluation of MR markers that predict survival in patients with newly diagnosed GBM prior to adjuvant therapy. J Neurooncol 2009;91(1):69–81.

54. Bowen BC. Glial neoplasms without elevated choline-creatine ratios. AJNR Am J Neuroradiol 2003;24(5):782–4.

55. Hwang JH, Egnaczyk GF, Ballard E, et al. Proton MR spectroscopic characteristics of pediatric pilocytic astrocytomas. AJNR Am J Neuroradiol 1998;19(3): 535–40.

56. Davies NP, Wilson M, Harris LM, et al. Identification and characterisation of childhood cerebellar

tumours by in vivo proton MRS. NMR Biomed 2008;
21(8):908–18.

57. Server A, Kulle B, Gadmar OB, et al. Measurements
of diagnostic examination performance using quantitative apparent diffusion coefficient and proton MR
spectroscopic imaging in the preoperative evaluation of tumor grade in cerebral gliomas. Eur J Radiol
2011;80(2):462–70.

58. Hattingen E, Raab P, Franz K, et al. Prognostic value
of choline and creatine in WHO grade II gliomas.
Neuroradiology 2008;50(9):759–67.

59. Castillo M, Smith JK, Kwock L. Correlation of myo-
inositol levels and grading of cerebral astrocytomas.
AJNR Am J Neuroradiol 2000;21(9):1645–9.

60. Mahvash M, Maslehaty H, Jansen O, et al. Functional magnetic resonance imaging of motor and
language for preoperative planning of neurosurgical
procedures adjacent to functional areas. Clin Neurol
Neurosurg 2014;123:72–7.

61. Petrella JR, Shah LM, Harris KM, et al. Preoperative
functional MR imaging localization of language and
motor areas: effect on therapeutic decision making
in patients with potentially resectable brain tumors.
Radiology 2006;240(3):793–802.

62. Wang LL, Leach JL, Breneman JC, et al. Critical role
of imaging in the neurosurgical and radiotherapeutic
management of brain tumors. Radiographics 2014;
34(3):702–21.

63. Bizzi A, Blasi V, Falini A, et al. Presurgical functional
MR imaging of language and motor functions: vali-
dation with intraoperative electrocortical mapping.
Radiology 2008;248(2):579–89.

64. Stippich C, Rapps N, Dreyhaupt J, et al. Localizing
and lateralizing language in patients with brain tumors: feasibility of routine preoperative functional
MR imaging in 81 consecutive patients. Radiology
2007;243(3):828–36.

65. Giussani C, Roux FE, Ojemann J, et al. Is preoperative functional magnetic resonance imaging reliable
for language areas mapping in brain tumor surgery?
Review of language functional magnetic resonance
imaging and direct cortical stimulation correlation
studies. Neurosurgery 2010;66(1):113–20.

66. Haberg A, Kvistad KA, Unsgard G, et al.
Preoperative blood oxygen level-dependent
functional magnetic resonance imaging in patients
with primary brain tumors: clinical application
and outcome. Neurosurgery 2004;54(4):902–14
[discussion: 14–5].

67. Smits M. functional magnetic resonance imaging
(fMRI) in brain tumour patients. European Association of Neurooncology Magazine 2012;123–8.

68. Kapsalakis IZ, Kapsalaki EZ, Gotsis ED, et al. Preoperative evaluation with FMRI of patients with intracranial gliomas. Radiol Res Pract 2012;2012:727810.

69. Spena G, Nava A, Cassini F, et al. Preoperative and
intraoperative brain mapping for the resection of

eloquent-area tumors. A prospective analysis of
methodology, correlation, and usefulness based on
clinical outcomes. Acta Neurochir 2010;152(11):
1835–46.

70. Holodny AI, Schulder M, Liu WC, et al. The effect of
brain tumors on BOLD functional MR imaging activation in the adjacent motor cortex: implications for
image-guided neurosurgery. AJNR Am J Neuroradiol 2000;21(8):1415–22.

71. Leclercq D, Delmaire C, de Champfleur NM, et al.
Diffusion tractography: methods, validation and ap-
plications in patients with neurosurgical lesions.
Neurosurg Clin N Am 2011;22(2):253–68, ix.

72. Price SJ, Burnet NG, Donovan T, et al. Diffusion
tensor imaging of brain tumours at 3T: a potential
tool for assessing white matter tract invasion? Clin
Radiol 2003;58(6):455–62.

73. Zhu FP, Wu JS, Song YY, et al. Clinical application of
motor pathway mapping using diffusion tensor imaging tractography and intraoperative direct subcortical stimulation in cerebral glioma surgery: a
prospective cohort study. Neurosurgery 2012;
71(6):1170–83 [discussion: 83–4].

74. Wu JS, Zhou LF, Tang WJ, et al. Clinical evaluation
and follow-up outcome of diffusion tensor imaging-
based functional neuronavigation: a prospective,
controlled study in patients with gliomas involving
pyramidal tracts. Neurosurgery 2007;61(5):935–48
[discussion 48–9].

75. Smits M, Vernooij MW, Wielopolski PA, et al. Incorporating functional MR imaging into diffusion tensor
tractography in the preoperative assessment of the
corticospinal tract in patients with brain tumors.
AJNR Am J Neuroradiol 2007;28(7):1354–61.

76. Potgieser AR, Wagemakers M, van Hulzen AL, et al.
The role of diffusion tensor imaging in brain tumor
surgery: a review of the literature. Clin Neurol Neurosurg 2014;124:51–8.

77. Kinoshita M, Hashimoto N, Goto T, et al. Fractional
anisotropy and tumor cell density of the tumor core
show positive correlation in diffusion tensor magnetic resonance imaging of malignant brain tumors.
Neuroimage 2008;43(1):29–35.

78. Lee HY, Na DG, Song IC, et al. Diffusion-tensor
imaging for glioma grading at 3-T magnetic resonance imaging: analysis of fractional anisotropy
and mean diffusivity. J Comput Assist Tomogr
2008;32(2):298–303.

79. Lu S, Ahn D, Johnson G, et al. Diffusion-tensor MR
imaging of intracranial neoplasia and associated
peritumoral edema: introduction of the tumor infiltration index. Radiology 2004;232(1):221–8.

80. Zou QG, Xu HB, Liu F, et al. In the assessment
of supratentorial glioma grade: the combined
role of multivoxel proton MR spectroscopy and
diffusion tensor imaging. Clin Radiol 2011;
66(10):953–60.

81. Alexander AL, Lee JE, Lazar M, et al. Diffusion tensor imaging of the brain. Neurotherapeutics 2007;4(3):316–29.

82. Steven AJ, Zhuo J, Melhem ER. Diffusion kurtosis imaging: an emerging technique for evaluating the microstructural environment of the brain. AJR Am J Roentgenol 2014;202(1):W26–33.

83. Raab P, Hattingen E, Franz K, et al. Cerebral gliomas: diffusional kurtosis imaging analysis of microstructural differences. Radiology 2010;254(3): 876–81.

84. Van Cauter S, Veraart J, Sijbers J, et al. Gliomas: diffusion kurtosis MR imaging in grading. Radiology 2012;263(2):492–501.

85. Dunet V, Pomoni A, Hottinger A, et al. Performance of 18F-FET versus 18F-FDG-PET for the diagnosis and grading of brain tumors: systematic review and meta-analysis. Neuro Oncol 2016;18(3):426–34.

86. la Fougere C, Suchorska B, Bartenstein P, et al. Molecular imaging of gliomas with PET: opportunities and limitations. Neuro Oncol 2011;13(8):806–19.

87. Chen W, Cloughesy T, Kamdar N, et al. Imaging proliferation in brain tumors with 18F-FLT PET: comparison with 18F-FDG. J Nucl Med 2005;46(6):945–52.

88. Calcagni ML, Galli G, Giordano A, et al. Dynamic O-(2-[18F]fluoroethyl)-L-tyrosine (F-18 FET) PET for glioma grading: assessment of individual probability of malignancy. Clin Nucl Med 2011;36(10):841–7.

89. Fueger BJ, Czernin J, Cloughesy T, et al. Correlation of 6-18F-fluoro-L-dopa PET uptake with proliferation and tumor grade in newly diagnosed and recurrent gliomas. J Nucl Med 2010;51(10):1532–8.

90. Collet S, Valable S, Constans JM, et al. [(18)F]-fluoro-L-thymidine PET and advanced MRI for preoperative grading of gliomas. Neuroimage Clin 2015;8: 448–54.

91. Bell C, Dowson N, Fay M, et al. Hypoxia imaging in gliomas with 18F-fluoromisonidazole PET: toward clinical translation. Semin Nucl Med 2015;45(2): 136–50.

92. Giovannini E, Lazzeri P, Milano A, et al. Clinical applications of choline PET/CT in brain tumors. Curr Pharm Des 2015;21(1):121–7.

93. Pauleit D, Floeth F, Hamacher K, et al. O-(2-[18F]fluoroethyl)-L-tyrosine PET combined with MRI improves the diagnostic assessment of cerebral gliomas. Brain 2005;128(Pt 3):678–87.

94. Niyazi M, Geisler J, Siefert A, et al. FET-PET for malignant glioma treatment planning. Radiother Oncol 2011;99(1):44–8.

95. Rieken S, Habermehl D, Giesel FL, et al. Analysis of FET-PET imaging for target volume definition in patients with gliomas treated with conformal radiotherapy. Radiother Oncol 2013;109(3):487–92.

96. Rockne RC, Trister AD, Jacobs J, et al. A patient-specific computational model of hypoxia-modulated radiation resistance in glioblastoma using 18F-FMISO-PET. J R Soc Interface 2015;12(103).

97. Bisdas S, Ritz R, Bender B, et al. Metabolic mapping of gliomas using hybrid MR-PET imaging: feasibility of the method and spatial distribution of metabolic changes. Invest Radiol 2013;48(5): 295–301.

Posttreatment Evaluation of Brain Gliomas

Mark F. Dalesandro, MD, Jalal B. Andre, MD*

KEYWORDS

- High-grade glioma • Glioblastoma • Treatment effects • Radiation necrosis • Pseudoprogression

KEY POINTS

- Clinical information is key to the correct interpretation of changes in imaging findings in treated gliomas.
- Subacute ischemia, blood–brain barrier breakdown related to recent surgery, pseudoprogression, and delayed radiation necrosis can cause increased or new foci of enhancement that do not reflect true progression of disease.
- Both antiangiogenic therapy and increases in steroid dosage can decrease tumor enhancement without affecting the underlying disease burden.
- Perfusion, spectroscopy, and PET can add specificity in differentiating treatment effects from true disease progression.

INTRODUCTION

Gliomas are the most common primary intracranial malignant neoplasm in adults. Among these, glioblastoma exhibits the greatest incidence, and simultaneously carries the highest grade and a dismal prognosis.[1,2] Lower grade glial neoplasms can range from nonaggressive lesions, amenable to curative treatment such as ganglioglioma, to infiltrative neoplasms with a high rate of transformation to higher grade disease. The World Health Organization classification segregates glial neoplasms into different grades based on resectability and proliferative potential.[3] The primary radiologic challenges are found in imaging gliomas of grade II or higher; the most commonly encountered such tumors include diffuse astrocytomas, oligodendrogliomas, anaplastic astrocytomas, and glioblastomas. These challenges are exacerbated in the posttreatment setting, particularly when imaging high-grade gliomas (World Health Organization grades III and IV lesions).

Complete surgical resection of diffuse gliomas is often compromised by the infiltrative nature of these tumors and the presence of tumor cells that lie beyond the tumor margin delineated by conventional imaging.[4–6] The current treatment paradigm for high-grade glial neoplasms begins with maximal safe resection of the enhancing portion of the tumor. If the entirety of the enhancing component can be resected safely, this is termed a gross total resection. This is followed by adjuvant therapy, the composition of which depends on the tumor's histology and cytogenetics. For glioblastoma, the current treatment paradigm status after primary resection is treatment with involved field radiation therapy and temozolomide, with recent possible consideration for the additional implementation of an alternating electric fields/tumor treating fields device.[7] Patients with primary treatment failure or recurrence may receive a variety of therapies; perhaps the most pertinent of these to the practicing radiologist is anti-vascular endothelial growth factor (VEGF) therapy, commonly undertaken with bevacizumab (an anti–VEGF-A antibody with the trade name Avastin). In this work, we explore a variety of current imaging approaches that attempt to

Funding Sources: None.
Conflict of Interest: None.
Department of Radiology, Harborview Medical Center, University of Washington, Box 357115, 1959 Northeast Pacific Street, NW011, Seattle, WA 98195-7115, USA
* Corresponding author.
E-mail address: drjalal@uw.edu

Neuroimag Clin N Am 26 (2016) 581–599
http://dx.doi.org/10.1016/j.nic.2016.06.007
1052-5149/16/© 2016 Elsevier Inc. All rights reserved.

distinguish posttreatment areas of true tumor progression from their common mimics.

TUMOR BIOLOGY

The typical high-grade glioma demonstrates 3 radiologic "zones." The first zone is defined by the enhancing core of the tumor, in which neoangiogenesis can result in a variety of aberrant vessel subtypes, ultimately leading to breakdown of the blood–brain barrier and leakage of radiologic contrast agent.[8,9] This *zone of neovascular proliferation* is important because it is both a cardinal feature of high-grade glioma as well as a potential target for antiangiogenic therapy, discussed in greater detail elsewhere in this article. The second zone is the perilesional area of T2/fluid attenuation inversion recovery (FLAIR) signal abnormality surrounding the core of the lesion, which comprises a mix of nonenhancing infiltrative tumor and vasogenic edema, sometimes referred to as *infiltrative edema*.[10,11] The third zone is the surrounding, normal-appearing brain parenchyma that harbors microscopic tumor at levels that are not currently detectable on conventional, routine 3T anatomic MR pulse sequences.[4,6] Although promising research is being undertaken currently to better define the extent of nonenhancing tumor burden using advanced imaging techniques such as quantitative magnetization transfer,[12] the full extent of the tumor is currently defined poorly in clinical practice. This is in part owing to the microscopic extensions of perilesional tumor that provide a mechanism for the apparent "skip lesions" identified when new sites of disease appear distant to previously perceived margins of the tumor, and help to explain the mechanism behind cases presenting with multifocal disease. Ultimately, it is the diffuse infiltrative nature of these lesions coupled with their relative resistance to chemoradiation that supports the observation that diffuse gliomas are largely, presently incurable.

In this context, tumor genetics is becoming increasingly relevant to the treatment of neoplasms. The recently released 2016 revision to the 4th edition of the World Health Organization (WHO) criteria for tumors of the Central Nervous System reflects an increasing emphasis on tumor genetics as they pertain to tumor behavior and therapeutic response.[13] A detailed discussion of tumor genetics is beyond the scope of this article, but the radiologist should be made aware of a few of the more relevant genetic markers for adult gliomas. The new WHO criteria place an emphasis on mutations of isocitrate dehygrogenase (IDH) and the codeletion of 1p and 19q loci as important determinants of tumor behavior.[14] IDH mutation, most commonly IDH-1, is positively correlated with survival versus the wild type gene product.[15–17] 1p 19q codeletion is also a mutant variant which demonstrates an improved survival; in addition, mutation of IDH-1 and codeletion of 1p 19q is now recognized as the genetic signature of an oligodendroglioma.[13,18] The gene, O6 methylguanine—DNA methyltransferase (MGMT), encodes an enzyme involved in DNA repair and has important therapeutic implications that can potentially impact radiological interpretation. Specifically, when the promoter of this gene is hypermethylated, its activity is downregulated and gliomas and other tumors are more susceptible to DNA damage from alkylating agents such as temozolomide.[2,14] Familiarity with these genetic marker subtypes and their effect on the behavior of high-grade gliomas is important for proper interpretation of imaging studies.

IMAGING TIME FRAME

Imaging is usually performed within the first 24 to 48 hours after maximal safe resection but should be undertaken within the first 72 hours to establish a new baseline while minimizing the confounding effects of postoperative changes.[19] The authors' institution currently performs follow-up imaging 4 weeks after the completion of chemoradiation to allow for the reduction of acute radiation- and chemotherapy-related changes before evaluation for a possible therapeutic response. However, it has been advocated that subsequent imaging may be delayed up to 12 weeks in nonenhancing tumors (eg, low-grade gliomas) to allow for complete resolution of postoperative edema and improved assessment of the true extend of tumor resection.[20]

CHALLENGES WITH IMAGING

In the untreated patient, the enhancing component of a tumor can represent a surrogate of high-grade disease with microvascular proliferation. However, once the patient has undergone treatment, a variety of therapeutic interventions can cloud this picture, causing increases or decreases in the amount of apparent contrast enhancement without a significant effect on the actual burden of high-grade disease. Because the amount of enhancing disease is a major criterion for therapeutic response in the currently implemented oncologic imaging criteria, the Response Assessment in Neuro-Oncology (RANO) criteria,[21] it is important to consider that changes in enhancement may not necessarily reflect changes in tumor burden.

Mimics of Progression (Increased Enhancement)

Subacute infarction and postoperative blood–brain barrier disruption

In the postoperative state, ischemia surrounding the resection cavity can demonstrate avid enhancement in the subacute phase, often mimicking residual, enhancing disease and result in an erroneous diagnosis of residual high-grade tumor.[22,23] To prevent this error, postoperative imaging is typically performed within the first 24 to 48 hours after tumor resection to establish a new baseline, while minimizing the confounding effects of evolving postoperative changes.[19]

Pseudoprogression

At the authors' institution, posttreatment imaging is generally performed 4 weeks after the completion of chemoradiation. In this early posttreatment stage, an increase in the contrast-enhancing portion of the tumor can represent 2 entities: (1) true early progression of disease or (2) an entity known as pseudoprogression. Pseudoprogression is a complex subacute treatment-related response in which abnormally enhancing tissue demonstrates transient increased vascular permeability, edema, and necrosis, with a reported incidence of 20% to 30%.[24,25] The cardinal feature of this entity that distinguishes it from true early progression on standard sequences is that it stabilizes and subsequently improves (and/or subsides) without any further treatment. Pseudoprogression is most commonly seen in the first 3 months after the conclusion of therapy, but can be seen up to 6 months after treatment (Fig. 1).[26] It is correlated positively with improved survival,[27] and hypermethylation (inactivation) of the MGMT promoter gene is associated with an increased incidence of pseudoprogression.[28]

In the face of increasing enhancement and in the appropriate time frame, it is the opinion of the authors that findings identified with advanced imaging techniques can often further differentiate a diagnosis of true early progression from that of pseudoprogression (discussed elsewhere in this paper), but follow-up imaging has historically been the preferred, noninvasive method to differentiate these respective diagnoses with clinical certainty, as demonstrated in Fig. 2.

Delayed radiation necrosis

This entity is most commonly seen 9 to 12 months after treatment but can be seen years after initial therapy. Radiation necrosis presents as a focus or curvilinear region of new contrast enhancement, often ringlike, within the field of prior radiation treatment.[29] As with pseudoprogression, differentiating radiation necrosis from recurrent tumor is often difficult using standard, conventional anatomic sequences, particularly if the enhancement is seen within the high dose portion of the radiation field. Perfusion imaging can be helpful (Fig. 3) but the disparity in published results, using a variety of "perfusion" techniques, each with a myriad imaging parameters and postprocessing methods, has resulted in significant heterogeneity in the literature; these observations make it difficult to draw concrete conclusions and accept associated discrete cutoff values that might otherwise be used to rule in or out the diagnosis of radiation necrosis.

Mimics of Improvement (Decreased Enhancement)

Pseudoresponse

Pseudoresponse is the radiologic term used to describe a decrease in the size of the enhancing component of a tumor in the setting of antiangiogenic therapy. In adult high-grade glioma therapy, the antiangiogenic medication of choice is currently bevacizumab. Bevacizumab is a monoclonal antibody against VEGF type A. It is used most commonly as a secondary therapy for glioblastoma progression after initial therapy has failed, although it is being investigated in other roles, including upfront, concomitant first-line therapy. When used as a secondary treatment, it can provide reported symptom improvements and often allows for reduction in simultaneous steroid dosage, but without a definite effect on prolonged overall survival.[30] This medication is known to produce striking improvements in the imaging "appearance" of the tumor, with marked decrease in tumoral enhancement.

Effects on perfusion are more complex depending on which technique and parameter are being investigated. Overall, cerebral blood volume (CBV), cerebral blood flow (CBF), and the transfer constant (K^{trans}, a measure of vascular permeability), all tend to decrease in response to initial antiangiogenic therapy, as illustrated with CBF in Figs. 4 and 5; this latter case is also illustrative of vessel co-option, in which there is a shift in tumor physiology such that tumors initially reliant on neoangiogenesis may shift to a more infiltrative nature, harnessing their blood supply by growing along perivascular spaces. As such, the effects of antiangiogenic medications on enhancement and perfusion parameters are owing to changes in the tumor vasculature, including decreased vascular permeability, decreased patency of preexisting blood vessels, and decreased vascular proliferation.[31,32] Although these changes can result in the improvement of reported patient

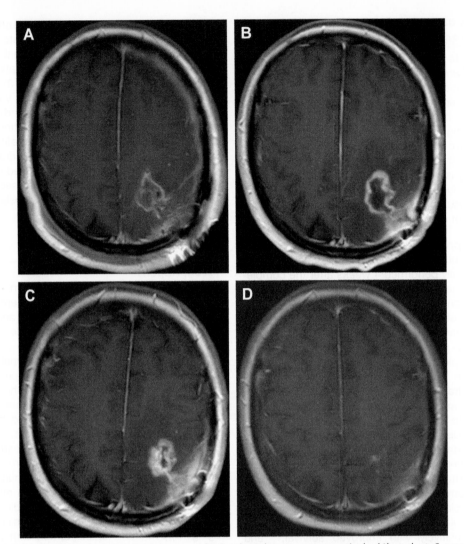

Fig. 1. Axial T1-weighted postcontrast images obtained 12 hours postoperatively (*A*) and at 6 months (*B*), 8 months (*C*), and 1 year (*D*) after the completion of radiation therapy. Irregular contrast enhancement around the margin initially increased after therapy with a peak between 6 and 8 months but nearly resolved at 1 year without additional therapy.

symptoms, it is important not to interpret the imaging changes as an antitumoral effect, but rather as a change in tumor vascularity and its associated imaging appearance. Other imaging biomarkers become more important in the setting of antiangiogenic therapy.[33,34] The use of apparent diffusion coefficient (ADC) values in the setting of antiangiogenic therapy has been extensively studied.

RADIOLOGIC INTERPRETATIONS BASED ON ROUTINE PULSE SEQUENCES
Response Assessment in Neuro-Oncology Criteria

The RANO criteria[21] are the imaging guidelines used to assess disease progression, stability,

and therapeutic response in current clinical trials and routine clinical care. Although rudimentary, these criteria should guide interpretations performed using standard pulse sequences acquired in postoperative brain tumors. The RANO imaging criteria are split into 2 distinct blocks of time, the first 12 weeks after completion of chemoradiotherapy and the time period after the first 12 weeks; this is done in recognition of the current difficulty that conventional imaging has in identifying true early progression in the immediate posttherapy period. Using these criteria, disease progression cannot be determined by conventional imaging alone in the first 12 weeks after completion of chemoradiation unless there is new enhancement outside the high-dose region of the radiation port.

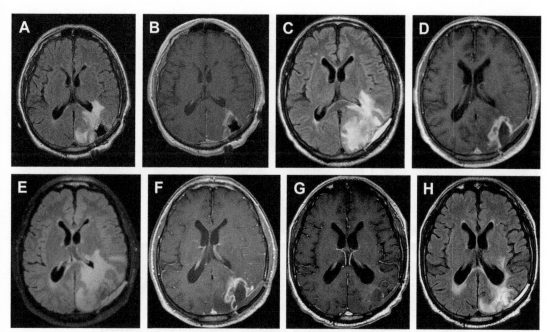

Fig. 2. Axial T2 fluid attenuation inversion recovery (FLAIR) and T1-weighted postcontrast images obtained immediately after resection (*A, B*) and at 2 months (*C, D*), 3 months (*E, F*), and 7 months (*G, H*) posttreatment demonstrate a marked initial worsening in enhancement and FLAIR hyperintensity around the resection cavity but with marked improvement by 7 months without additional therapy, compatible with pseudoprogression.

After 12 weeks, the guidelines become more complex, but take into account information that may not be easily obtainable by the radiologist, including clinical status and changes in corticosteroid doses. However, the 2 main imaging surrogates of disease recognized by the RANO criteria are the enhancing component and the T2/FLAIR component of disease. **Table 1** summarizes these important imaging criteria.

Clinical data to gather before beginning interpretation
There are several key pieces of clinical data that should shape the interpretation of the imaging findings in a posttreatment glioma, summarized in **Table 2**. The most crucial piece of information is the date when radiotherapy was completed; without this piece of data, interpretation of the significance of an increase in enhancement is

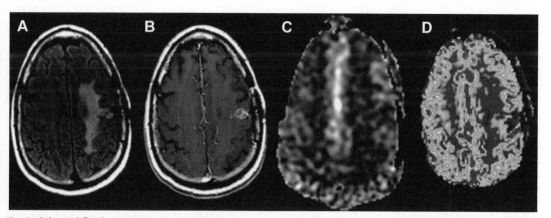

Fig. 3. (*A*) Axial fluid attenuation inversion recovery, (*B*) T1-weighted postcontrast, (*C*) pseudocontinuous arterial spin labeling, and (*D*) dynamic susceptibility contrast images obtained 10 months after the completion of chemoradiotherapy. There is a focus of ring enhancement in the region of the resection cavity, which does not demonstrate increased cerebral blood flow or relative cerebral blood volume, suggesting delayed radiation necrosis over recurrent tumor. This diagnosis was confirmed with biopsy.

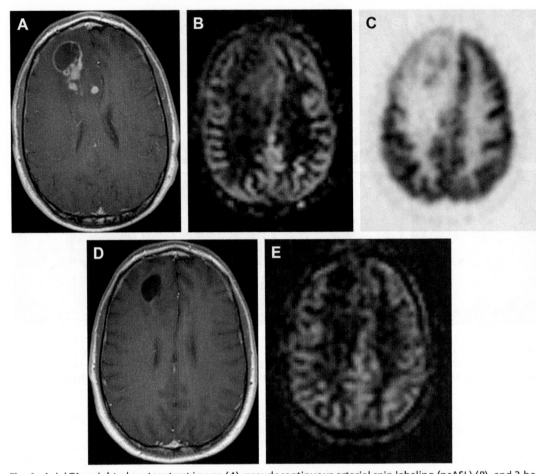

Fig. 4. Axial T1-weighted postcontrast image (*A*), pseudocontinuous arterial spin labeling (pcASL) (*B*), and 3-hour delay ^{18}fludeoxyglucose (FDG) PET (*C*) images at a location superior to the resection cavity (not shown) demonstrating an area of ring enhancement with elevated cerebral blood flow (CBF) and FDG uptake relative to the contralateral white matter, concerning for progression of high-grade disease. Bevacizumab therapy was initiated. One month after therapy was initiated, repeat T1-weighted postcontrast (*D*) and pcASL (*E*) images demonstrate a marked reduction in contrast enhancement and CBF.

problematic. It is also imperative to establish if the patient is currently on antiangiogenic therapy or was receiving the medication previously, at the time a prior comparison examination was acquired, owing to the drastic effects of this class of medications on the enhancement pattern of the tumor. Knowledge of the patient's current steroid dose and any changes in dosage from the most recent comparison can also help interpretation of changes in T2/FLAIR signal and enhancement. Although often technically challenging from an information technology perspective, it can also be extremely useful to have the radiation treatment field available in PACS (picture archiving and communication system) to determine whether new enhancing foci are within the high dose zone of the radiation treatment field. Finally, knowledge of the MGMT methylation status of the evaluated tumor is important from an imaging perspective, because MGMT hypermethylated (deactivated) tumors are more likely to undergo pseudoprogression[28] and attempting to differentiate pseudoprogression from true early progression using dynamic susceptibility contrast (DSC)-based relative CBV (rCBV) may be less useful in MGMT hypermethylated tumors.[35]

Enhancement

Any new foci of enhancement beyond the high-dose radiation zone are concerning for spread of high-grade tumor regardless of the time frame. Using the RANO criteria, an increase by 25% or more in the enhancing component of a tumor (including new foci within the radiation field) after the first 12 weeks after completion of chemoradiation is

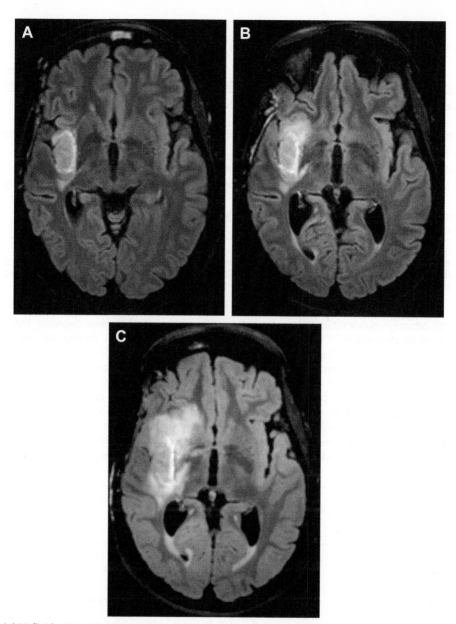

Fig. 5. Axial T2 fluid attenuation inversion recovery images obtained immediately postoperatively (*A*) and at 2 (*B*) and 6 (*C*) months after treatment demonstrate increasing masslike hyperintensity anterior and medial to the resection cavity. Postcontrast T1-weighted images (not shown) demonstrated no appreciable enhancement. This was confirmed to represent disease progression by further follow-up and ultimately patient demise.

seen as disease progression. In practice, however, new areas of enhancement within the radiation field must be interpreted with caution as these areas could also represent pseudoprogression/radiation necrosis. Advanced imaging techniques can help to differentiate these entities but ultimately the determination becomes clinical. As with any other area of suspected enhancement, it is crucial to check for T1 signal on the unenhanced sequence because posttreatment changes can result in blood

products and mineralization with intrinsic T1 hyperintensity that can easily simulate enhancement on the postcontrast sequence.

T2/Fluid Attenuation Inversion Recovery Imaging

Unlike contrast enhancement, the common clinical interpretation of T2/FLAIR imaging changes currently invokes more of a qualitative

Table 1
Response Assessment in Neuro-Oncology Working Group (RANO) criteria

Criterion	Complete Response	Partial Response	Stable Disease	Progressive Disease[a]
Enhancement	None	≥50% decrease	<50% decrease but >25% increase	≥25% increase
T2/FLAIR	Stable to decreased	Stable to decreased	Stable to decreased	Increased
New lesion	No	No	No	Yes
Corticosteroid dose	None	Stable to decreased	Stable to decreased	N/A
Clinical status	Stable or improved	Stable or improved	Stable or improved	Declining
Requirement for response	All of the above	All of the above	All of the above	Any

Abbreviation: FLAR, fluid attenuation inversion recovery.
[a] In the first 12 weeks, only histology or new enhancement outside the radiation field can indicate progression.
Adapted from Wen PY, Macdonald DR, Reardon DA, et al. Updated response assessment criteria for high-grade gliomas: Response Assessment in Neuro-Oncology Working Group. J Clin Oncol 2010;28(11):1963–72.

assessment, although quantitative volumetry has been successfully performed.[36,37] As discussed, the T2/FLAIR changes surrounding the enhancing component of a tumor typically represent a combination of vasogenic edema and infiltrative tumor without discrete microvascular proliferation that is typical of blood–brain barrier breakdown and associated tumoral enhancement. This is further complicated in the posttreatment setting by treatment-related changes including tissue injury and concomitant laminar necrosis. Differentiating between changes in edema, gliosis, and other treatment-related effects is difficult, but signs that suggest tumor involvement include a bulky, masslike component and new signal alteration that extends into the cortex (see **Fig. 5**). A variety of advanced imaging techniques have been investigated that attempt to differentiate treatment related changes from definite tumor infiltration and are discussed elsewhere in this paper.

Table 2
Clinical information to gather prior to image interpretation

Clinical Parameter	Imaging Effect(s)
Date of completion of chemoradiotherapy	Alters interpretation of areas of increasing or new enhancement in the radiation field: pseudoprogression in the first 6 mo and delayed radiation necrosis from 9 mo on.
Antiangiogenic therapy	Alters interpretations of areas of increasing or decreasing enhancement. Alters what the radiologist should monitor for disease progression: restricted diffusion becomes much more important and T2/FLAIR becomes more important than enhancement.
Radiation field	Helps to decide if a new focus of enhancement represents multifocal disease or could possibly be owing to radiation necrosis.
MGMT status of tumor	MGMT hypermethylated tumors more often undergo pseudoprogression. Pseudoprogression in MGMT hypermethylated tumors have a better outcome. rCBV may be less useful to differentiate pseudoprogression from true early progression in MGMT hypermethylated tumors.
Change in steroid dose from prior imaging study	Changes in steroid doses can affect the size of the T2/FLAIR component of the lesion as well as the size of the enhancing component of disease.

Abbreviations: FLAIR, fluid attenuation inversion recovery; MGMT, O^6methylguanine–DNA methyltransferase; rCBV, relative cerebral blood volume.

Diffusion Signal

A basic diffusion-weighted sequence is commonly obtained in most MR imaging protocols and should be obtained as part of a basic glioma follow-up. The usefulness of the ADC map has been investigated in a variety of settings, including estimating the grade of a primary brain neoplasm,[38] differentiating between treatment changes and true progression,[39] and evaluating for disease progression in the setting of antiangiogenic therapy.[33,40] In these studies, high-grade tumor was shown to have lower ADC values than treatment-related effects when compared with contralateral white matter owing to the hypercellularity of high-grade tumor. The ADC, then, can be useful in suggesting that nonenhancing T2/FLAIR changes are tumor related rather than treatment related and are also useful in monitoring a patient in the setting of antiangiogenic therapy when the degree of enhancement will no longer reliably identify active, high-grade tumor. More advanced analyses of ADC values have also been performed. A lower mean ADC was found to correlate to decreased survival when segmented using a double Gaussian mixture model.[41] In the setting of antiangiogenic therapies, a thresholded voxel-based analysis of the ADC has been shown to predict outcomes.[42,43] Serial ADC maps have also been used to generate maps of cell invasion, motility, and proliferation level estimate.[43,44] In these studies, cell invasion, motility, and proliferation level estimate maps were able to predict areas of tumor recurrence and predict progression free-survival. However, the significance of diffusion-restricting tissue may differ in the setting of antiangiogenic therapy, as illustrated in a study by Mong and colleagues,[45] in which increased overall survival was observed in patients treated with bevacizumab in whom persistent diffusion-restricting tissue was identified. This observation lead the authors to postulate that the diffusion restriction may represent hypoxic tissue rather than hypercellular, aggressive tumor.

ADVANCED MR IMAGING TECHNIQUES

A variety of advanced MR imaging techniques have been investigated that attempt to differentiate treatment-related changes from true tumor progression. Some of the more clinically relevant techniques are discussed here. Although these techniques may be currently considered optional in evaluation of the posttreatment glioma, they can provide valuable clinical input. It is the opinion of the authors that these techniques should be implemented whenever possible, with the caveat that resultant interpretations should be limited to the recognized strengths and experience within a given institution.

Dynamic Susceptibility Contrast-Enhanced Perfusion

DSC perfusion-weighted imaging (PWI) is a technique that uses the T2* effects of gadolinium-based contrast agents (GBCA) to estimate cerebral perfusion. The reader is referred to an excellent review by Willats and Calamante[46] for the implementation of optimal DSC technique. Until recently, initial models of DSC PWI assumed a completely intravascular contrast agent, without any correction for extravascular leakage of GBCA. In the absence of correcting for extravascular GBCA leakage, the use of DSC PWI can be suboptimal in brain regions where the blood–brain barrier has broken down, particularly involving areas of high-grade, enhancing tumor and enhancing foci of treated disease. Quantitative perfusion assessment in such areas can result in both artifactual decreases and artifactual increases[47] in calculated CBV if leakage correction techniques are not used. The historical lack of correcting for extravascular GBCA leakage, which was initially unrecognized as problematic, has rendered inconclusive the results of several years of prior publications, including the usefulness of previously published DSC PWI cutoff values in identifying true tumor progression.

The most commonly used parameter in DSC perfusion in tumor imaging is the rCBV, a parameter that also has the benefit of being clinically friendly, because it requires relatively little postprocessing. Unfortunately, the literature is quite heterogeneous with regard to DSC perfusion, because a variety of techniques and protocols have been used, making it difficult to discern a clear, numerical value to distinguish tumor progression from pseudoprogression or radiation necrosis. The critical dependence on specific DSC PWI techniques and postprocessing methods is summarized nicely in an excellent paper by Paulson and Schmainda.[48] Although a substantial body of literature has demonstrated that rCBV values are significantly lower in the latter entities than in high-grade tumor, there is considerable overlap between the values of treatment-related changes and recurrent tumor,[49–52] which may in part be secondary to the relative lack of correction for leakage effects among many of the earlier studies. Sensitivity and specificity are strongly dependent on the technique used but have been reported to be greater than 90% in some studies.

Dynamic Contrast-Enhanced Perfusion

Dynamic contrast-enhanced (DCE) perfusion is a technique that uses the T1-shortening effect of GBCAs to estimate cerebral perfusion parameters. The most common parameter used in tumor imaging is the K^{trans}, which is a measure of vascular permeability. Unlike the rCBV parameter of DSC, calculating the K^{trans} requires substantial postprocessing. The K^{trans} has been shown to be increased in recurrent glioma and decreased in radiation necrosis in many studies.[53–55] The K^{trans} tends to normalize in response to antiangiogenic therapy, but this response alone has not been shown to be useful in predicting outcomes.[56] Like DSC, the reported sensitivity and specificity of DCE depends on the technique used and there is overlap between the ranges of K^{trans} values in treatment-related effects and recurrent tumor.

Arterial Spin Labeling Perfusion

Arterial spin labeling (ASL) perfusion, unlike DSC and DCE, does not require administration of any exogenous contrast agent. In ASL, intravascular water is labeled magnetically and used as the contrast agent to measure perfusion. The most commonly used ASL parameter for imaging gliomas is relative CBF, although absolute CBF can be obtained readily. Literature describing the use of ASL in tumor imaging is sparse compared with that of DSC and DCE. Although one of the primary advantages of ASL is the lack of administration of an exogenous contrast agent, this benefit is currently less relevant when imaging a high-grade glioma; changes to the contrast-enhancing component of the tumor are still considered a primary method to evaluate therapeutic response, although with sometimes uncertain results, as discussed. Like the other perfusion techniques, differences in relative CBF obtained from ASL experiments have suggested usefulness in differentiating treatment effects from tumor progression (Fig. 6), and correlation with overall and progression-free survival,[57] including evaluation of response to antiangiogenic therapies such as cediranib, found to correlate with increased progression-free and overall survival.[58] It is the experience of the current authors that recurrent GBM is typically associated with initially increased intratumoral relative CBF that then subsequently decreases after antiangiogenic (bevacizumab) therapy, as documented by pseudocontinuous ASL, when performed without vascular crushing gradients,[59] the same technique used by Qiao and associates,[57] and advocated by a coalition of several prominent international perfusion groups.[60] Although it has been suggested that ASL may be

more accurate than DSC PWI in distinguishing predominantly recurrent high-grade glioma from radiation necrosis,[61] this study did not correct for leakage of GBCA, rendering the results somewhat inconclusive, and underscoring the critical importance of incorporating leakage correction techniques when performing a DSC PWI experiment.

Choosing a Perfusion Technique

Each of these perfusion techniques has its own advantages and disadvantages. DSC is the most widely used in clinical practice owing to a relatively rapid acquisition time and the perception that there is little need for postprocessing, although this has been shown to be erroneous.[48] In addition, DSC is prone to errors in the setting of blood–brain barrier breakdown, as discussed, so appropriate leakage-correction techniques must be performed.[47] Table 3 summarizes the advantages and disadvantages of common perfusion techniques.

Diffusion Tensor Imaging

Diffusion tensor imaging (DTI) evaluates the directionality of water diffusion. The number of directions of sampling can vary from the most basic 6 directional study (anterior–posterior, left–right, cranial–caudal) up to 256 or more directions. The tradeoff between accuracy in directionality and scanning time is a major determinant in deciding how many directions to obtain. In the brain, the primary structural component that imparts directionality in water diffusion is the axon bundle that comprises the white matter tracts. Fractional anisotropy is the parameter that measures the directionality of this water diffusion. Its usefulness in distinguishing tumor progression from radiation necrosis varies, based on the study, from no significant differentiation between the 2 entities (using 25 directions)[62] to significantly increased fractional anisotropy in tumor progression versus radiation necrosis, with a sensitivity and specificity of 85% and 86.7%, respectively (using 64 directions).[51] Although valuable in the initial evaluation of tumors, the usefulness of DTI in evaluating posttreatment changes remains unclear. The ADC can also be derived from DTI and is discussed elsewhere in this paper.

Spectroscopy

Proton MR spectroscopy uses the resonant frequency of protons in different organic compounds to identify and quantify the ratios of various metabolites within a sampled tissue. MR spectroscopy can aid in differentiating among a variety of disease processes and has been investigated extensively in tumor imaging. The main metabolites

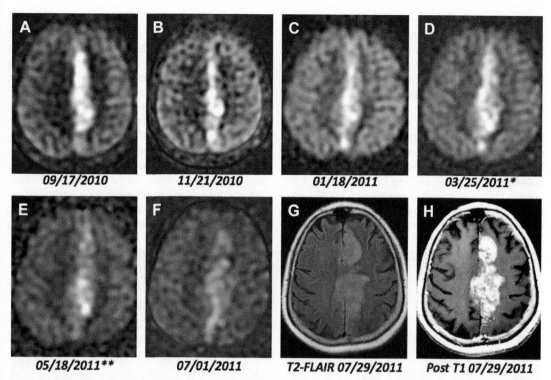

Fig. 6. A 54-year-old patient with biopsy-proven glioblastoma multiforme (GBM) initially treated with chemoradiation only owing to unresectability. First available pseudocontinuous arterial spin labeling (pCASL) MR imaging on September 17, 2010 (*A*) demonstrates significantly increased cerebral blood flow (CBF) in the left paramedian frontal lobe. Two follow-up scans demonstrate continued decreased in elevated CBF, albeit with slight increased in area of regional CBF alteration on November 21, 2010 (*B*) and January 18, 2011 (*C*), respectively. Interval increase in size and extent of elevated CBF is identified on the scan performed on March 25, 2011 (*D*), interpreted as GBM progression, representing the final imaging data obtained prior to bevacizumab administration (denoted by *), which was subsequently administered later that same day. Initial post-bevacizumab pCASL examination (denoted by **) performed on May 18, 2011 (*E*) demonstrates interval reduction in CBF, and decreased regional involvement, although continued follow-up on July 1, 2011 (*F*) suggests increased size of altered CBF, still decreased in value compared with prebevacizumab pCASL (*D*). Axial T2- fluid attenuation inversion recovery (*G*) and postgadolinium T1-weighted (*H*) images both obtained on July 29, 2011, demonstrate marked progression of disease. The patient was placed in hospice care and shortly thereafter expired.

Table 3
Advantages and disadvantages of MRI perfusion techniques

Technique	Advantage	Disadvantage
DSC	Shortest overall acquisition time of MR perfusion techniques Simple postprocessing if rCBV is the chosen parameter	Vulnerable to primarily false-negatives (underestimation of CBV) if leakage correction is not performed
DCE	Simpler evaluation of endothelial permeability	Long acquisition time (5–10 min)
ASL	No exogenous contrast agent is needed Insensitive to disruption of blood brain barrier Theoretically infinitely repeatable	Low signal to noise ratio Long acquisition time (5–10 min) CBV difficult to reliably obtain

Abbreviations: ASL, arterial spin labeling; CBV, cerebral blood volume; DCE, dynamic contrast-enhanced; DSC, dynamic susceptibility contrast; rCBV, relative cerebral blood volume.

used in tumor imaging in the postoperative setting are N-acetyl aspartate (NAA), a marker of neuronal health, choline (Cho), a marker of cell turnover, and creatine (Cr), a relatively constant metabolite. Lactate and mobile lipids, among a variety of other minor metabolites, can also be of use in certain situations. The cornerstone of tumor imaging is the so-called Hunter's angle, a reference to the relative concentrations of Cho, Cr, and NAA in the normal adult brain. In tumors with high cell proliferation, these concentrations change, with the ratio between Cho to NAA shifting from less than 1 to greater than 1, suggesting an increase in cell turnover and decrease in neuronal health. In very rapidly proliferating tumors, areas of necrosis can cause the release of mobile lipids and areas of ischemia can result in lactate peaks. Various ratios of the metabolites comprising Hunter's angle have suggested an ability to differentiate treatment effects from tumor progression, including Cho:NAA (elevated in recurrence), Cho:Cr (elevated in recurrence), and NAA:Cr (decreased in recurrence).[63–66] Fig. 7 provides an example of the clinical usefulness of spectroscopy. Other metabolites such as lactate (seen in tissue ischemia) and free lipids (seen in necrosis) are useful in the initial evaluation of neoplasms, but are less useful in differentiating treatment effects from tumor progression because both can be related to hypoxia and necrosis. In the setting

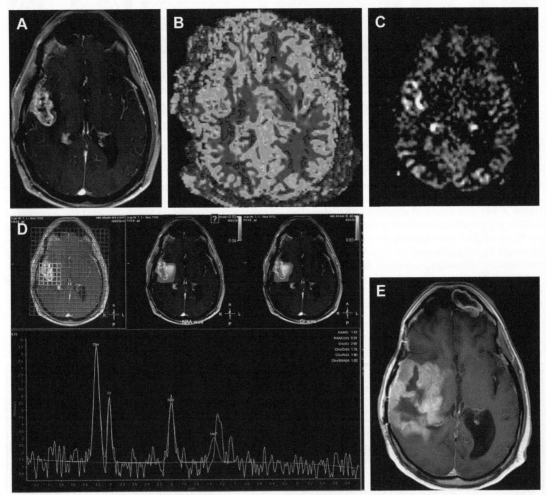

Fig. 7. Patient with promoter unmethylated glioblastoma who demonstrates progressive worsening enhancement seen 1 and 2 months after the completion of radiotherapy. Axial T1-weighted postcontrast image (A) demonstrates a thick, irregular rim of enhancement around the margin of the resection cavity. Dynamic susceptibility contrast (B) and pseudocontinuous arterial spin labeling (C) reveal an increased relative cerebral blood volume and cerebral blood flow. Two-dimensional multivoxel spectroscopy (D) demonstrates markedly increased choline relative to creatine and N-acetyl aspartate. These findings were suspicious for true early progression. Histopathologic confirmation was not obtained, but the enhancing component of disease continued to enlarge up to 18 months after the completion of therapy (E), consistent with disease progression.

of antiangiogenic therapy, evaluation of the NAA:Cho ratio in serial examinations can be useful for predicting outcomes: high values of this ratio correlate positively with 6-month overall survival in patients being treated with cediranib[39] and correlate with 6-month progression-free survival in patients being treated with bevacizumab.[67,68] The results of another study evaluating 53 subjects suggest that [1]H-MR spectroscopy indices taken from "hyperperfused" regions of gliomas, as detected by ASL, can be useful in distinguishing high-grade from low-grade gliomas.[69] However, additional studies are limited by small sample sizes and further studies and technique homogenization are needed before mainstream clinical integration.

NUCLEAR MEDICINE TECHNIQUES
[18]Fludeoxyglucose PET

[18]Fludeoxyglucose (FDG) is a glucose analog that provides a rough estimate of tissue-specific energy utilization and is used in PET imaging of a wide variety of neoplasms throughout the body. In theory, radiation necrosis should show decreased FDG uptake compared with hypermetabolic, rapidly proliferating tumor cells (see **Fig. 5**; **Fig. 8**); in practice, however, FDG PET has shown

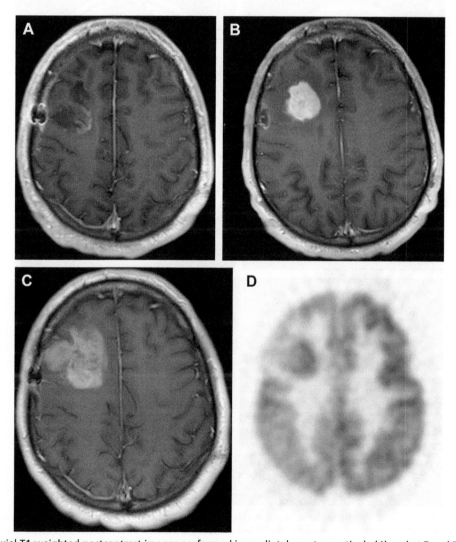

Fig. 8. Axial T1-weighted postcontrast images performed immediately postoperatively (*A*) and at 5 and 7 months (*B*, *C*) after the completion of radiotherapy demonstrate a large focus of enhancement around the resection cavity with progressive enlargement. This was concerning for true early progression of disease. Axial [18]fludeoxyglucose PET images obtained with a 3-hour delay (*D*) showing intense uptake in the region of enhancement on MR imaging, suggestive of tumor progression over treatment effects.

limited efficacy in differentiating tumor progression from radiation necrosis.[70–72] The widespread use of FDG in imaging other corporeal neoplasms is evidence of its availability in clinical imaging. However, its use in imaging posttreatment gliomas should be interpreted with caution; a metaanalysis of prior studies demonstrated an overall sensitivity of 78% and specificity of 78%, lower than many other imaging modalities.

Other PET Agents

A variety of PET agents other than FDG have been investigated to differentiate treatment effects from

tumor progression. ^{11}C-methionine has shown promise in studies,[73–76] but its short half-life (20.334 minutes) necessitates a cyclotron near the site of radiopharmaceutical administration, limiting its clinical usefulness; 3-deoxy-3-^{18}F-fluorothymidine is a thymidine analog, which is theorized to provide an imaging biomarker for areas of cell division. However, use of this agent is limited in the central nervous system because uptake is primarily seen in areas of blood–brain barrier breakdown.[77] To compensate for this, a kinetic analysis of the 3-deoxy-3-^{18}F-fluorothymidine flux compensates for the leakage across the blood barrier and has shown some promise in

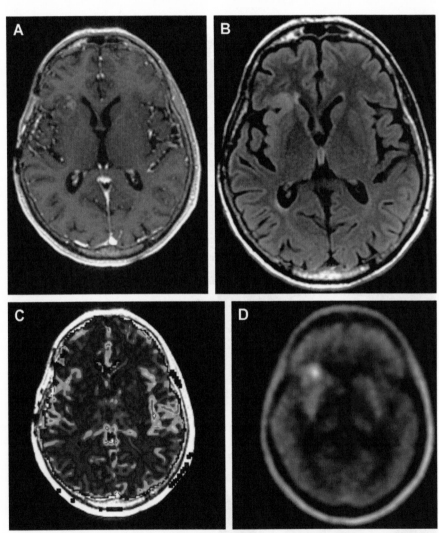

Fig. 9. Patient with a history of anaplastic oligodendroglioma who underwent subtotal resection and developed a new contrast-enhancing focus superior to the resection cavity 5 months after the completion of radiotherapy. T1-weighted postcontrast (A) and T2 fluid attenuation inversion recovery (B) images demonstrate a focal signal abnormality in the region of the right frontal operculum. Dynamic susceptibility contrast (C) demonstrates an increased relative cerebral blood volume in the region of enhancement. F-DOPA (3,4-dihydroxy-6-18F-fluoro-l-phenylalanine) PET (D) demonstrates focal increased uptake. Findings were concerning for disease progression, confirmed by resection which showed transformation to glioblastoma.

distinguishing tumor recurrence from treatment effects.[78] 18F-Fluoroethyl-L-tyrosine[79] and 3,4-dihydroxy-6-18F-fluoro-L-phenylaline[80] have also shown promising results in the evaluation of posttreatment gliomas (Fig. 9).

WHAT THE REFERRING CLINICIAN NEEDS TO KNOW

A key to preparing a clinically relevant report in the setting of posttreatment gliomata is to carefully consider and integrate the relevant clinical information that can impact image interpretation. Knowledge of the timing of radiation therapy relative to the current imaging study and any concurrent or prior antiangiogenic therapy is crucial. If using primarily conventional imaging only, look for subtle changes in T2/FLAIR signal alteration over the temporal course of multiple prior examinations, particularly if they exhibit a masslike quality or infiltrate the cortex. Measurable enhancing disease should be quantified by RANO criteria and reported with the appropriate RANO qualifiers. Appropriately choosing and implementing advanced imaging techniques to increase specificity can be of notable benefit.

SUMMARY

Some additional investigational imaging techniques and modalities have shown early promise, but have not yet been widely adopted into clinical practice. Ferumoxytol is an MR imaging contrast agent that is less susceptible to leakage across the blood brain barrier than GBCAs. Although it has shown promise in distinguishing treatment effects from tumor progression,[26,50,81] it carries a black box warning for anaphylactic-type reactions and its clinical adoption has been halted at many institutions owing to often life-threatening complications.

Computer-aided analysis of MR imaging data is another promising field. The majority of the changes in the T2/FLAIR area on MR imaging are very subtle, such that making a summative assessment, incorporating changes on all pulse sequences rather than focusing on a particular sequence, can be difficult. Akbari and colleagues[82] used computer learning on retrospective cases to form a model of tumor infiltration using standard pulse sequences, DSC, and DTI, and then applied this computer model prospectively to evaluate for early infiltrative recurrence, achieving a sensitivity of 91% and specificity of 92%. Although not clinically implementable at this time, if future studies confirm this method of analysis, a commercially available software package could expand the diagnostic usefulness of MR imaging data.

The infiltrative nature of gliomas and difficulties distinguishing treatment effects from tumor progression on standard MR imaging pulse sequences renders the follow-up imaging of treated gliomas a diagnostic challenge. Obtaining the appropriate clinical information and adding advanced imaging techniques to supplement standard pulse sequences can add specificity and help avoid pitfalls (Box 1). A standardization

---

Box 1
Pearls and pitfalls

- Changes in enhancement must be interpreted in the context of clinical information, including time from completion of radiation therapy, field of radiation therapy, and medication history.

- Differentiating pseudoprogression or radiation necrosis from disease progression is usually not possible on standard anatomic sequences obtained at a single timepoint. Use of advanced imaging techniques can add specificity to diagnosis.

- Key anatomic imaging findings that are specific for disease progression include (1) an increased, expansile, masslike region of T2/FLAIR signal, (2) T2/FLAIR signal that infiltrates and expands the cortex, and (3) subependymal spread of enhancing disease.

- Owing to the infiltrative nature of gliomas, there is often microscopic tumor involvement in normal-appearing brain. Be aware of the possibility of "skip lesions," which are new foci of disease separated from the main burden of disease surrounding the resection cavity.

- Marked improvement in the enhancing component of disease and decrease in perfusion parameters is common in antiangiogenic therapy and does not necessarily represent an antitumoral effect but rather a "normalization" of tumor vasculature.

- Leakage correction is essential to obtaining useful dynamic susceptibility contrast perfusion data.

Abbreviation: FLAIR, fluid attenuation inversion recovery.

of advanced imaging technique parameters to aid in reproducibility is needed before widespread incorporation of these techniques into routine clinical practice.

REFERENCES

1. Bag AK, Cezayirli PC, Davenport JJ, et al. Survival analysis in patients with newly diagnosed primary glioblastoma multiforme using pre- and post-treatment peritumoral perfusion imaging parameters. J Neurooncol 2014;120(2):361–70.
2. Stupp R, Mason WP, Van DB, et al. Radiotherapy plus concomitant and adjuvant temozolomide for glioblastoma. N Engl J Med 2005;352(10):987–96.
3. Louis DN, Ohgaki H, Wiestler OD, et al. The 2007 WHO classification of tumours of the central nervous system. Acta Neuropathol 2007;114(2):97–109.
4. Silbergeld DL, Chicoine MR. Isolation and characterization of human malignant glioma cells from histologically normal brain. J Neurosurg 1997;86(3):525–31.
5. Kelly PJ, Daumas-Duport C, Kispert DB, et al. Imaging-based stereotaxic serial biopsies in untreated intracranial glial neoplasms. J Neurosurg 1987;66(6):865–74.
6. Johnson PC, Drayer BP, Rigamonti D, et al. Defining the extent of infiltrating glioblastoma multiforme (GBM): a comparison of postmortem magnetic resonance imaging (MRI) with histopathology. J Neuropathol Exp Neurol 1987;46(3):389.
7. Zhang I, Knisely JS. Tumor-treating fields—a fundamental change in locoregional management for glioblastoma. JAMA Oncol 2016;2(6):813–4.
8. Nagy JA, Feng D, Vasile E, et al. Permeability properties of tumor surrogate blood vessels induced by VEGF-A. Lab Invest 2006;86(8):767–80.
9. Nagy JA, Dvorak AM, Dvorak HF. VEGF-A and the induction of pathological angiogenesis. Annu Rev Pathol 2007;2:251–75.
10. Cha S, Knopp EA, Johnson G, et al. Intracranial mass lesions: dynamic contrast-enhanced susceptibility-weighted echo-planar perfusion MR imaging. Radiology 2002;223(1):11–29.
11. Strugar JG, Criscuolo GR, Rothbart D, et al. Vascular endothelial growth/permeability factor expression in human glioma specimens: correlation with vasogenic brain edema and tumor-associated cysts. J Neurosurg 1995;83(4):682–9.
12. Underhill HR, Rostomily RC, Mikheev AM, et al. Fast bound pool fraction imaging of the in vivo rat brain: Association with myelin content and validation in the C6 glioma model. Neuroimage 2011;54(3):2052–65.
13. Louis DN, Perry A, Reifenberger G, et al. The 2016 World Health Organization Classification of Tumors of the Central Nervous System: a summary. Acta Neuropathol 2016;131:803–20.
14. Stupp R, Hegi ME, Mason WP, et al. Effects of radiotherapy with concomitant and adjuvant temozolomide versus radiotherapy alone on survival in glioblastoma in a randomised phase III study: 5-year analysis of the EORTC-NCIC trial. Lancet Oncol 2009;10(5):459–66.
15. Wick W, Hartmann C, Engel C, et al. NOA-04 randomized phase III trial of sequential radiochemotherapy of anaplastic glioma with procarbazine, lomustine, and vincristine or temozolomide. J Clin Oncol 2009;27(35):5874–80.
16. van den Bent MJ, Dubbink HJ, Marie Y, et al. IDH1 and IDH2 mutations are prognostic but not predictive for outcome in anaplastic oligodendroglial tumors: a report of the European Organization for Research and Treatment of Cancer Brain Tumor Group. Clin Cancer Res 2010;16(5):1597–604.
17. Weller M, Felsberg J, Hartmann C, et al. Molecular predictors of progression-free and overall survival in patients with newly diagnosed glioblastoma: a prospective translational study of the German Glioma Network. J Clin Oncol 2009;27(34):5743–50.
18. Lassman AB, Iwamoto FM, Cloughesy TF, et al. International retrospective study of over 1000 adults with anaplastic oligodendroglial tumors. Neuro Oncol 2011;13(6):649–59.
19. Vogelbaum MA, Jost S, Aghi MK, et al. Application of novel response/progression measures for surgically delivered therapies for gliomas: Response Assessment in Neuro-Oncology (RANO) Working Group. Neurosurgery 2012;70(1):234–43 [discussion: 243–244].
20. Shiroishi MS, Booker MT, Agarwal M, et al. Posttreatment evaluation of central nervous system gliomas. Magn Reson Imaging Clin N Am 2013;21(2):241–68.
21. Wen PY, Macdonald DR, Reardon DA, et al. Updated response assessment criteria for high-grade gliomas: Response Assessment in Neuro-Oncology Working Group. J Clin Oncol 2010;28(11):1963–72.
22. Henegar MM, Moran CJ, Silbergeld DL. Early postoperative magnetic resonance imaging following nonneoplastic cortical resection. J Neurosurg 1996;84(2):174–9.
23. Cairncross JG, Pexman JH, Rathbone MP, et al. Postoperative contrast enhancement in patients with brain tumor. Ann Neurol 1985;17(6):570–2.
24. Chamberlain MC, Glantz MJ, Chalmers L, et al. Early necrosis following concurrent Temodar and radiotherapy in patients with glioblastoma. J Neurooncol 2007;82(1):81–3.
25. Yoo RE, Choi SH. Recent application of advanced MR imaging to predict pseudoprogression in high-grade glioma patients. Magn Reson Med Sci 2016;15(2):165–77.
26. Nasseri M, Gahramanov S, Netto JP, et al. Evaluation of pseudoprogression in patients with glioblastoma multiforme using dynamic magnetic resonance

imaging with ferumoxytol calls RANO criteria into question. Neuro Oncol 2014;16(8):1146–54.

27. Brandsma D, Stalpers L, Taal W, et al. Clinical features, mechanisms, and management of pseudoprogression in malignant gliomas. Lancet Oncol 2008;9(5):453–61.

28. Brandes AA, Franceschi E, Tosoni A, et al. MGMT Promoter methylation status can predict the incidence and outcome of pseudoprogression after concomitant radiochemotherapy in newly diagnosed glioblastoma patients. J Clin Oncol 2008; 26(13):2192–7.

29. Kumar AJ, Leeds NE, Fuller GN, et al. Malignant gliomas: MR imaging spectrum of radiation therapy- and chemotherapy-induced necrosis of the brain after treatment. Radiology 2000;217(2):377–84.

30. Seystahl K, Wick W, Weller M. Therapeutic options in recurrent glioblastoma—An update. Crit Rev Oncol Hematol 2016;99:389–408.

31. Sitohy B, Nagy JA, Dvorak HF. Anti-VEGF/VEGFR therapy for cancer: reassessing the target. Cancer Res 2012;72(8):1909–14.

32. Inai T, Mancuso M, Hashizume H, et al. Inhibition of vascular endothelial growth factor (VEGF) signaling in cancer causes loss of endothelial fenestrations, regression of tumor vessels, and appearance of basement membrane ghosts. Am J Pathol 2004; 165(1):35–52.

33. Gerstner ER, Chen P-J, Wen PY, et al. Infiltrative patterns of glioblastoma spread detected via diffusion MRI after treatment with cediranib. Neuro Oncol 2010;12(5):466–72.

34. Norden AD, Young GS, Setayesh K, et al. Bevacizumab for recurrent malignant gliomas Efficacy, toxicity, and patterns of recurrence. Neurology 2008;70(10):779–87.

35. Kong D-S, Kim ST, Kim E-H, et al. Diagnostic dilemma of pseudoprogression in the treatment of newly diagnosed glioblastomas: the role of assessing relative cerebral blood flow volume and oxygen-6-methylguanine-DNA methyltransferase promoter methylation status. AJNR Am J Neuroradiol 2011;32(2):382–7.

36. Zhang Z, Jiang H, Chen X, et al. Identifying the survival subtypes of glioblastoma by quantitative volumetric analysis of MRI. J Neurooncol 2014;119(1): 207–14.

37. Grabowski MM, Recinos PF, Nowacki AS, et al. Residual tumor volume versus extent of resection: predictors of survival after surgery for glioblastoma. J Neurosurg 2014;121(5):1115–23.

38. Castillo M, Smith JK, Kwock L, et al. Apparent diffusion coefficients in the evaluation of high-grade cerebral gliomas. AJNR Am J Neuroradiol 2001; 22(1):60–4.

39. Hein PA, Eskey CJ, Dunn JF, et al. Diffusion-weighted imaging in the follow-up of treated high-grade gliomas: tumor recurrence versus radiation injury. AJNR Am J Neuroradiol 2004;25(2):201–9.

40. Andre JB, Lu S, Spearman K, et al. Peritumoral apparent diffusion coefficient as a metric of response in patients with recurrent glioblastoma multiforme treated with bevacizumab and irinotecan. Neuroradiol J 2008;21(3):350–61.

41. Pope WB, Qiao XJ, Kim HJ, et al. Apparent diffusion coefficient histogram analysis stratifies progression-free and overall survival in patients with recurrent GBM treated with bevacizumab: a multi-center study. J Neurooncol 2012;108(3):491–8.

42. Ellingson BM, Cloughesy TF, Lai A, et al. Graded functional diffusion map-defined characteristics of apparent diffusion coefficients predict overall survival in recurrent glioblastoma treated with bevacizumab. Neuro Oncol 2011;13(10):1151–61.

43. Ellingson BM, LaViolette PS, Rand SD, et al. Spatially quantifying microscopic tumor invasion and proliferation using a voxel-wise solution to a glioma growth model and serial diffusion MRI. Magn Reson Med 2011;65(4):1131–43.

44. Ellingson BM, Cloughesy TF, Lai A, et al. Cell invasion, motility, and proliferation level estimate (CIMPLE) maps derived from serial diffusion MR images in recurrent glioblastoma treated with bevacizumab. J Neurooncol 2011;105(1):91–101.

45. Mong S, Ellingson BM, Nghiemphu PL, et al. Persistent diffusion-restricted lesions in bevacizumab-treated malignant gliomas are associated with improved survival compared with matched controls. AJNR Am J Neuroradiol 2012;33(9):1763–70.

46. Willats L, Calamante F. The 39 steps: evading error and deciphering the secrets for accurate dynamic susceptibility contrast MRI. NMR Biomed 2013; 26(8):913–31.

47. Schmiedeskamp H, Andre JB, Straka M, et al. Simultaneous perfusion and permeability measurements using combined spin- and gradient-echo MRI. J Cereb Blood Flow Metab 2013;33(5):732–43.

48. Paulson ES, Schmainda KM. Comparison of dynamic susceptibility-weighted contrast-enhanced MR methods: recommendations for measuring relative cerebral blood volume in brain tumors. Radiology 2008;249(2):601–13.

49. Hu LS, Baxter LC, Smith KA, et al. Relative cerebral blood volume values to differentiate high-grade glioma recurrence from posttreatment radiation effect: direct correlation between image-guided tissue histopathology and localized dynamic susceptibility-weighted contrast-enhanced perfusion MR Imaging measurements. AJNR Am J Neuroradiol 2009;30(3): 552–8.

50. Gahramanov S, Muldoon LL, Varallyay CG, et al. Pseudoprogression of glioblastoma after chemo- and radiation therapy: diagnosis by using dynamic susceptibility-weighted contrast-enhanced perfusion

MR imaging with ferumoxytol versus gadoteridol and correlation with survival. Radiology 2013; 266(3):842–52.

51. Xu J-L, Li Y-L, Lian J-M, et al. Distinction between postoperative recurrent glioma and radiation injury using MR diffusion tensor imaging. Neuroradiology 2010;52(12):1193–9.

52. Barajas RF, Chang JS, Segal MR, et al. Differentiation of recurrent glioblastoma multiforme from radiation necrosis after external beam radiation therapy with dynamic susceptibility-weighted contrast-enhanced perfusion MR imaging. Radiology 2009; 253(2):486–96.

53. Hazle JD, Jackson EF, Schomer DF, et al. Dynamic imaging of intracranial lesions using fast spin-echo imaging: differentiation of brain tumors and treatment effects. J Magn Reson Imaging 1997;7(6):1084–93.

54. Bisdas S, Naegele T, Ritz R, et al. Distinguishing recurrent high-grade gliomas from radiation injury: a pilot study using dynamic contrast-enhanced MR imaging. Acad Radiol 2011;18(5):575–83.

55. Narang J, Jain R, Arbab AS, et al. Differentiating treatment-induced necrosis from recurrent/progressive brain tumor using nonmodel-based semiquantitative indices derived from dynamic contrast-enhanced T1-weighted MR perfusion. Neuro Oncol 2011;13(9): 1037–46.

56. Kreisl TN, Zhang W, Odia Y, et al. A phase II trial of single-agent bevacizumab in patients with recurrent anaplastic glioma. Neuro Oncol 2011;13(10): 1143–50.

57. Qiao XJ, Ellingson BM, Kim HJ, et al. Arterial spin-labeling perfusion MRI stratifies progression-free survival and correlates with epidermal growth factor receptor status in glioblastoma. AJNR Am J Neuroradiol 2015;36(4):672–7.

58. Sorensen AG, Emblem KE, Polaskova P, et al. Increased survival of glioblastoma patients who respond to anti-angiogenic therapy with elevated blood perfusion. Cancer Res 2012;72(2):402–7.

59. Andre JB, Nagpal S, Hippe DS, et al. Cerebral blood flow changes in glioblastoma patients undergoing bevacizumab treatment are seen in both tumor and normal brain. Neuroradiol J 2015;28(2):112–9.

60. Alsop DC, Detre JA, Golay X, et al. Recommended implementation of arterial spin-labeled perfusion MRI for clinical applications: a consensus of the ISMRM perfusion study group and the European consortium for ASL in dementia. Magn Reson Med 2015;73(1):102–16.

61. Ozsunar Y, Mullins ME, Kwong K, et al. Glioma recurrence versus radiation necrosis? A pilot comparison of arterial spin-labeled, dynamic susceptibility contrast enhanced MRI, and FDG-PET imaging. Acad Radiol 2010;17(3):282–90.

62. Agarwal A, Kumar S, Narang J, et al. Morphologic MRI features, diffusion tensor imaging and radiation dosimetric analysis to differentiate pseudo-progression from early tumor progression. J Neurooncol 2013;112(3):413–20.

63. Zeng Q-S, Li C-F, Zhang K, et al. Multivoxel 3D proton MR spectroscopy in the distinction of recurrent glioma from radiation injury. J Neurooncol 2007; 84(1):63–9.

64. Elias AE, Carlos RC, Smith EA, et al. MR spectroscopy using normalized and non-normalized metabolite ratios for differentiating recurrent brain tumor from radiation injury. Acad Radiol 2011;18(9):1101–8.

65. Rock JP, Hearshen D, Scarpace L, et al. Correlations between magnetic resonance spectroscopy and image-guided histopathology, with special attention to radiation necrosis. Neurosurgery 2002;51(4): 912–9 [discussion: 919–20].

66. Einstein DB, Wessels B, Bangert B, et al. Phase II trial of radiosurgery to magnetic resonance spectroscopy-defined high-risk tumor volumes in patients with glioblastoma multiforme. Int J Radiat Oncol Biol Phys 2012;84(3):668–74.

67. Kim H, Catana C, Ratai E-M, et al. Serial MR spectroscopy reveals a direct metabolic effect of cediranib in glioblastoma. Cancer Res 2011;71(11):3745–52.

68. Ratai E-M, Zhang Z, Snyder BS, et al. Magnetic resonance spectroscopy as an early indicator of response to anti-angiogenic therapy in patients with recurrent glioblastoma: RTOG 0625/ACRIN 6677. Neuro Oncol 2013;15(7):936–44.

69. Chawla S, Wang S, Wolf RL, et al. Arterial spin-labeling and MR spectroscopy in the differentiation of gliomas. AJNR Am J Neuroradiol 2007;28(9): 1683–9.

70. Nihashi T, Dahabreh IJ, Terasawa T. Diagnostic accuracy of PET for recurrent glioma diagnosis: a meta-analysis. AJNR Am J Neuroradiol 2013;34(5): 944–50.

71. Ricci PE, Karis JP, Heiserman JE, et al. Differentiating recurrent tumor from radiation necrosis: time for re-evaluation of positron emission tomography? AJNR Am J Neuroradiol 1998;19(3):407–13.

72. Valk PE, Dillon WP. Radiation injury of the brain. AJNR Am J Neuroradiol 1991;12(1):45–62.

73. Chung J-K, Kim YK, Kim S, et al. Usefulness of 11C-methionine PET in the evaluation of brain lesions that are hypo- or isometabolic on 18F-FDG PET. Eur J Nucl Med Mol Imaging 2002;29(2):176–82.

74. Kim YH, Oh SW, Lim YJ, et al. Differentiating radiation necrosis from tumor recurrence in high-grade gliomas: assessing the efficacy of 18F-FDG PET, 11C-methionine PET and perfusion MRI. Clin Neurol Neurosurg 2010;112(9):758–65.

75. Van Laere K, Ceyssens S, Van Calenbergh F, et al. Direct comparison of 18F-FDG and 11C-methionine PET in suspected recurrence of glioma: sensitivity, inter-observer variability and prognostic value. Eur J Nucl Med Mol Imaging 2005;32(1):39–51.

76. Tripathi M, Sharma R, Varshney R, et al. Comparison of F-18 FDG and C-11 methionine PET/CT for the evaluation of recurrent primary brain tumors. Clin Nucl Med 2012;37(2):158–63.

77. Muzi M, Spence AM, O'Sullivan F, et al. Kinetic analysis of 3'-Deoxy-3'-18F-Fluorothymidine in patients with gliomas. J Nucl Med 2006;47(10):1612–21.

78. Spence AM, Muzi M, Link JM, et al. NCI-sponsored trial for the evaluation of safety and preliminary efficacy of 3'-deoxy-3'-[18F]fluorothymidine (FLT) as a marker of proliferation in patients with recurrent gliomas: preliminary efficacy studies. Mol Imaging Biol 2009;11(5):343–55.

79. Galldiks N, Rapp M, Stoffels G, et al. Response assessment of bevacizumab in patients with recurrent malignant glioma using [18F]Fluoroethyl-L-tyrosine PET in comparison to MRI. Eur J Nucl Med Mol Imaging 2013;40(1):22–33.

80. Chen W, Silverman DHS, Delaloye S, et al. 18F-FDOPA PET imaging of brain tumors: comparison study with 18F-FDG PET and evaluation of diagnostic accuracy. J Nucl Med 2006;47(6):904–11.

81. Gahramanov S, Raslan AM, Muldoon LL, et al. Potential for differentiation of pseudoprogression from true tumor progression with dynamic susceptibility-weighted contrast-enhanced magnetic resonance imaging using ferumoxytol vs. gadoteridol: a pilot study. Int J Radiat Oncol 2011;79(2):514–23.

82. Akbari H, Macyszyn L, Da X, et al. Imaging surrogates of infiltration obtained via multiparametric imaging pattern analysis predict subsequent location of recurrence of glioblastoma. Neurosurgery 2016; 78(4):572–80.

Metastasis in Adult Brain Tumors

Ramon Francisco Barajas Jr, MD[a], Soonmee Cha, MD[b],*

KEYWORDS

- Metastasis • MR Imaging • DSC perfusion • Brain

KEY POINTS

- CT imaging of metastatic disease is largely used as a tool for screening of life-threatening complications, such as hemorrhage, herniation, and hydrocephalus.
- Contrast-enhanced MR imaging is currently viewed as the ideal imaging modality for the diagnosis of metastatic disease to the central nervous system (CNS), monitoring of therapeutic response, and assessment for disease progression following chemoradiotherapy.
- Parenchymal spread of disease is the most common form of CNS metastasis. Contrast-enhanced MR imaging is superior to CT at the detection of brain metastasis.
- Dynamic T2* susceptibility-weighted contrast-enhanced (DSC) perfusion MR imaging has been shown to improve the diagnostic capabilities of differentiating solitary brain metastasis from high-grade glioma and radiation necrosis from recurrent metastatic disease after stereotactic radiosurgery.

INTRODUCTION

Noninvasive imaging techniques play a critical role in the diagnosis and management of patients with metastatic disease to the CNS (Boxes 1–5). Up to 40% of all adult cancer patients are diagnosed with metastatic disease, with approximately 25% involving the brain.[1] The presence of metastatic disease to the CNS portends a poor prognosis and is a leading cause of morbidity and mortality. The predilection for metastatic CNS involvement greatly varies by disease origin: as high as 40% for lung, 20% for breast, 10% for cutaneous, and 6% for enteric primaries. The disease origin also plays an important role in the preferential anatomic site seeding outside of the brain parenchyma. For instance, metastatic prostate cancer is rarely observed within the brain parenchyma; however, it often involves the calvarium or pachymeninges.[2,3]

Patients with neurologic symptoms often undergo noncontrast CT as an initial screening tool for the diagnosis of metastatic disease. The presence of a mass lesion by CT may be the first clue to the presence of a previously unidentified systemic neoplastic process. Conversely, asymptomatic patients with known systemic malignancy often undergo staging of the CNS prior to the initiation of medical therapy using MR imaging.

The aim of this article is to review the imaging assessment of metastatic tumors to the brain and its surrounding structures. First, technical considerations for imaging patients with

Disclosures: None.
[a] Departments of Radiology and Advanced Imaging Research Center, Oregon Health and Science University, 3181 South West Sam Jackson Park Road, Portland, OR 97239, USA; [b] Departments of Neurological Surgery, Radiology and Biomedical Imaging, University of California, San Francisco, 505 Parnassus Avenue, Long L200B, Box 0628, San Francisco, CA 94143, USA
* Corresponding author. Departments of Neurological Surgery, Radiology and Biomedical Imaging, University of California, San Francisco, 505 Parnassus Avenue, Long L200B, Box 0628, San Francisco, CA 94143.
E-mail address: soonmee.cha@ucsf.edu

1052-5149/16/© 2016 Elsevier Inc. All rights reserved.

Box 1
MR imaging protocol

Indication	Key Imaging Sequences
Initial diagnosis/screening	Axial T2 3-D FLAIR T2*/SWI Diffusion Spin-echo axial T1 precontrast Spin-echo T1 postcontrast[a] 3-D gradient T1 postcontrast
Preoperative stereotactic[b]	3-D T2 3-D T1 postcontrast
Follow-up/high clinical suspicion[c]	DSC perfusion

[a] The number and planes of imaging vary based on whether a 3-D gradient T1 postcontrast is obtained. If no gradient sequence, then minimum 2 planes is recommended.
[b] The exact stereotactic sequence used by the intraoperative guidance machine varies by manufacturer and imaging vendor. Generally, a 3-D acquisition protocol is required.
[c] Follow-up/high clinical suspicion imaging indication is similar to the initial diagnosis/screening indication; however, DSC perfusion can be added to provide additional diagnostic information.

---

metastatic CNS disease are introduced. Next, the varied imaging appearance of metastatic CNS tumors are reviewed. Finally, how advanced physiologic MR sequences can provide additional diagnostic capabilities to standard morphologic T1-weighted and T2-weighted imaging when evaluating for progression of metastatic disease after therapeutic intervention and in differentiating metastatic disease from primary high-grade glial neoplasms is discussed.

NORMAL ANATOMY AND IMAGING TECHNIQUES
Anatomy of the Cranial Meninges

In general terms, metastatic disease can involve any CNS compartment. Most commonly, metastatic disease affects the brain parenchyma, spine parenchyma, and calvarium. Metastatic disease, however, can also involve the brain parenchymal coverings: leptomeninges and pachymeninges (Table 1). The pachymeninges form the outermost

---

Box 2
Diagnostic criteria

	Criteria	
CNS Location	**CT**	**MR Imaging**
Calvarium	Focal lytic or sclerotic lesion	Marrow replacing process with focal enhancement
Pachymeninges	Isodense to hyperdense dural thickening with enhancement. Often difficult to appreciate by noncontrast examinations	Sheet or nodular dural thickening and enhancement
Leptomeninges	Sulcal or basilar cisternal enhancement. Often difficult to appreciate by CT unless florid disease	Sulcal, cisternal, or cranial nerve FLAIR hyperintensity and enhancement. Often diffuse and linear
Parenchyma	Regional hypodenisty sparing the cortical margin. Variable degrees of enhancement after intravenous contrast. Nonhemorrhagic metastatic foci are often occult by noncontrast CT.	Focal enhancing mass at the gray–white matter junction associated with robust vasogenic edema. Edema spares the surrounding gray matter.

Common CT and MR imaging appearance by location. Metastatic disease can appear varied based on disease etiology.

Box 3
Differential diagnosis in adult metastatic tumors

Central Nervous System Location	Differential Diagnosis	
	Neoplastic	Non-Neoplastic
Calvarium	Secondary leukemia/lymphoma Multiple myeloma Interoseous meningioma	Paget disease Fibrous dysplasia Histiocytosis Aneurysmal bone cyst Venous lakes/arachnoid granulations Osteomyelitis
Pachymeninges	Meningioma Hemangioma Hemangiopericytoma Secondary leukemia/lymphoma Osteoma	Intracranial hypotension Extramedullary hematopoiesis
Leptomeninges	Germinoma Choroid plexus carcinoma Primary glial Secondary leukemia/lymphoma	Infectious/chemical meningitis Neurosarcoidosis
Parenchyma	High-grade astrocytoma Hemangioblastoma	Embolic abscesses Subacute embolic infarctions Chronic microvascular oschemia Tumefactive demyelination Cavernous angiomas Metastatic pseuodoprogression

Common, but not complete, list.

layer of the cranial meninges, composed of the dura matter. The dura mater is a 3-layered fibrous membrane that lines the bony coverings of the CNS. The leptomeninges form the 2 innermost layers of the cranial meninges, composed of the arachnoid and pia mater. The arachnoid mater is the middle layer of cranial meninges, composed of a thin membrane interpositioned between the dura matter and pia matter. The arachnoid matter is loosely attached to the overlying dura matter, allowing it to follow the dura matter contour within the calvarium. The pia mater is the inner most layer of cranial meninges composed of a thin membrane directly adherent to the brain parenchymal cortex.

Preferential Locations of Central Nervous System Metastasis

CNS metastasis can occur via direct geographic invasion or hematogenous spread. Although much less common than hematogenous spread, direct geographic invasion of the CNS typically occurs by perineural or perivascular extension. Direct geographic invasion is the preferential route of spread into the CNS for primary head and neck tumors (**Fig. 1**). A second, rarer,

form of direct geographic invasion is found in multifocal glioblastoma (**Fig. 2**). High-grade glial neoplasms can spread both locally and distantly via direct extension along white matter tracts to involve cranial nerves, ventricular ependymal surfaces, pial surfaces, and even the dura matter (**Fig. 3**).

The most common method of metastasis to the CNS is via hematogenous spread. Metastasis spread via the circulatory system within the CNS occurs through a series of events that begins with detachment of neoplastic cells from the primary tumor mass into the circulatory system, hematogenous spread of disease to the metastatic site, extravasation through the vascular wall, and perivascular or brain parenchymal proliferation.[4] The neurovascular unit (blood-brain barrier) plays a significant role in the pathogenesis of metastasis. The neurovascular unit is a selectively permeable tissue found around most CNS blood vessels that limits the movement of molecules from the blood based on molecular size and charge. The ability to regulate metabolite entry into the CNS can result in the exclusion of hydrophilic molecules, such as chemotherapeutics. This tightly controlled microenvironment facilitates early metastatic

Box 4

Pearls, pitfalls, and variants

- Parenchymal metastatic disease can have a varied appearance, however, most likely involving the gray–white matter junction with vasogenic edema that spares the surrounding gray matter.

- Metastatic disease lacks a neurovascular unit. As a result, it has reduced recovery values compared with high-grade glioma on DSC perfusion MR imaging analysis.

- Small subacute ischemic infarctions can have a similar appearance to metastatic disease. Older subacute infarcts can demonstrate gyriform T1 hyperintensity in a vascular pattern on precontrast imaging suggesting laminar necrosis. Short follow-up MR imaging should show improved vasogenic edema and enhancement in patients with prior infarctions.

- Tumefactive demyelination can have a similar appearance to metastatic disease. Acute lesions can have leading rim of reduced diffusion with incomplete rim of contrast enhancement and often have evidence of prior demyelinating lesions. Short follow-up MR imaging should show improvement.

- Septic emboli can have a similar appearance to metastatic disease. Abscesses demonstrate centrally reduced diffusion with rim of susceptibility. Ring enhancement can be incomplete. Patients are often very ill at time of presentation.

- Metastatic melanoma can demonstrate T1 hyperintensity and marked susceptibility on noncontrast imaging due to the melanin content.

Table 1

Common anatomic localization of central nervous system metastatic tumor burden

Location	Histologic Origin
Common	
Calvarium	Breast, lung, prostate, renal
Leptomeninges (arachnoid and subarachnoid)	Breast, melanoma, lung, leukemia, lymphoma
Parenchyma (gray–white matter junction)	Lung, breast, melanoma, colon, renal
Rare	
Pachymeningeal carcinomatosis (dura)	Breast, lymphoma, prostate, lung, neuroblastoma
Leptomeninges (isolated subpial; milliary)	Melanoma

Data from Nussbaum ES, Djalilian HR, Cho KH, et al. Brain metastases. Histology, multiplicity, surgery, and survival. Cancer 1996;78(8):1781–8; and Das A, Hochberg FH. Clinical presentation of intracranial metastases. Neurosurg Clin N Am 1996;7(3):377–91.

the types of neoplastic cells that can more easily proliferate within its confines. For instance, the high chloride content of the brain's interstitial fluid enables neoplastic cells of neuroepithelial origin, such as small cell carcinoma of the lung or melanoma, to proliferate.[4,5] Many factors, both inherent to the tumor origin and microenvironment about the CNS deposition site, influence the location of metastatic disease observed on imaging.

Neuroimaging Approach and Techniques

Neuroimaging plays a critical role in patients with metastatic disease to the CNS. The imaging modality depends on the particular clinical setting and the clinical information needed to make treatment decisions. Neuroimaging of metastatic disease can be divided into 3 broad categories, each serving specific clinical questions: (1) diagnosis, (2) preoperative or therapy planning, and (3) post-treatment evaluation.

Initial Diagnosis

In the initial diagnostic work-up for metastatic disease, the choice of imaging modality is largely dependent on a clinician's pretest probability, the information needed to make immediate treatment decisions, and a patient's overall clinical status.

tumor growth, allowing for the establishment of a foothold within the bounds of the perivascular space.[4] Additionally, the metabolic environment established by the neurovascular unit influences

Box 5

What the referring physician needs to know

- Selection of initial imaging modality is dependent on the clinical question that needs answering.

- Noncontrast CT excludes the presence of a neurosurgical emergencies: hemorrhage, herniation, and hydrocephalus.

- Unless otherwise contraindicated, contrast-enhanced MR imaging is the screening modality of choice to exclude the presence of brain parenchymal metastatic disease.

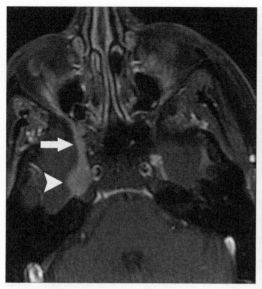
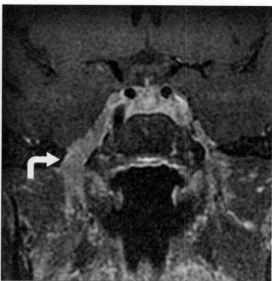

Fig. 1. Direct geographic invasion of primary head and neck cancer. A 56-year-old woman with no significant past medical history presented with 3 months' right facial pain. Axial (*left*) and coronal (*right*) T1-weighted fat saturated postcontrast MR imaging of the skull base demonstrates nodular enhancement of the right trigeminal nerve ganglion (*arrowhead*) with mass like expansion of Meckel cave. Linear thickening and enhancement is noted to extend through foramen rotundum (*straight arrow*) and foramen ovale (*curved arrow*). Tissue sampling of the lesion demonstrated adenoid cystic carcinoma of the trigeminal nerve ganglion.

If high clinical suspicion exists for the presence of metastatic disease and the patient's clinical status permits, an extended imaging examination, such as MR imaging with intravenous gadolinium-based contrast, is the recommended first-line imaging modality.[6]

In an emergent situation where, for example, a patient presents with new-onset neurologic symptoms, CT is often used as a first-pass screening modality for CNS disease due to its fast examination time, wide availability, and ability to detect acute intracranial hemorrhage (**Fig. 4**).

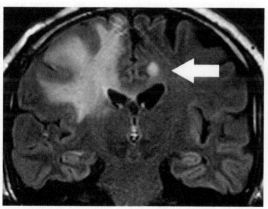
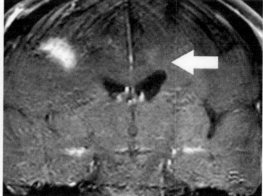

Fig. 2. Direct geographic invasion of glioblastoma. A 63-year-old man with altered mental status presented for MR imaging. Coronal FLAIR (*left*) and T1-weighted postcontrast (*right*) MR imaging of the brain demonstrates extensive FLAIR signal within the right cingulate, superior frontal, middle frontal, and inferior frontal gyri that extends across the corpus callosum to involve the contralateral cingulate gryus (*arrows*). Focal enhancement is noted within the ipsilateral mass and contralateral cingulate gyrus lesion. Subsequent resection of the right frontal mass demonstrated glioblastoma. Multifocal glioma can occur at initial presentation with metastatic disease occurring via direct perineural infiltration.

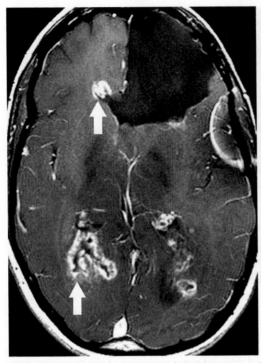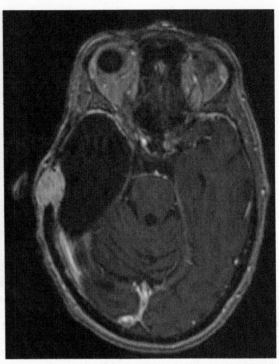

Fig. 3. Direct geographic invasion of glioblastoma. Axial T1-weighted postcontrast MR imaging in 2 patients with prior brain parenchymal resection for glioblastoma demonstrate direct geographic invasion of disease along the ependymal margins of the lateral ventricular system (*left, arrows*) and dura (*right*). Although rare, systemic or primary metastatic tumor can demonstrate direct invasion along any CNS surface.

As such, noncontrast CT imaging is sensitive in detecting acute life-threatening sequelae of metastatic disease: hemorrhage, hydrocephalus, and herniation. Because of these factors, CT imaging is commonly performed even though it is less sensitive than MR imaging in tumor detection and characterization. In situations where MR imaging is not possible, contrast-enhanced CT can be helpful in detecting areas of neurovascular unit disruption and defining the contrast-enhancing tumor burden for large areas of disease (Fig. 5). Despite CT's usefulness in acute situations, it suffers from important limitations due to intrinsically low soft tissue contrast resolution, which prevents the detection of nonenhancing tumor margin; limited ability to provide multiplanar acquisitions; and lack of physiologic imaging capabilities.

Once it has been established that a patient has metastatic disease to the CNS, MR imaging is currently viewed as the ideal imaging modality for monitoring of therapeutic response and assessment for disease progression. There are numerous MR imaging protocols that can be used in the diagnosis of CNS metastatic disease. The most widely accepted standard imaging protocol for this purpose includes pre–contrast-enhanced and post–contrast-enhanced T1-weighted, T2-weighted, and fluid-attenuated inversion recovery (FLAIR) imaging sequences.

Contrast-enhanced T1-weighted imaging is among the most important MR imaging sequences for characterization of metastatic CNS tumor. The administration of gadolinium-based contrast agent allows for the detection of neurovascular unit breakdown, a hallmark of aggressive neoplasia. The interpretation of contrast enhancement should be done in conjunction with nonenhanced T1-weighted images to evaluate for inherent T1 shorting that is suggestive of blood products, fat, melanin, or proteinaceous fluid (Fig. 6).

The lack of a neurovascular unit within the metastatic microvasculature is often manifested by the robust production of vasogenic edema. The evaluation of edema can be subtle on T1-weighted sequences; however, on T2-weighted sequences, vasogenic edema is readily apparent due to higher sensitivity to changes in water content of the brain. FLAIR imaging has signal from CSF suppressed to increase the conspicuity of lesions adjacent to ventricles or sulci. FLAIR imaging is sensitive to subtle differences in soft tissue T2 prolongation and can depict the full extent of tumor and surrounding tumor-related changes far

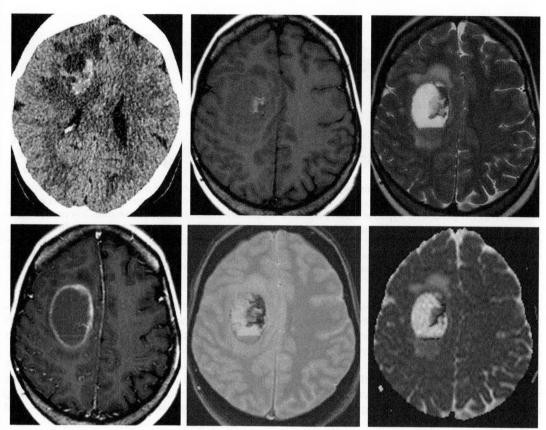

Fig. 4. Hemorrhagic brain metastasis. A 58-year-old woman with history of metastatic breast cancer presents with right sided weakness. Noncontrast CT imaging (*top left*) was used as a screening modality given the patients acute presentation demonstrates a hyperdense hemorrhagic mass with surrounding edema that spares the cortex centered within the deep right fontal white matter. Subsequent contrast-enhanced T1-weighted MR imaging (*bottom left*) demonstrated a mixed solid and cystic rim-enhancing mass with layering blood products of differing ages on gradient T2*-weighted imaging (*bottom middle*). Susceptibility from the blood products mimics the appearance of reduced diffusion on ADC map (*bottom right*). The age of blood products can be delineated by using T1 (*top middle*) and T2 (*top right*) signal intensity. Acute blood products are noted to layer within the dependent portion of the lesion. Early subacute blood products are noted within the midmedial aspect of the lesion.

better than contrast-enhanced T1-weighted imaging. In addition, FLAIR imaging has been shown superior to contrast-enhanced T1-weighted imaging in detecting subtle leptomeningeal spread of tumor as well as in demonstrating low-contrast lesions and subarachnoid hemorrhage (**Fig. 7**).[7,8]

Preoperative and Therapy Planning

Noncontrast CT has limited utility in the preoperative imaging of patients with metastatic CNS tumor due to its low resolution for differences in soft tissue contrast (see **Fig. 5**). The mainstay of CT imaging is for intraoperative guidance during stereotactic tissue sampling in patients with contraindication to MR imaging. MR imaging is widely used as the preoperative imaging modality of choice. Neurosurgical and radiotherapy planning is often benefitted

by MR imaging in all 3 orthogonal planes after the administration of contrast media.

Post-Treatment Evaluation

Despite their superb soft tissue contrast resolution and multiplanar capability, T1-weighted and T2-weighted MR imaging sequences are limited to depicting morphologic abnormalities. This limitation results in decreased specificity for the diagnosis of metastatic disease progression after standard therapies. Various disease processes can appear similar on morphologic MR sequences. Ideally, the physiologic process occurring within the CNS would be able to be directly imaged using noninvasive techniques. To that end, several physiology-based MR imaging methods have been developed to improve tissue characterization.

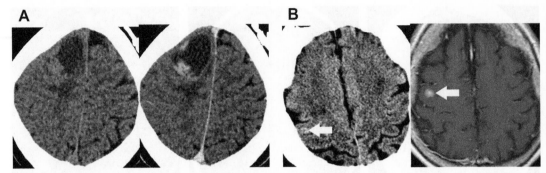

Fig. 5. CT imaging of brain metastasis. (*A*) Most brain metastases are hypodense or isodense by noncontrast CT imaging (*left*). On contrast administration, the solid nodular tissue within the lesion often is seen to enhance (*middle left*). The peripheral hypodense component on CT presents vasogenic edema whereas any central hypodensity represents cystic fluid collection. (*B*) Occasionally, brain metastasis can appear hyperdense (*middle right* [*arrow*]) on noncontrast CT, however, these lesions are often subtle, given the propensity to involve the gray–white matter junction. Subsequent contrast-enhanced MR imaging (*right*) easily delineates the same lesion. This example highlights the improved sensitivity at detecting CNS metastatic disease by MR imaging.

MR sequences, such as diffusion-weighted imaging (DWI), DSC perfusion, and susceptibility-weighted imaging (SWI) techniques, allow for the characterization of certain physiologic properties within metastatic disease to the CNS. Although still largely investigational, these physiologic MR imaging techniques are increasingly becoming an integral part of post-treatment brain tumor imaging.

DWI is now the MR standard of care in patients who present with acute neurologic symptoms and is increasingly used to characterize tumor biological properties. This sequence takes advantage of the diffusion of water molecules within the brain, which is affected by complex interactions within the extracellular compartment, including the cytoarchitecture of the microstructures and

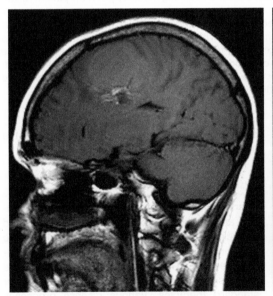
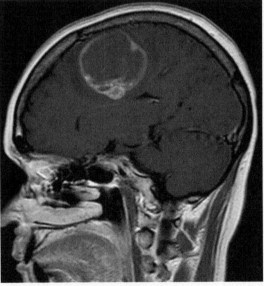

Fig. 6. Examination of T1-weighted noncontrast sequence. T1-weighted contrast-enhanced images (*right*) should always be compared with precontrast images (*left*). Several substances, including gadolinium contrast, blood products, fat, melanin, and proteinaceous fluid, induce T1 hyperintensity. Sagittal T1 precontrast image demonstrates T1 shortening within the caudal component of the lesion consistent with blood products. Contrast-enhanced image demonstrates a rim-enhancing mass. Note the similar T1 signal intensity in the caudal component of the lesion on both images. Failure to examine the precontrast images with the contrast-enhanced images can lead to the misidentification of contrast enhancement.

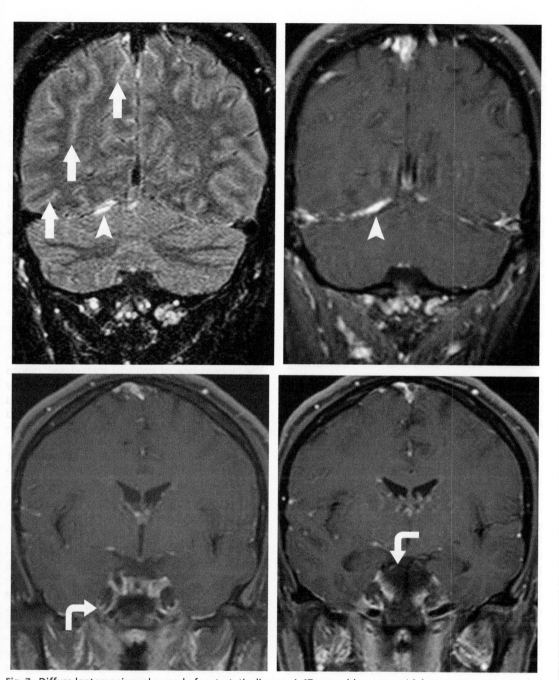

Fig. 7. Diffuse leptomeningeal spread of metastatic disease. A 47-year-old woman with known systemic spread of metastatic breast cancer presented for follow-up MR imaging. Diffuse leptomeningeal spread of disease is noted to involve multiple cranial nerves (*curved arrows*) including right trigeminal nerve as it courses through Meckel cave (*bottom left*) and the right oculomotor nerve (*bottom right*). FLAIR imaging can be helpful in delineating subtle leptomeningeal metastatic disease (*top left*). FLAIR hyperintensity within multiple sulci (*arrows*) is nonspecific but in this patient suggests sites of disease burden. The right tentorium also demonstrates FLAIR hyperintensity and enhancement (*top; arrowhead*) suggesting metastatic focus.

permeability barriers. The variation of water diffusion characteristics by disease processes and the ability to quantify these diffusion characteristics form the foundation for the use of DWI in the

clinical setting. Echoplanar imaging (EPI) is the most widely used MR Imaging technique in clinical application of DWI. EPI allows for the fast generation of echoes needed to form an image within a single acquisition period of 25 ms to 100 ms. The diffusion sensitivity parameter, the b-value, is related to duration, strength, and time interval between the diffusion-sensitizing gradients. A typical b-value used in clinical imaging is in the range of 900 s/mm^2 to 1000 s/mm^2. The higher the b-value, the more sensitive the diffusion imaging is in obtaining greater contrast and detecting areas of reduced water motion. The apparent diffusion coefficient (ADC) value characterizes the rate of diffusional motion (in millimeters squared per second). ADC values take into consideration the heterogeneous environment of brain cytoarchitecture temperature that can affect the measurement of thermally induced water molecular motion. High ADC implies relatively little reduced water motion, such as found in a sample of water placed in the magnetic field. Low ADC indicates reduced diffusional motion, as seen in acute cerebral ischemia or cellular tumor microenvironment.

The application of DSC perfusion MR imaging in clinical neuro-oncology hinges on the differential expression of angiogenic processes within neoplastic tissues compared with surrounding normal brain. DSC perfusion MR imaging uses the rapid changes in susceptibility induced by the intravascular bolus of paramagnetic contrast agents to calculate physiologic values, such as cerebral blood volume (CBV) and percentage of signal intensity recovery (PSR). DSC MR imaging is a straightforward methodology that can be completed within several minutes. The typical imaging approach for T2* data collection is to use a fast-imaging technique, such as single or multishot EPI, to produce a temporal resolution of 1 to 2 seconds per imaging pass before, during, and after the contrast agent bolus injection. During this acquisition period, a time course series of spatially registered images must be collected without significant motion artifact. The use of EPI techniques is essential to facilitating the imaging process because it allows for the generation of approximately 10 MR imaging sections every second, which is ideal for covering a large heterogeneous tumor in a rapid dynamic fashion. Measuring the area under the contrast concentration–time curve allows for the calculation of CBV. Other quantitative DSC perfusion MR imaging parameters, including PSR, have been characterized from the signal intensity–time curve and show promise in characterizing brain tumors (Fig. 8). The degree of residual signal loss (PSR) is estimated using the signal intensity during the recirculation phase of the perfusion curve, the minimum signal intensity of the perfusion curve, and baseline signal intensity at the time of contrast bolus arrival. In principle, the estimation of DSC perfusion parameters is a simple process; however, the clinical application of these principles is fraught with difficulty due to the presence of contrast bolus recirculation and leakage into the tumor interstitium via disrupted neurovascular unit. Given these confounding variables, optimization of the imaging sequence by reducing T1 weighting and use of low spin angle, among many others, can be implemented in an attempt to produce physiologically accurate DSC perfusion metrics. Alternatively, prebolus contrast loading has also been suggested as a means of reducing variability of CBV metrics by reducing the degree of signal loss in the postbolus phase of imaging. This methodology, however, limits the determination of other DSC metrics, such as PSR. Finally, various postprocessing methods that mathematically account for disruption of the neurovascular unit can more accurately quantify CBV.

IMAGING FINDINGS AND PATHOLOGY
Skull Metastases

The appearance of calvarial metastases ranges from easily identified lesions with extensive bony destruction to subtle lesions within the diploic space (Figs. 9 and 10).[9,10] Hematogenous spread from primary sites within the breast and lung is the most common etiology of calvarial metastases. Lytic and blastic lesions are best observed on CT bone reconstructions with wide window settings; however, contrast-enhanced MR imaging is superior at detecting lesion extension to dura, brain, or diploic space (see Fig. 10).

Pachymeningeal Carcinomatosis

The development of solitary dural-based metastatic disease is uncommon. This metastatic pattern typically involves direct invasion from an adjacent calvarial metastasis (see Fig. 10). If a solitary dural-based lesion is identified in a patient with a known systemic malignancy, it can be extraordinarily difficult to determine if the lesion represents a primary dural process, such as meningioma or malignant metastasis, using imaging alone.[11] In this situation, comparison with prior CNS imaging and clinical history of primary cancer can be useful in determining the etiology of focal dural metastases.

The most common manifestation of metastatic disease to the dura is the presence of multifocal dural-based enhancing lesions. Although rare, hematogenous spread is the most common route by which pachymeningeal carcinomatosis occurs in cancers outside the CNS.[12] Frequent causes of pachymeningeal carcinomatosis include metastatic breast, lung, prostate, and lymphoma.

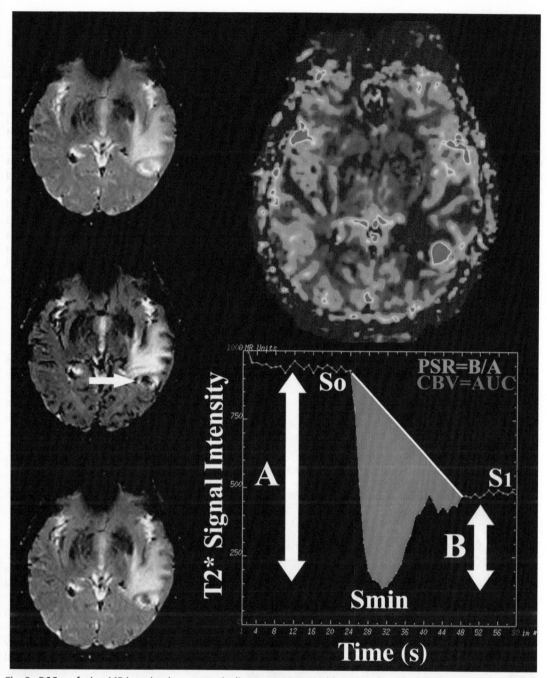

Fig. 8. DSC perfusion MR imaging in metastatic disease. A 55-year-old man with metastatic lung cancer presented for preoperative perfusion MR imaging. Sequential T2*-weighted imaging prior to (*top left*), concurrent with (*middle left*), and after (*bottom left*) bolus intravenous power injection of gadiolinum contrast allows for the generation of signal intensity-time curve (*bottom right*) of intraparenchymal metastatic disease (*arrow*). Integration of the area under the curve (*pink shaded area*) allows for calculation of CBV metrics. PSR is calculated by dividing the relative postbolus signal intensity value (B) by the relative prebolus signal intensity value (A). Elevated CBV (*top right*) within the enhancing component of the enhancing focus is nonspecific for the diagnosis of neoplastic etiology (high-grade glioma vs metastatic). Reduced PSR values have been shown to be specific for the initial diagnosis and subsequent recurrence of intraparenchymal metastatic disease after standard therapy. AUC, area under the curve; S1, post bolus signal intensity; So, baseline signal intensity; Smin, minimum signal intensity.

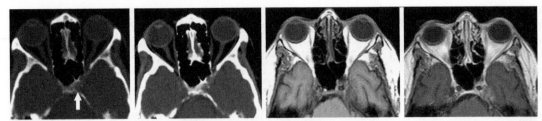

Fig. 9. Lytic metastatic disease of the skull base. Noncontrast CT in bone (*left*) and soft tissue (*middle left*) windows demonstrates a subcentimeter lytic mass within the left lateral aspect of the clivus (*arrow*). Precontrast (*middle right*) and postcontrast (*right*) T1-weighted MR imaging in the same patient demonstrates enhancing mass extending from the left aspect of the clivus to involve the cavernous sinus. CT and MR imaging can complement different biological manifestations of metastatic disease. CT is superior at delineating the destructive lysis of the clivus. Conversely, MR better delineates the degree of soft tissue invasion of the adjacent cavernous sinus.

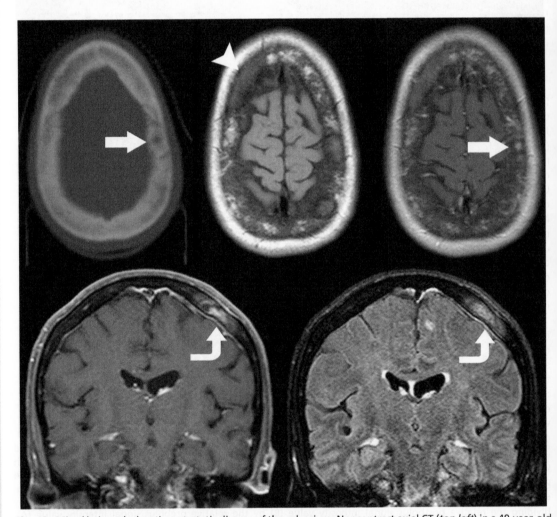

Fig. 10. Mixed lytic and sclerotic metastatic disease of the calvarium. Noncontrast axial CT (*top left*) in a 49-year-old woman with metastatic breast cancer demonstrates a mixed lytic sclerotic diploic space mass (*arrow*). Subsequent precontrast (*top middle*) and post–contrast-enhanced (*top right*) MR imaging demonstrates extensive loss of fatty diploic space marrow (*arrowhead*) with evidence of focal contrast-enhancing mass (*arrow*). Coronal T1-weighted postcontrast (*bottom left*) and FLAIR (*bottom right*) MR imaging demonstrates the enhancing diploic space mass with direct extension to the subjacent dura (*curved arrows*) suggesting parchymeningeal involvement. Contrast-enhanced MR imaging is superior to CT in the detection of metastatic disease within the diploic space, dura, and brain.

Common imaging findings of pachymeningeal carcinomatosis include noncommunicating hydrocephalus and dural-based enhancement. The dural enhancement pattern can appear as multiple nodules, diffuse dural thickening, or a combination of the 2 morphologies (Figs. 11 and 12).[11,12] The varying appearance of dural enhancement is due to the meningeal fibrous layer of the dura becoming diffusely infiltrated by neoplastic cells, which results in the formation of thickened and nodular appearing dura sparing the subarachnoid space. CT has limited sensitivity for the detection of dural-based metastatic disease (see Fig. 11). Contrast-enhanced MR imaging is the modality of choice when dural metastases are suspected. FLAIR and postcontrast T1-weighted images are far superior to CT at demonstrating dural enhancement and thickening, which spares the subarachnoid space.

Leptomeningeal Carcinomatosis

Diffuse multifocal tumor infiltration and thickening of the leptomeninges is not an uncommon manifestation of metastatic disease involving the CNS (see Fig. 7).[12,13] Hematogenous spread is the most common route by which leptomeningeal carcinomatosis occurs in cancers outside the CNS. Direct invasion, however, can occur, most commonly in primary head and neck cancers. Metastatic tumors spread via hematogenous route become implanted within the subarachnoid space and can spread to other meningeal surfaces by direct extension or indirect extension via the shedding of cells that are then carried to different parts of the neuroaxis by CSF flow, resulting in leptomeningeal carcinomatosis.

Nodular, miliary, and sheetlike enhancing imaging patterns have been described in the setting of leptomeningeal carcinomatosis. Arachnoid and subarachnoid metastases with or without pial infiltration often demonstrate sheet and/or nodular patterns of leptomeningeal tumor growth. Local extension of disease spread along the pial surface with a secondary inflammatory reaction from adjacent intraparnchymal tumor can appear as a sheetlike thickening of the leptomeninges (Fig. 13). Conversely, nodular leptomeningeal disease is often the result of diffuse CSF seeding with metastatic cells (see Fig. 13). The basal cisterns are the most common site of leptomeningeal carcinomatosis; however, nodular growth appearance is typically seen within the cerebellar folia or cerebral sulci and can easily be mistaken for intraparenchymal metastases. As discussed previously, pial infiltration often occurs as a result of direct extension from arachnoid and subarachnoid metastatic

tumor. A rarer form of leptomeningeal metastatic involvement is isolated direct pial infiltration by metastatic tumor that is seen when disease is spread in a cortical and perivascular subpial distribution without formation of macroscopic masses—carcinomatous encephalitis.[14–16] This pattern of leptomeningeal carcinomatosis is evidenced on MR Imaging by innumerable military-appearing submillimeter nodules and can be easily mistaken for an infectious CSF process.

Parenchymal Metastases

Parenchymal spread of disease is the most common form of CNS metastasis. Although, direct invasion can occur most commonly in primary head and neck cancers, the most common route by which parenchymal disease occurs is hematogenous spread. The most common primary tumors to metastasize to the brain parenchyma are lung, breast, melanoma, colon, pancreas, renal, testes, ovary, and cervix.[2,3] At autopsy, parenchymal metastases are typically well-circumscribed nodules with varying internal contents, including hemorrhagic fluid, mucinous material, or necrotic debris. The absence of a neurovascular unit within metastatic disease results in extensive peritumoral vasogenic edema. This edema can be differentiated from invasive tumoral edema associated with primary glioma in that metastatic vasogenic edema spears cortical gray matter and is disproportionate to the size of the contrast-enhancing lesion.

Any region of the brain parenchyma can be affected by metastatic tumor; however, the most common site of disease involvement is the corticomedullary junction. Hematogenous spread of disease is multifocal in up to 85% of patients.[2,3] The degree of disease burden and propensity to have multiple lesions can often be traced to histologic origin with breast, renal, colon, and thyroid commonly presenting as single metastatic lesions. Conversely, metastatic melanoma or lung-brain parenchymal metastasis is frequently multifocal.[2,3]

Patients with metastatic parenchymal disease can present as asymptomatic to acutely obtunded with severe neurologic deficits. A majority of patients, up to 60%, with brain metastases have progressive subacute symptoms that are directly related to the anatomic location of tumor deposition.[2,3] Headache and new-onset seizure are the 2 most common presenting symptoms. Asymptomatic patients typically have lesions detected during imaging staging.

The detection of metastatic parenchymal disease forebodes a poor prognosis and often necessitates a change in therapeutic strategy; therefore, the accurate characterization of disease burden

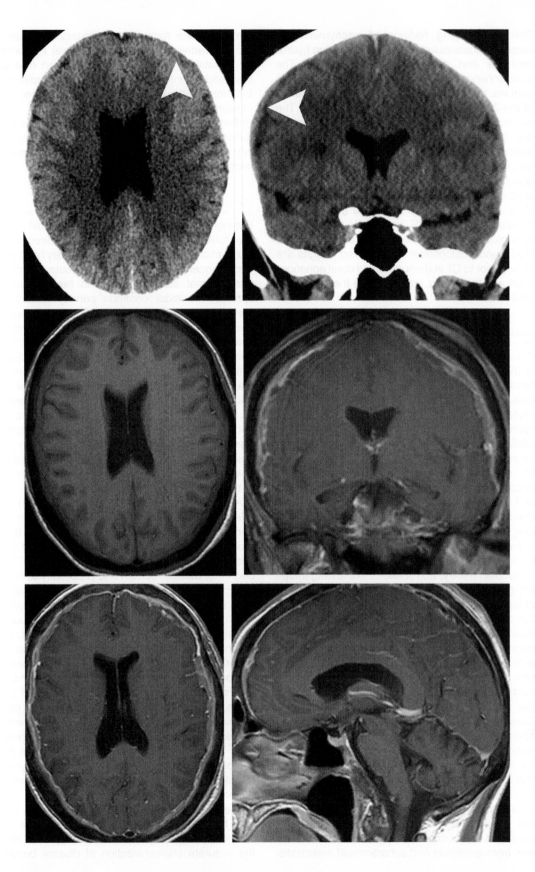

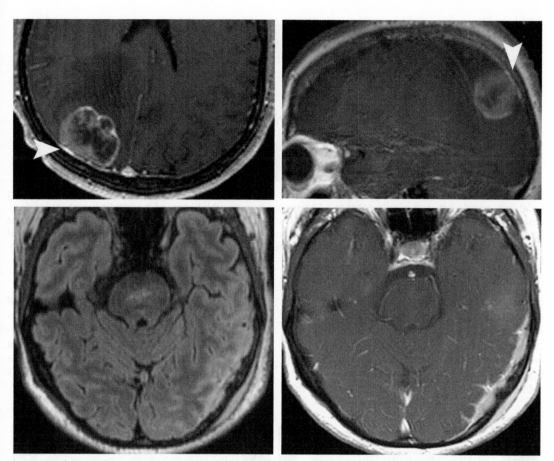

Fig. 12. Nodular pachymeningeal metastatic disease. A 68-year-old man with history of lung cancer presents with progressive altered mental status and right-sided weakness. Contrast-enhanced MR imaging (*top*) demonstrates mixed solid and cystic right parietal lobe mass with subjacent nodular dural thickening suggesting metastatic disease (*arrowhead*). Another site of pachymeningeal and leptomeningeal disease is evidenced by nodular dural and pial thickening, FLAIR hyperintensity (*bottom left*) and enhancement (*bottom right*) are noted in the same patient.

is clinically important. As discussed previously, noncontrast CT of the head is typically the first imaging modality for patients presenting with acute-onset neurologic dysfunction. CT imaging remains the standard of care to rule out life-threatening sequelae of metastatic disease, including hemorrhage, herniation, and hydrocephalus. Knowledge of these 3 potential neurosurgical emergencies allows for patient triage.

Depending on the histologic origin, cerebral metastases can present with varying attenuation on noncontrast CT.[17] A majority of metastases are hypodense to isodense compared with adjacent brain parenchyma (see **Fig. 5**). Tumors with a high nuclear to cytoplasmic ratio often present as a hyperdense lesion without the underlying presence of hemorrhage (see **Fig. 5**; **Fig. 14**). Acute hemorrhage also characteristically makes cerebral

Fig. 11. Diffuse pachymeningeal carcinomatosis. Noncontrast axial (*top left*) and coronal (*top right*) CT imaging in a 52-year-old woman with 4 months' new-onset headaches demonstrates a nonspecific subtle holohemispheric extra-axial isodensity (*arrowheads*). Subsequent precontrast (*middle left*) and post–contrast-enhanced MR imaging (*middle right and bottom*) demonstrates extensive dural thickening and enhancement. The lack of findings suggesting intracranial hypotension (enlarged pituitary gland, brainstem sagging, and downward tonsillar displacement) suggested the presence of pachymeningeal carcinomatosis from an undiagnosed primary neoplasm. Whole-body cancer screening, which included mammography and tissue sampling of right breast mass, revealed the underlying diagnosis of breast cancer as the etiology of pachymeningeal carcinomatosis.

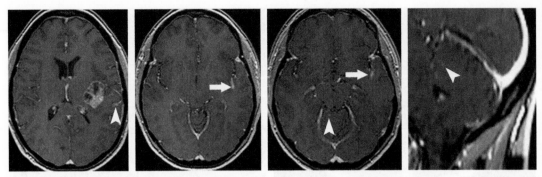

Fig. 13. Nodular and sheet leptomeningeal metastatic disease-enhancing patterns. Preoperative MR imaging (axial; left, middle left, and middle right) in a 56-year-old woman with history of metastatic breast cancer demonstrates mixed solid and cystic left subinsular mass with local sheetlike extension of leptomeningeal disease involving the adjacent sylvian fissure (*arrows*). Multifocal nodular leptomeningeal disease was also observed within the adjacent brain sulci and distantly in the cerebellar follia (*arrowheads*); left and right suggesting diffuse CSF seeding with metastatic cells.

metastasis appear hyperdense on CT (see **Fig. 4**). Hemorrhage can occur in any metastatic tumor; however, the most likely histologic origin to demonstrate blood products includes melanoma, breast, thyroid, and renal cell carcinoma. Calcified cystic masses are rare; however, primary breast, colorectal, and lung neoplasia can assume this imaging appearance. The predominant feature of cerebral metastases is the appearance of vasogenic edema as evidenced by peritumoral hypodensity abutting gray matter peripherally. Often a disproportionate degree of vasogenic edema is the only abnormality identified on noncontrast CT imaging (**Fig. 15**).

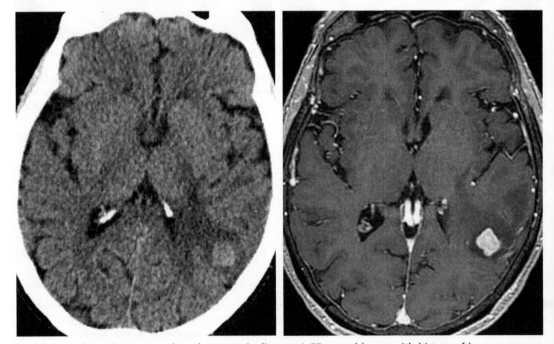

Fig. 14. Hyperdense brain parenchymal metastatic disease. A 55-year-old man with history of lung cancer presents for CT imaging with acute left sided weakness. Noncontrast CT (*left*) demonstrates a left temporal hyperdense mass with surrounding white matter hypodensity. Subsequent contrast-enhanced MR imaging (*right*) demonstrated an enhancing mass with surrounding vasogenic edema consistent with metastatic disease. A majority of intraparenchymal metastatic lesions appears isodense to hypodense on noncontrast CT imaging. Lesions with a high nuclear to cytoplasmic ratio often appear hyperdense on noncontrast CT despite the lack of underlying hemorrhage.

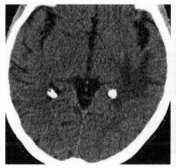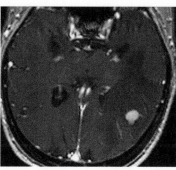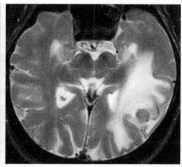

Fig. 15. Disproportionate vasogenic edema observed in metastatic disease. A 63-year-old woman with history breast cancer presented for CT imaging in the setting of acute-onset altered mental status. Noncontrast CT (*left*) demonstrated extensive left temporal occipital lobe white matter hypodensity without loss of gray–white differentiation. Subsequent MR imaging demonstrates a nodular intraparenchymal enhancing mass on T1-weighted postcontrast imaging (*middle*) with disproportionate white matter T2 hyperintensity for the size of the lesion (*right*). A common imaging appearance of intraparenchymal metastatic disease is the presence of robust peritumoral vasogenic edema that preserves the gray–white matter interface.

After the administration of contrast media, most parenchymal metastases avidly enhance due to the lack of neurovascular unit.[17] Two predominant patterns of enhancement include solid nodular and ring enhancing with nodular components (see **Figs. 4–6**, **14** and **15**). CT imaging, however, incompletely evaluates for the extent of disease burden, thereby underestimating of the number of brain lesions due to the inherent limitations of soft tissue contrast resolution.

Contrast-enhanced MR imaging is the modality of choice for diagnostic examination of brain parenchymal metastasis.[5,17] The inherent T1-weighted signal of brain metastases can vary. A majority of nonhemorrhagic parenchymal lesions are slightly hypointense relative to normal brain. One exception is malignant melanoma, which can appear hyperintense on non–contrast-enhanced T1-weighted imaging due to the T1 shortening effects of melanin (**Fig. 16**). Hemorrhagic parenchymal lesions can have variable inherent T1-weighted signal depending on the time period in which the blood products are imaged (see **Fig. 4**; **Table 2**).[18–20] A majority of cerebral metastases demonstrate prolonged T2 relation times and are, therefore, hyperintense on T2-weighted sequences. Mucin-secreting neoplasms or densely cellular tumors can appear hypointense on T2-weighted imaging. T2-weighted

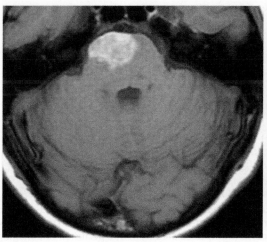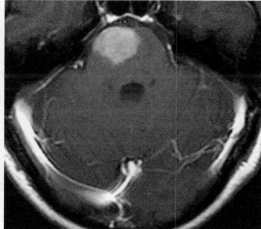

Fig. 16. Intrinsic T1 hyperintensity of melanoma metastasis. A 43-year-old woman with history of cutaneous melanoma presented with acute-onset weakness. Precontrast (*left*) and postcontrast (*right*) T1-weighted MR imaging demonstrates intrinsic T1 hyperintensity in a right pontine lesion consistent with metastatic melanoma. Hyperintensity on precontrast T1-weighted MR imaging can occur as a result of late subacute hemorrhage, protenaceous fluid, focal macrocellular fat, or melanin deposition.

Table 2
Aging of blood products on MR imaging

Stage	Time	Hemoglobin State	T1 Signal Intensity	T2 Signal Intensity
Hyperacute	<24 h	Intracellular oxyhemoglobin	Isointense	Hyperintense
Acute	<48 h	Intracellular deoxyhemoglobin	Isointense	Hypointense
Early subactue	2–14 d	Intracellular methemoglobin	Hyperintense	Hypointense
Late subacute	10–21 d	Extracellular methaemoglobin	Hyperintense	Hyperintense
Chronic	>21 d	Hemosiderin	Hypointense	Hypointense

Data from Refs.[18–20]

FLAIR images are particularly useful for evaluating the extent of peritumoral vasogenic edema.

Physiologic MR imaging can also be helpful in characterizing parenchymal metastatic foci. ADC values obtained by DWI sequences can be markedly reduced in the setting of highly cellular lesions or the presence of intralesional mucin deposition.[21] DSC perfusion MR imaging typically demonstrates elevated CBV with reduced PSR compared with normal-appearing white matter (see **Fig. 8**; **Fig. 17**).[22,23]

Differentiating Progression of Disease from Effects of Stereotactic Radiation Therapy

Standard of care therapy for intraparenchymal metastatic disease includes chemoradiotherapy. After stereotactic radiosurgery, the treated lesion can demonstrate increased contrast-enhancing volume. Distinguishing progression of parenchymal metastatic disease from the effects of stereotactic radiosurgery can present a major clinical conundrum. Several studies have focused on the noninvasive characterization of progressive contrast-enhancing lesions after radiosurgery for cerebral metastasis using DSC perfusion-weighted MR imaging.[24] Barajas and colleagues[24] demonstrated that quantitative analysis of DSC signal-intensity time curves can be helpful in increasing specificity of distinguishing metastatic tumor recurrence. In this retrospective study, PSR measurements reliably distinguished metastatic tumor recurrence from radiation necrosis with 96% sensitivity and 100% specificity with disease progression demonstrating significantly lower recovery metrics (**Fig. 18**).

Distinguishing Solitary Metastasis from High-Grade Glioma

Approximately 30% of patients with metastatic disease to the CNS present with a solitary

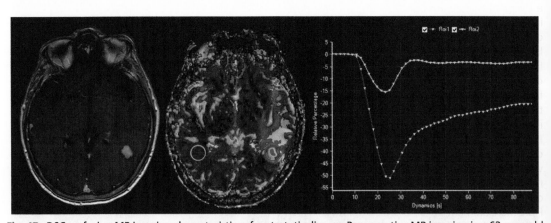

Fig. 17. DSC perfusion MR imaging characteristics of metastatic disease. Preoperative MR imaging in a 63-year-old woman with history of metastatic breast cancer demonstrates a contrast-enhancing mass (*left*) within the left temporal lobe. CVB map (*middle*) and signal intensity/time curve (*right*) calculated from DSC perfusion MR imaging sequence (not shown) demonstrate elevated CBV with reduced PSR metrics (blue region of interest [Roi1]) compared with contralateral normal appearing white matter (orange region of interest [Roi2]). Prior investigators have demonstrated that elevated CBV within an enhancing mass is nonspecific for either high-grade glioma or metastatic disease. Reduced PSR values have been shown, however, specific for the diagnosis of intraparenchymal metastatic disease.

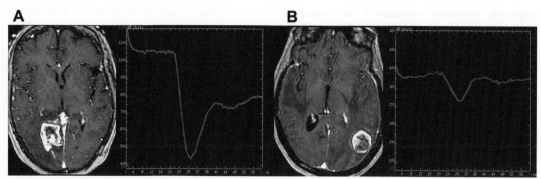

Fig. 18. Differentiating recurrent metastatic disease from the effects of stereotactic radiation therapy. Distinguishing progression of metastatic disease in patients who have previously undergone stereotactic radiation therapy can be markedly challenging because the effects of radiation therapy can have nearly identical morphologic appearance on contrast-enhanced MR imaging. DSC perfusion MR imaging has been shown to help in this diagnostic dilemma. Lesion wide analysis of recurrent metastatic disease (A) tends to demonstrate elevated CBV with reduced PSR. Radiation necrosis (B), although appearing similarly as a progressively enhancing lesion, tends to have normal to minimally elevated CBV with near-normal recovery metrics. Prior retrospective studies have suggested signal intensity recovery measurements are reliable to distinguish metastatic tumor recurrence from radiation necrosis with 96% sensitivity and 100% specificity.

brain parenchymal lesion. Differentiating a solitary metastasis from high-grade glioma can often pose a diagnostic dilemma on contrast-enhanced MR imaging. It is clinically important to distinguish between these disease processes because medical staging, surgical planning, and therapeutic decisions are drastically different. The capillaries of brain metastasis resemble those from the site of the original systemic cancer and thus have no similarity to the normal brain capillaries and completely lack neurovascular unit components resulting in the uniformly increased production of vasogenic edema. Conversely, high-grade glioma often demonstrates a dysfunctional neurovascular unit associated with invasive tumor. The use of DSC MR imaging sequences allows for the interrogation of tumor vasculature.[22,23] The DSC hemodynamic metrics peak height and PSR have been shown to add further diagnostic information, which complements conventional contrast-enhanced MR imaging sequences, thereby allowing for the reliable differentiation of solitary brain metastases from high-grade glioma (see **Figs. 8** and 17). Cha and colleagues[22] previously demonstrated that peak height measurements were significantly lower within nonenhancing peritumoral T2 regions of solitary brain metastasis compared with high-grade glioma. Additionally, PSR measurements were significantly lower within contrast-enhancing regions of solitary brain metastasis when compared to high-grade glioma.

Pearls, Pitfalls, and Variants

Non-neoplastic hematomas

Hemorrhagic intracranial neoplasms are often mistaken for non-neoplastic hematomas. Differentiating non-neoplastic hematomas from hemorrhagic intracranial neoplasms can be difficult because of their considerable overlap in imaging characteristics; however, subtle clues can aid in the correct diagnosis.[25] On MR imaging, non-neoplastic hematomas often have a well-delineated rim of hemosiderin that undergoes characteristic metabolism of blood products. Additionally, vasogenic edema and mass effect that results from a benign hemorrhage resolve on serial MR imaging (see **Table 2**). Conversely, hemorrhagic neoplasms appear heterogeneous with incomplete hemosiderin rim and nonhemorrhagic enhancing regions. Hemorrhagic intracranial neoplasms also continue to demonstrate robust vasogenic edema and mass effect on follow-up examinations.

Remote microvascular ischemia

Multifocal white matter and corticomedullary metastases often demonstrate similar T2-weighted imaging characteristics as white matter microvascular ischemia. In elderly patients, it can initially be difficult to differentiate multifocal metastases from small vessel disease; however, T2 hyperintense foci along with enhancement on T1-weighted sequences after the administration of contrast media are highly suggestive of a malignant lesion in patients with a known primary site of neoplasia.

Ischemic infarction

Patients with metastatic intracranial neoplasms often present with focal neurologic deficits, which are clinically indistinguishable from acute cerebral infarction. To further confuse the clinical diagnosis, metastatic neoplasms can resemble cerebral ischemia on initial imaging examinations. CT findings that favor the diagnosis of metastatic intracranial neoplasms include round hypodensity that preferentially involves the white matter with sparing of cortical gray matter that is not confined to a specific vascular territory. MR imaging is markedly useful in the evaluation of lesions initially detected by noncontrast CT imaging. Evolving subacute infarctions with normalizing ADC metrics should not demonstrate elevated CBV by DSC perfusion imaging.

SUMMARY

The identification and classification of metastatic tumor can be a challenging task; however, with advanced CT and MR imaging of the CNS, multiple tools are available to correctly achieve this objective. DWI and DSC MR imaging, although currently investigational to some degree, add additional diagnostic information, allowing for improved tumor characterization.

REFERENCES

1. Barnholtz-Sloan JS, Sloan AE, Davis FG, et al. Incidence proportions of brain metastases in patients diagnosed (1973 to 2001) in the metropolitan Detroit cancer surveillance system. J Clin Oncol 2004;22: 2865–72.

2. Nussbaum ES, Djalilian HR, Cho KH, et al. Brain metastases. Histology, multiplicity, surgery, and survival. Cancer 1996;78(8):1781–8.

3. Das A, Hochberg FH. Clinical presentation of intracranial metastases. Neurosurg Clin N Am 1996; 7(3):377–91.

4. Svokos KA, Salhia B, Toms SA. Molecular biology of brain metastasis. Int J Mol Sci 2014;15(6):9519–30.

5. Beasley KD, Toms SA. The molecular pathobiology of metastasis to the brain: a review. Neurosurg Clin N Am 2011;22:7–14.

6. Cha S. Neuroimaging in neuro-oncology. Neurotherapeutics 2009;6(3):465–77.

7. Ercan N, Gultekin S, Celik H, et al. Diagnostic value of contrast-enhanced fluid-attenuated inversion recovery MR imaging of intracranial metastases. AJNR Am J Neuroradiol 2004;25:761–5.

8. Singer MB, Atlas SW, Drayer BP. Subarachnoid space disease: diagnosis with fluid-attenuated inversion-recovery MR imaging and comparison with gadolinium-enhanced spin-echo MR imaging– blinded reader study. Radiology 1998;208:417–22.

9. Lloret I, Server A, Taksdal I. Calvarial lesions: a radiological approach to diagnosis. Acta Radiol 2009;50(5):531–42.

10. Garfinkle J, Melançon D, Cortes M, et al. Imaging pattern of calvarial lesions in adults. Skeletal Radiol 2010;40(10):1261–73.

11. Tyrrell RL 2nd, Bundschuh CV, Modic MT. Dural carcinomatosis: MR demonstration. J Comput Assist Tomogr 1987;11(2):329–32.

12. Mahendru G, Chong V. Meninges in cancer imaging. Cancer Imaging 2009;9:S14–21.

13. Demopoulos A. Leptomeningeal metastases. Curr Neurol Neurosci Rep 2004;4(3):196–204.

14. Ribeiro HB, Paiva TF Jr, Mamprin GP, et al. Carcinomatous encephalitis as clinical presentation of occult lung adenocarcinoma: case report. Arq Neuropsiquiatr 2007;65(3B):841–4.

15. Olsen WL, Winkler ML, Ross DA. Carcinomatous encephalitis: CT and MR findings. AJNR Am J Neuroradiol 1987;8:553–4.

16. Nemzek W, Poirier V, Salamat MD, et al. Carcinomatous encephalitis (miliary metastases): lack of contrast enhancement. AJNR Am J Neuroradiol 1993;14:540–2.

17. Walker MT, Kapoor V. Neuroimaging of parenchymal brain metastases. Cancer Treat Res 2007;136:31–51.

18. Chalela JA, Gomes J. Magnetic resonance imaging in the evaluation of intracranial hemorrhage. Expert Rev Neurother 2004;4(2):267–73.

19. Aygun N, Masaryk TJ. Diagnostic imaging for intracerebral hemorrhage. Neurosurg Clin N Am 2002; 13(3):313–34.

20. Bradley WG. MR appearance of hemorrhage in the brain. Radiology 1993;189(1):15–26.

21. Hayashida Y, Hirai T, Morishita S, et al. Diffusion-weighted imaging of metastatic brain tumors: comparison with histologic type and tumor cellularity. AJNR Am J Neuroradiol 2006;27(7):1419–25.

22. Cha S, Lupo JM, Chen MH, et al. Differentiation of glioblastoma multiforme and single brain metastasis by peak height and percentage of signal intensity recovery derived from dynamic susceptibility-weighted contrast-enhanced perfusion MR imaging. AJNR Am J Neuroradiol 2007;28(6):1078–84.

23. Wang S, Kim S, Chawla S, et al. Differentiation between glioblastomas, solitary brain metastases, and primary cerebral lymphomas using diffusion tensor and dynamic susceptibility contrast-enhanced MR imaging. AJNR Am J Neuroradiol 2011;32(3):507–14.

24. Barajas RF, Chang JS, Sneed PK, et al. Distinguishing recurrent intra-axial metastatic tumor from radiation necrosis following gamma knife radiosurgery using dynamic susceptibility-weighted contrast-enhanced perfusion MR imaging. AJNR Am J Neuroradiol 2009;30(2):367–72.

25. Bronen RA, Fulbright RK, Spencer DD, et al. MR characteristics of neoplasms and vascular malformations associated with epilepsy. Magn Reson Imaging 1995;13(8):1153–62.

Extraparenchymal Lesions in Adults

Marta Drake-Pérez, MD[a],*, James G. Smirniotopoulos, MD[b,c]

KEYWORDS

- Extra-axial • Tumors • Neoplasm • Cyst • Imaging • Meningioma • Hemangiopericytoma
- Pituitary

KEY POINTS

- Meningiomas are the most common extra-axial tumor. They have a typical radiologic appearance 75% of the time, including well-demarcated, homogeneous enhancement in extra-axial supratentorial mass, with peritumoral vasogenic edema, hyperostosis, and a dural tail.
- Hemangiopericytomas (HPCs) are extra-axial mesenchymal tumors, characterized by high vascularization and cellularity. Radiologically they often appear as lobulated noncalcified masses with heterogeneous MR imaging signal, internal signal voids, and associated bone erosion. Several granulomatous diseases, such as sarcoidosis, Langerhans cells histiocytosis, and Rosai-Dorfman disease (RDD), can present as extra-axial masses and may mimic meningioma.
- In adults, masses localized in the sellar region are mainly pituitary adenomas and craniopharyngiomas — the squamous and papillary subtype, besides other lesions, such as meningiomas or granulomatous diseases, may also be suprasellar.
- Epidermoids, dermoids, colloid, arachnoid, Rathke cleft, and craniopharyngiomas are all epithelial-lined cystic masses that can present as extra-axial lesions in adults. Location and fluid-attenuated inversion recovery (FLAIR)/diffusion-weighted imaging (DWI) features help in the differential diagnosis.
- A practical approach for pineal masses is differentiating germ cell tumors (GCTs) (germinoma and teratoma) from pineal parenchymal tumors. Germinoma is by far the most common pineal tumor, showing typically homogenous attenuation and enhancement and central calcification.

MENINGIOMA

Meningiomas are nonglial and extra-axial dural-based tumors. They are the most common nonglial primary brain and central nervous system (CNS) tumor, accounting for 35% of all histologic reports.[1] The autopsy prevalence is estimated at 1% to 1.5%, and meningiomas are frequent incidentalomas in 1% to 3% of adults screened as volunteers for MR imaging research or during executive physicals that include neuroimaging.

Meningiomas arise from arachnoid meningothelial (cap) cells, especially where arachnoid granulations are numerous (along the dural sinuses).

Classic or typical meningiomas, which account for more than 90% of all meningiomas, including several subtypes (transitional, fibroblastic, and meningothelial), are World Health Organization (WHO) grade 1 neoplasms. Less than 1 in 10 (8.3%) of all meningiomas are atypical meningioma, which are WHO grade 2. Less than 1% are classified as malignant or anaplastic meningioma,

The authors have nothing to disclose.
[a] Department of Radiology, Marqués de Valdecilla University Hospital/IDIVAL, Avda. Valdecilla n° 25, Santander 39008, Cantabria, Spain; [b] MedPix, National Library of Medicine, 8600 Rockville Pike, Bethesda, MD 20894, USA; [c] Department of Radiology, George Washington University, 2121 Eye Street Northwest, Washington, DC 20052, USA
* Corresponding author.
E-mail address: drake.marta@gmail.com

neuroimaging.theclinics.com

WHO grade 3. The subtype of papillary meningioma is also included in WHO grade 3.[2]

Inherited susceptibility to meningioma is suggested by multiplicity, family history (NF2), and sporadic mutations in tumor suppressor genes (chromosome 22q). Atypical and malignant meningiomas incur additional genetic alterations; malignant meningioma typically has reactivation of telomerase or inactivation of CDKN2A.[3]

Ionizing radiation exposure is an established risk factor, and meningiomas are the most common radiation-induced tumors, with a latency of 20 to 35 years after initial radiotherapy.

Because women are twice as likely as men to develop meningiomas, these tumors show a correlation with breast cancer, and they may increase size and/or present during pregnancy. They harbor hormone receptors (progesterone receptors in 66%–88% and estrogen receptors are less common). An etiologic role for female sex hormones (both endogenous and exogenous) has been hypothesized.

Obesity has newly been related to enhanced risk for meningioma.[4]

Head trauma and cell phone use have also been suggested as a risk factor for meningioma, although the results across studies are not consistent in proving these controversial associations.[5]

Approximately 90% of all meningiomas are located above the tentorium. The most common locations include the cerebral convexity, parasagittal/falx, the sphenoid ridge, the olfactory groove, or parasellar-like tuberculum sella. The cerebellopontine angle is the most common place for infratentorial meningiomas, accounting for 8% to 10% of them, and the paranasal sinuses are the most common extracranial location. Meningiomas also represent approximately 25% of all intraspinal tumors.[6]

Data from the Central Brain Tumor Registry of the United States demonstrate more than 2-fold higher incidence among women. Age-specific incidence rates reveal increasing risk with age in both men and women (typically arising after age 40). Malignant meningioma occurs 10 years earlier than typical meningiomas. Regarding ethnicity, meningiomas are more common in African Americans.

Meningiomas are usually slow growing and indolent (90%). Small tumors near eloquent cortex may present when small (<3 cm) whereas larger tumors are seen in other locations, such as subfrontal/olfactory groove. Symptoms are dependent on location, and include: seizures, headache, paresis, change in mental status, and sometimes focal neurologic deficits.

There are 2 basic morphologies for meningiomas: globose (well-demarcated spherical/hemispherical mass with a wide dural attachment and convex toward the brain) and en plaque — a carpet-like thickening of the dura, without parenchymal invagination. On gross inspection, the tumors are usually homogenous and often reddish-brown in color (Fig. 1).

There is a wide range of histologic subtypes. Meningothelial is the most common, characterized by uniform tumor cells, collagenous septa, and psammomatous calcifications (Fig. 2). Other common subtypes include fibrous, transitional, lipoblastic, and microcystic (also called humid).

Typical diagnostic features are seen on imaging in 75% of all meningiomas (Box 1), including a sharply circumscribed and homogenous extra-axial mass with a broad-based dural attachment (Fig. 3). Calcification is occasionally seen in approximately 25%. Necrosis, cysts, and hemorrhage are less frequently present. Most meningiomas have a clearly demonstrable cleavage plane that separates them from underlying brain and facilitates surgery. On MR imaging, especially, trapped cerebrospinal fluid (CSF) or vessels are often seen in a cleft between the mass and the brain.

On noncontrast CT, typical meningioma is isodense (25%) or hyperdense (75%) to gray matter. Most (>90%) show intense, homogeneous enhancement on postcontrast CT imaging, with a dural tail (on both CT and MR imaging). The dural

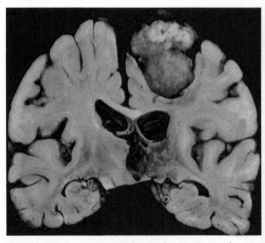

Fig. 1. Meningioma WHO grade 1. Coronal gross photograph. There is a clearly demarcated extra-axial lesion displacing the brain — but without invading into the gray matter. The whitish region along the superior part of the tumor contains more dense calcifications.

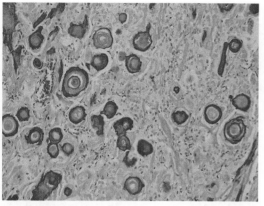

Fig. 2. Meningioma WHO grade 1 hematoxylin-eosin, original magnification ×200 photomicrograph showing multiple gray-purple rounded calcospherites (psammoma bodies).

tail is not a specific feature but is typical of meningiomas and it usually represents reactive vascular changes and dural edema (Fig. 4A).

Intraosseous extension may be evidenced by irregular cortical margins in the skull, hyperostosis, and increased bone vascularity (Fig. 5). Hyperostosis is present in 25% to 60% (or more) of meningiomas and may occur with or without microscopic invasion of the bone.

On MR imaging, meningioma is typically isointense to slightly hypointense to gray matter on T1W-weighted (T1W) images. Gray matter buckling can be seen, a sign of extra-axial location of the tumor (Fig. 6).

On T2W-weighted (T2W) imaging, signal intensity is variable; a central sunburst pattern may be present, which is often correlated with a radial or spoke-wheel pattern of tumor neovascularity. Approximately 80% demonstrate internal flow voids on MR. A variable degree of peritumoral vasogenic edema within the overlying brain (Fig. 7) is common on T2W or FLAIR. This is not directly related to the histology or WHO grade of the tumor but it is indirectly related to prognosis due to its relation to more difficult surgical resectability (the more edema, the more difficult to resect).

Diffusion signal is variable with reports of reduced diffusion in more cellular and/or more aggressive meningioma. Magnetic resonance venography may show occlusion of adjacent dural venous sinuses, especially when the tumor is in proximity to the superior sagittal sinus (Fig. 4B).

On angiogram, meningiomas are usually fed primarily by branches of the external carotid but may have dual supply (external > internal carotid), and it is characteristic for an early arterial stain, yet a

---

Box 1
Meningioma key points

Imaging tips

Best modality: MR imaging with contrast. CT: look for typical bone hyperostosis and calcium within the lesion. MRS: might be useful in uncertain cases (ALA peak for well-differentiated and lower ADC with increased cellularity).

Differential diagnosis

HPC: bone destruction, not calcified, lobulated, and narrow dural based

Dural metastasis: skull first affected, multifocal

Granulomatous diseases: multifocal

Pearls, pitfalls, and variants

Atypical meningioma: invasion of brain (shallow/microscopic)

Anaplastic meningioma: intratumoral cystic change, prominent tumor pannus extending away from mass (mushrooming), extracranial extension through foramina

Atypical imaging features do not correspond to atypical histology.

What the referring physician needs to know

Vascular supply: plan need of presurgical embolization

Bone/dural extension and relation between meningioma and brain parenchyma (CSF cleft? Apparent infiltration?): plan surgical strategy to achieve a complete tumoral resection (including bone and dura affected).

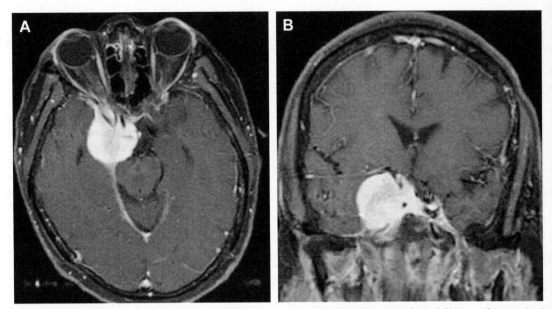

Fig. 3. Meningioma. WHO grade 1. (*A*) Axial and (*B*) Coronal T1W MR imaging with gadolinium. This meningioma of the right cavernous sinus is bulging both medially into the suprasellar cistern and laterally into the middle fossa — where it is pressing on the uncus and temporal lobe. The edge of the tentorium enhances all the way back to the posterior margin of the falx.

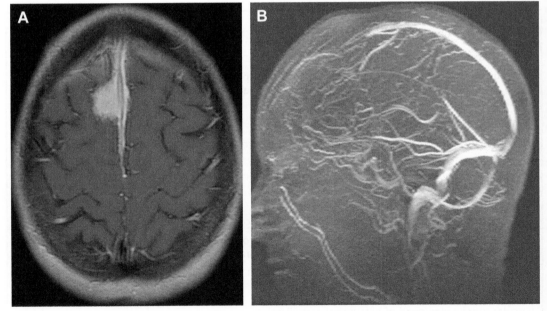

Fig. 4. Meningioma. WHO grade 1. (*A*) Axial T1W MR imaging with gadolinium. There is a hemispheric extra-axial lesion, broad-based on the falx, and convex toward the medial aspect of the right frontal lobe. The falx is slightly thickened and enhancing adjacent to the tumor — the dural tail. (*B*) Magnetic resonance venography shows a ball-like arrangement of abnormal vessels ateriorly, and poor filling of the anterior superior sagittal sinus. This is from infiltration and obstruction of the sinus by the meningioma.

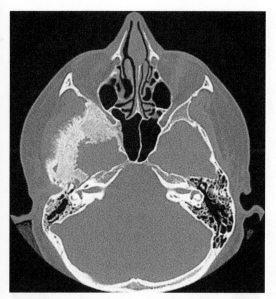

Fig. 5. Meningioma. WHO grade 1. This noncontrast CT, with bone window, shows extensive hyperostosis of the right temporal bone. Hyperostosis in meningioma is often associated with slower growth. In less than half of cases, the hyperostosis is related to intraosseus extension of tumor — in the remainder, the bone is stimulated to thicken, but without any microscopic involvement.

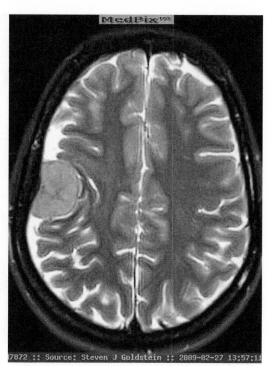

Fig. 6. Meningioma. WHO grade 1. Axial T2W MR imaging clearly demonstrates this hemispheric extra-axial lesion, convex toward the brain. There is widening of the subarachnoid space both anterior and posterior to the greatest convexity of the tumor. The inner table of the skull is thickened — hyperostosis caused by the meningioma. (*Courtesy of* SJ Goldstein, MD.)

prominent and persistent tumor blush into the venous phase.

Well-differentiated meningiomas show alanine (ALA) peak on magnetic resonance spectroscopy (MRS) (Fig. 8).[7]

On PET, typical meningiomas are usually hypometabolic compared with cortex. Typical meningiomas, however, may become hypermetabolic after radiation therapy, despite benign histology.

In general, the various imaging features of meningiomas may not accurately reflect the specific histologic subtypes: atypical imaging features do not correspond to atypical histology regarding meningiomas, and typical imaging findings do not exclude atypical variants. But attempts at differentiating typical from atypical/malignant meningioma can be useful for preoperative planning, so attempts must be done from the radiologic viewpoint. Invasion of dura, bone, or scalp; hyperostosis or bone destruction; arterial encasement (often with a narrowed lumen); and peritumoral brain edema are not considered signs of malignant histology but alter the prognosis. Invasion of brain (shallow/microscopic) is considered a grade 2 feature according to WHO 2007 (Fig. 9).

Intratumoral cystic change, prominent tumor lobules extending away from the primary mass (mushrooming) and extracranial extension through foramina are features associated with high-grade (WHO 2–3) meningioma.[8] Elevated relative cerebral blood volume in peritumoral edema on perfusion MR imaging, restricted diffusion with low signal on ADC, low ALA peak on MRS, and hypermetabolic activity in relation to the cortex on PET may be all suggestive of atypical or anaplastic meningioma.

Prognosis depends on WHO grade, tumor location, and completeness of resection. Typical meningioma is a WHO grade 1 tumor that usually follows a benign clinical course. The tumor is slow growing and may grow slowly to compress adjacent structures. The tumor may spread along the dura, invading the adjacent bone, and parasagittal tumors may invade and occlude the superior sagittal sinus. Hematogenous metastases are extremely rare (in 0.1%–0.2%).

Standard treatment is surgical resection. Rarely radiation, including stereotactic radiosurgery for small lesions, may be used. Prognosis is good. Grade 1 meningiomas have a 5-year survival rate of more than 90%. Resection, if complete, is

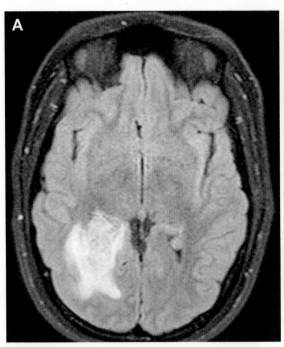
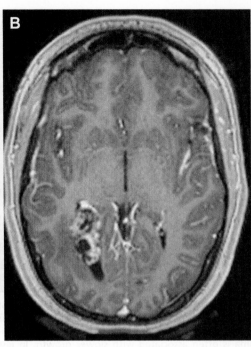

Fig. 7. Meningioma. WHO grade 1 intraventricular. (*A*) FLAIR (*B*) gadolinium-enhanced T1W show a heterogeneous intraventricular mass in the right atrium (trigone). There is surrounding intra-axial vasogenic edema — seen best on the FLAIR.

curative without risk of metastatic disease. Local recurrence is estimated at 9% within a median presentation time of 7.5 years.[9] Poor prognostic indicators include local invasion, high rate of mitosis, and anaplastic features.

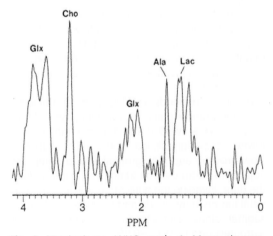

Fig. 8. Meningioma. WHO grade 1. Magnetic resonance spectroscopy — from a voxel entirely within the tumor — shows an ALA peak @ 1.6 ppm, characteristic for meningioma. Glx, Glutamate-Glutamine; Cho, Choline; Ala, Alanine; Lac, Lactate; PPM, parts per million.

Atypical histology in meningiomas implies both a higher incidence and shorter time to recurrence: 30% total recurrence rate, with a median time to recurrence of 3 years for atypical meningiomas, and 75% of total recurrence rate with a median time to recurrence of 2 years for anaplastic meningiomas (all less than typical meningioma).[10]

HEMANGIOPERICYTOMA

HPC is an extradural mesenchymal tumor, unrelated to meningioma, and characterized by its high cellularity and irregular vascularization. They represent less than 1% of all primary CNS tumors.

HPC arises from primitive mesenchymal cells. The definitive cell of origin is still controversial, but it is thought to be the Zimmermann pericytes, which are modified smooth muscle contractile cells surrounding capillaries and postcapillary venules. HPC may occur in any part of the body where capillaries are found, and HPCs are more common in the skin and musculoskeletal system (especially in lower extremities, pelvis, and retroperitoneum). Contemporary pathologic classifications have described most non-CNS HPC as part of a spectrum with solitary fibrous tumor (SFT).[11]

Theses lesions are classified as WHO grade 2 or as grade 3 for the anaplastic form of HPC.

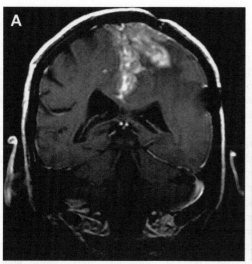
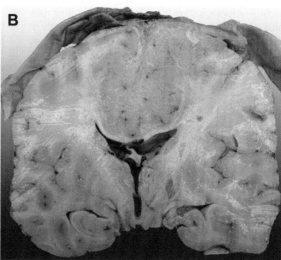

Fig. 9. Meningioma. WHO grade 1 recurrent meningioma. (*A*) Coronal T1W MR imaging with gadolinium shows extensive involvement of the falx, and the dura of the left vertex. The tumor, which was previously partially resected (left parietal craniectomy), is clearly invaginating into the brain, with mass effect with depression of the corpus callosum and compression of the ventricle. There are 2 scalp lesions, indicating a previous craniotomy. (*B*) Autopsy gross photograph shows the tumor has grown (since the last MR image, on the *left*). This particular meningioma does not show a clear CSF cleft nor plane of separation from the brain.

In some of the older literature HPC was called angioblastic meningioma, hemangiopericytic type, but the name was changed in 1993 to reflect its closer relation to soft tissue HPCs and as distinct from meningiomas.[12]

There is currently no known consistent chromosomal loss or gain. There have been reports, however, of abnormalities of chromosomes 12 and 3.

The most common location is supratentorial, in the occipital region; and, HPC — like meningioma — may involve falx, tentorium, or dural sinuses.

Although HPCs can occur at any age, they are rare in children. Mean age of diagnosis and presentation is 43 years old (earlier age than meningioma). There is a slight male predominance (male-to-female ratio = 1.4:1).[13]

Macroscopically they are well circumscribed, encapsulated, and extremely vascular tumors attached to the dura that tend to bleed at surgery. HPC is a highly cellular and vascular monotonous tumor with randomly oriented plump cells with scant cytoplasm, surrounded by a dense reticulin network. Lobules of tumor cells surrounded by capillaries with angular branches give it the characteristic staghorn vascular pattern. Immunohistochemistry may help differentiate HPCs from other tumors, such as solitary fibrous tumors and synovial sarcomas, with positive reactivity to CD34, Leu-7, and factor XIIIa antibodies. It is also vimentin positive and epithelial membrane antigen negative.

The anaplastic form has a prominent mitotic activity, with a median Ki-67 of 5% to 10%, or necrosis, along with at least 2 of the following: hemorrhage, nuclear atypia, and cellularity (**Fig. 10**).

On CT, HPCs appear as hyperdense, noncalcified, extra-axial masses with surrounding intra-axial vasogenic edema and often with homogeneous enhancement of solid areas. They may have associated calvarial erosion, but hyperostosis does not occur. Because many — if not

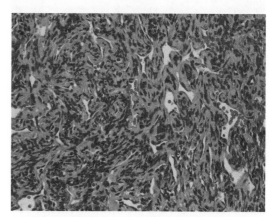

Fig. 10. HPC WHO grade 3. Photomicrograph. Highly cellular neoplasm with irregular stag-horn vessels — characteristic for HPC (hematoxylin-eosin, original magnification ×200).

most — meningiomas have hyperostosis, this may be a useful differential feature. Inner low-density or necrotic areas are frequent. On MR imaging, they are usually heterogeneous, isointense to gray matter, on multiple sequences, with prominent internal signal voids (often irregular and multiple) (Fig. 11), and surrounding brain edema with mass effect or hydrocephalus.

HPCs are hypervascular on angiography, with many randomly oriented irregular vessels, and they may show a prolonged and dense tumor pattern and contrast stain.

They enhance heterogeneously on contrast-enhanced MR imaging and usually show a dural tail sign — a feature shared with meningioma. HPC may produce occlusion of dural sinuses. On MRS, HPC has been reported to show an elevation of myoinositol (Fig. 12).[14]

Typical features that help differentiate HPCs from meningiomas are (Box 2): absence of hyperostosis and commonly bone destruction, no calcification within the tumor, a lobulated (not hemispheric) shape, and, typically, a relatively narrow dural base (mushrooming).

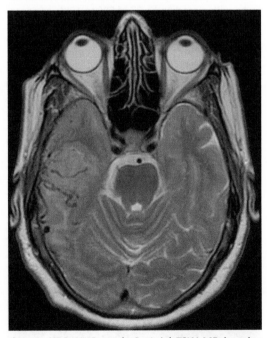

Fig. 11. HPC WHO grade 2. Axial T2W MR imaging shows this right middle fossa extra-axial mass to be more spherical (than hemispherical) with a narrower base of attachment and prominent flow voids from intratumoral vessels. These features are suggestive of HPC. There is asymmetric widening of the right lateral pontine cistern, from early lateral herniation of the cerebral hemisphere.

The current treatment options include preoperative embolization followed by surgical resection of the tumor—often with adjuvant radiation therapy (50–60 Gy). Chemotherapy may improve survival in patients with disease recurrence. Long-term follow-up is necessary due to probable local recurrence and metastases many years after initial diagnosis.

In comparison to meningioma, HPC is a much more aggressive lesion with a significantly diminished long-term prognosis. Local recurrence is common, with a rate of 50% to 90% and a median time of 3 to 6 years. The reported 5-year survival, however, is greater than 90% in the modern era.[15] Approximately 20% of patients have extracranial metastases with the liver, lymph nodes, lungs, and bones the most common sites. Mean survival among patients with extracranial metastatic disease is 2 years. Overall, hemangiopericytomas have a higher incidence of recurrence and shorter time to recurrence compared with meningioma.

NEUROSARCOIDOSIS

Other extra-axial diseases include granulomatous and hematopoietic lesions.

Sarcoidosis is a chronic, multisystem inflammatory disease characterized by the formation of noncaseating epithelioid-cell granulomas. It has neurologic findings in approximately 5% of patients, and, usually, patients have presenting symptoms suggestive of systemic sarcoidosis. Primary isolated CNS sarcoidosis is rare (<1%).[16]

The etiology remains unknown, but it is considered related to an abnormal immune response. Associated conditions include Löfgren syndrome and Heerfordt syndrome.

Sarcoidosis has a bimodal age distribution, with an initial peak at approximately 25 years old and a late peak in women over 50 years old. It is more frequent in women,[17] and it is more common among African Americans, Swedish, and Danes.[18]

The most typical location in the CNS is dural-leptomeningeal, especially in the basal cisterns, optic chiasm, hypothalamus, and infundibulum. But it can also present as an intra-axial lesion.

The common gross appearance is a granulomatous leptomeningitis or a dural-based solitary (and usually infiltrating) mass. Histologically there are noncaseating granulomas (pale nuclei– epithelioid cells, compact and radially arranged, with large multinucleated giant cells surrounding them), with accumulation of fibrocollagenous tissue. They can invade the arterial walls.

The radiologic findings include T1W-isointense and T2W-hypointense dural-based lesions and/or

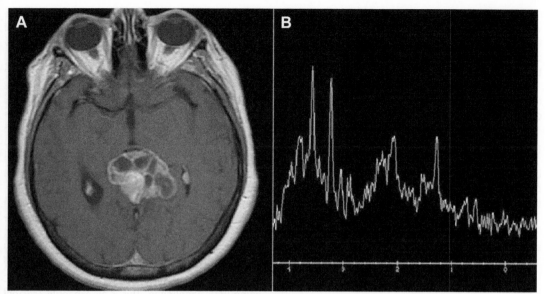

Fig. 12. (A) HPC WHO grade 2. Axial T1W MR imaging with gadolinium. Tectal (quadrigeminal) cistern extra-axial mass. Heterogeneous, with multiple nonenhancing regions. (B) HPC grade 2 MR imaging spectroscopy shows a myoinositol peak, which is suggestive of HPC but should not be present with a meningioma.

Box 2
Hemangiopericytoma key points

Imaging tips

Best modality: multiplanar MR imaging with contrast. CT: assessing bone erosion. MRS might be useful differentiating from meningiomas (myoinositol peak).

Diagnostic criteria

Lobulated, narrow base of attachment

Differential diagnosis

Meningioma: hyperostosis, calcium within the tumor, spherical, broad dural based

Dural metastasis: multifocal, usually skull is first affected.

Granulomatous diseases: multifocal, no bone involvement

Pearls, pitfalls, and variants

Where: extra-axial, supratentorial, occipital

When: earlier than meningeal tumors (mean: 40 years old)

How: lobulated noncalcified mass with heterogeneous MR imaging signal, internal signal voids, dural tail, and associating bone erosion

What the referring physician needs to know

Vascular supply: plan need of presurgical embolization

Bone/dural extension and relation between HPC and brain parenchyma (CSF cleft? Apparent infiltration?): plan surgical strategy to achieve a complete tumoral resection (including bone and dura affected).

material within the subdural space that enhance with contrast. Cranial nerve enhancement may be the only sign in some patients. There might be associated parenchymal enhancing lesions and periventricular T2W hyperintense abnormalities too.[19]

Systemic sarcoidosis usually responds to steroid therapy, but CNS disease responds less often, only in approximately half of cases.

LANGERHANS CELL HISTIOCYTOSIS

Langerhans cell histiocytosis is considered in-between a neoplasm and an inflammatory process that implies clonal proliferation of Langerhan cells.

Langerhans cells are abnormal cells deriving from bone marrow but capable of migrating to skin and lymph nodes.

Previously it was known as histiocytosis X, Letterer-Siwe disease, or Hand-Schüller-Christian disease.

It is more common in the pediatric population, with a peak presentation age of 1 to 3 years.

Grossly, the lesions are yellow-grey-brown masses formed by Langerhans cells with Birbeck granules seen on microscopy.

The skull is the most frequent cranial site involved. Involvement of the pituitary infundibulum and hypothalamus, however, may also occur, presenting with endocrine dysfunction, including diabetes insipidus.[20]

Classic calvarial lesions are purely lytic defects — with a sharp margin — and with a small soft tissue mass (Fig. 13).

ROSAI-DORFMAN DISEASE

Rosai-Dorfman disease (RDD) is a benign and progressive lymphohistiocytosis. It usually involves lymph nodes, presenting with lymphadenopathies and polyclonal hypergammaglobulinemia. The CNS is involved in less than 5% of all cases reported.

Postulated causes for RDD include infection, immunodeficiency, and autoimmune processes and it has also been reported after bone marrow transplant for precursor-B acute lymphoblastic leukemia and concurrently or after Hodgkin and non-Hodgkin lymphoma.

RDD usually presents in children and young adults, although it can occur at any age. Patients presenting with isolated intracranial disease tend to be older. RDD is more common in men and in individuals of African descent.

RDD is a benign and progressive disease with good prognosis. The clinical course of RDD is unpredictable, however, with episodes of exacerbation and remissions that could last many years.

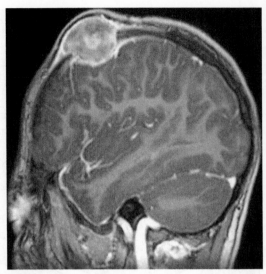

Fig. 13. Langerhan histiocytosis. Sagittal T1W MR imaging with gadolinium. This is an expansile calvarial lesion, extending both outward and bulging the scalp; and, protruding inward displacing the frontal lobe. There is some thickening and pachymeningeal enhancement.

In a majority of the cases, RDD is often self-limiting with a very good outcome; nevertheless, 5% to 11% of patients die from their disease.

Involvement of neck soft tissues is characteristic of RDD but may or may not be visible on imaging limited to the brain. Common sites of involvement include the salivary glands, orbits, globe, and eyelids. When RDD involves the CNS, up to 70% of patients show no associated lymphadenopathy. The most common site of CNS involvement is the dura as well as the parasellar, cavernous sinus, petroclival, and parafalcine regions — the cerebellopontine angle and posterior fossa.

Histologic examination shows infiltration of the meninges by large pale cells mixed with lymphocytes and plasma cells. The specific histologic finding to diagnose RDD is emperipolesis — seeing one intact cell within another. In RDD, this is the engulfment of lymphocytes, plasma cells, erythrocytes, or polymorphonuclear leukocytes by RDD histiocytes. It may be associated with dense fibrosis, which gives the lesion a nodular appearance. Occasionally small clusters of menengothelial cells and psammoma bodies are present. Immunohistochemistry stains are positive for S100, CD68, and vimentin (Fig. 14).

Radiologically, RDD may mimic meningiomas as a dural-based enhancing mass (or masses), which appear as slightly hyperattenuating on CT. MR imaging demonstrates a T1W hypointense or

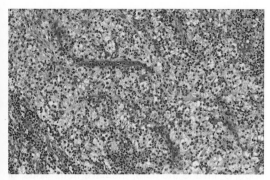

Fig. 14. RDD photomicrograph. Hematoxylin-eosin, original magnification ×200 demonstrates a lymphocytic infiltrate, along with plasma cells and histiocytes.

isointense and T2W hypointense lesion with edema in the underlying brain. Postcontrast MR imaging usually demonstrates diffuse, homogeneous enhancement. Presurgical imaging is usually given a diagnosis of meningioma (Fig. 15).

Although RDD demonstrates similar imaging findings to those of meningiomas, a discriminator may be very low signal intensity on T2W images on RDD. The authors speculate it has a similar mechanism to that reported for abscess — free radicals released by inflammatory macrophages.[21] The lack of hypervascularity on angiography (including magnetic resonance angiography and CT angiography), which is more typically seen

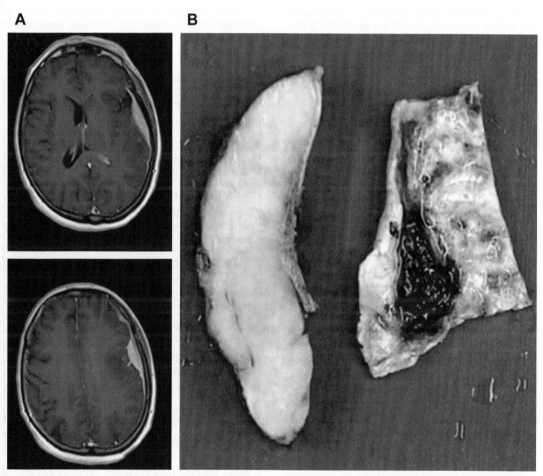

A   **B**

Fig. 15. RDD. (A) Axial T1W MR imaging with gadolinium. There is a shallow hemispheric extra-axial lesion with a dural tail. Looking carefully, some leptomenigeal enhancement within several sulci are seen, in addition to the pachymeningeal mass. Meningiomas usually do not extend into the sulci like this, rather, they push them away. (B) Gross photograph of the surgical mass, arising from the dura.

with meningiomas, may also distinguish RDD in the preoperative diagnosis.

Treatment options are varied and usually include surgery with debulking of the mass. Other treatment modalities used for RDD include radiation therapy, steroids, and chemotherapy.[22]

PITUITARY MASSES

The sellar, parasellar, and suprasellar regions are other common locations for extra-axial tumors. In adults, the most common neoplasms are pituitary adenomas and craniopharyngiomas (squamous and papillary subtype) in addition to tumors described elsewhere (meningiomas, granulomatous diseases, germinomas, epithelial cysts, and so forth).

Pituitary adenomas arise from the different endocrine cells secreting the hypophyseal hormones (ACTH — corticotrophs; thyroid-stimulating hormone — thyrotrophs; growth hormone — somatotrophs; prolactin — lactotrophs; and follicle-stimulating hormone–luteinizing hormone — gonadotrophs). They are almost always WHO grade 1 tumors — primary pituitary carcinoma is rare. Adenomas probably form due to either an over-hyperplastic stimulation (hypophysiotrophic hormone or growth factor excess) or a genomic change that leads to an abnormal proliferation.[23] They can occur in association with multiple endocrine neoplasia type I or Carney complex.

Adenomas are morphologically subdivided by size into microadenomas (<10 mm) or macroadenomas (>10 mm). Macroadenomas represent up to 10% of intracranial tumors and are the most frequent suprasellar neoplastic mass in adults.

A majority (60%) of patients with functioning pituitary tumors have prolactinomas (prolactin-secreting adenomas). Clinical symptoms in women of reproductive age include oligomenorrhea/amenorrhea, infertility, and galactorrhea. Men and postmenopausal women usually present with symptoms of a pituitary or suprasellar mass (headache and visual abnormalities: bitemporal hemianopsia). Serum prolactin levels always exceed 200 µg/L in patients with macroadenomas but may be only moderately increased in patients with microprolactinomas. Mild elevations (50–200 ng/mL) of serum prolactin may also occur with other sella/suprasellar masses due to the stalk effect, theoretically from interference with prolactin inhibitory factor, which travels down the stalk from the hypothalamus.[24]

Macroscopically, adenomas are nodules, formed by monotonous sheets of uniform cells that may be specifically stained depending on their cellular origin or type of hormone produced.

The imaging features of pituitary adenomas include (**Box 3**) microadenoma lesions that enhance slower than the rest of the pituitary gland and macroadenomas that may have degenerative features, including necrosis, hemorrhage and cystic components, and extension upward through the diaphragma sella (figure-of-8 or snowman shape), and usually enlarge the sella turcica, displace the posterior pituitary (posterior bright spot), or invade the dura, the cavernous sinus, or the sphenoid sinus. If there is compression of the optic chiasm and pathways, those structures may show hyperintensity from edema. These changes are more common in macroadenomas (**Fig. 16**).

Microadenomas are — by definition — small and, therefore, more difficult to identify on routine brain imaging. High-resolution (512 × 512), small field-of-view (12 cm), and thin-section (<1 mm) imaging is usually required. Dynamic contrast enhancement may increase detection.[25]

Box 3
Pituitary key points

Imaging tips

Best modality: MR imaging with small field of view (16–18) and thin sections (3 mm). Gadolinium and 3-D T1W increase yield.

Diagnostic criteria

Deviation of stalk, deviation of sella floor, and differential enhancement of the tumor vs normal gland

Differential diagnosis

Pituitary adenoma: hypoenhancing mass, ± hemorrhage, cysts. Pituitary stalk deviation from the lesion

Craniopharyngioma (squamous/papillary): solid, heterogeneous.

Other: meningiomas, granulomatous diseases, germinomas, cysts, and so forth

Pearls, pitfalls, and variants

If there is going to be a surgical approach (macroadenoma compressing the optic chiasm or ACTH-secreting tumor), necessary to find the tumor.

What the referring physician needs to know

Rule out cavernous sinus invasion.

Compression of the optic path

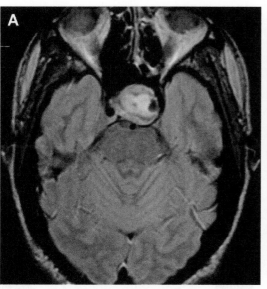
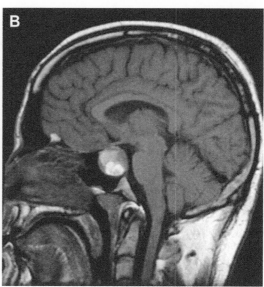

Fig. 16. Pituitary macroadenoma. (*A*) Axial FLAIR shows an expansile heterogeneous intrasellar mass from a macroadenoma, bulging into the left cavernous sinus. (*B*) Sagittal T12 MR image. This large macroadenoma, slowly growing, has ballooned the sella turcica and is now extending upward into the cistern to press on the optic nerves and chiasm. Multiple bright areas of T1W shortening from blood products (methemoglobin). Large pituitary macroadenomas are often complicated by internal hemorrhage that may be asymptomatic or apoplectic.

Prolactin-secreting tumors — even some macroadenomas — are often treated medically with dopamine agonists like bromocriptine. Finding microadenomas producing Cushing disease becomes a task that is especially relevant when there is an elevated ACTH because these require surgery. Approximately 20% of all microadenomas can only be seen in dynamic scans (recommended: imaging acquisition every 10–15 s for 3–4 sequences) (**Fig. 17**).[26] Radiologists have to be aware, however, that these thin-slice techniques might increase false-positive results (showing incidentalomas).

In macroadenomas, the MRA shows displacement, without occlusion, of the internal carotid arteries. In contrast, cavernous sinus and other

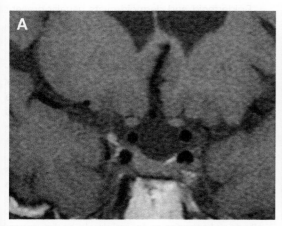
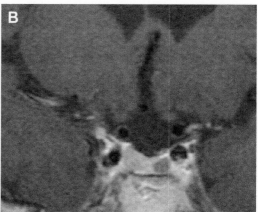

Fig. 17. Pituitary microadenoma. Both images are sagittal T1W, (*A*) without and (*B*) with gadolinium contrast. The lesion is not actually discernable on (*A*) but after contrast appears as the small round nonenhancing lesion in the left half of the pituitary gland.

nearby meningiomas may show constriction or compression of these arteries and can produce ischemia.

Surgery is performed for macroadenomas causing mass effect symptoms and in ACTH-microadenomas that can lead to Cushing syndrome. Prolactin-secreting microadenomas are usually treated with dopamine agonists (bromocriptine and cabergoline). Prognosis is good. Pituitary adenomas are slow-growing tumors, and recurrence after resection is low (15% recurrence at 8 years).

Craniopharyngiomas are the most common extra-axial suprasellar mass in children. But they have a bimodal age range, with a second incidence peak at approximately 50 to 60 years old.[27] They represent WHO grade 1 tumors.

They are usually located in the suprasellar region but may have an intrasellar component or other cranial fossae extension. In adults, the squamous and papillary is the most frequent subtype, whereas in children, the adamantinomatous type predominates. Histologically, the squamous and papillary represent sheets of squamous (no palisading) epithelium, forming (pseudo) papillary structures, in a villous fibrovascular stroma.

They are usually solid masses, often partially isointense and heterogeneous in T2W imaging, without cholesterol and no wet keratin and they calcify far less frequently than the adamantinomatous type that is typical in children (**Fig. 18**).[28]

Squamous and papillary types are also easier to resect than the pediatric type because they are less adherent to the adjacent hypothalamus and optic nerves. Their recurrence rates mainly depend on their size at presentation and extent of resection.

EPIDERMOID AND DERMOID

Epidermoids and dermoids are ectoderm-lined inclusion cysts that differ in complexity (**Table 1**): epidermoids have only squamous epithelium and are filled with keratin debris; dermoid cysts also have squamous epithelium but include dermal adnexa (hair, sebaceous, and sweat glands). Both may arise from developmental trapped pouches of surface ectoderm. There are different hypotheses to explain their formation: a failure to separate surface ectoderm from the neural tube between 3 and 5 weeks of gestation, abnormal invagination or sequestration of ectoderm at sites of normal folding (eye, ear, branchial cleft, and so forth), and implantation after lumbar puncture, surgery, or trauma.[29,30]

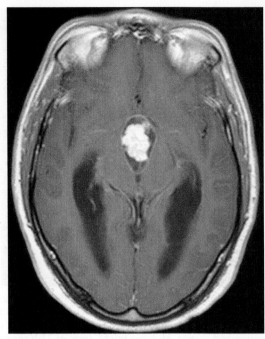

Fig. 18. Craniopharyngioma papillary type. Axial T1W MR with gadolinium. There is a heterogeneous — partly solid and partly fluid — midline mass, projecting in the anterior to the third ventricle.

Epidermoid cysts represent approximately 1% of all primary intracranial tumors and are 4 to 9 times more frequent than dermoid cysts.

The most common location for epidermoid cysts is the cerebellopontine angle, followed by the middle cranial fossa, suprasellar cistern, or fourth ventricle. They are usually placed off the midline, whereas dermoids are typically more midline lesions situated retroclival, suprasellar, or infracerebellar as their most characteristic places.

Epidermoid and dermoid cysts usually present in middle-aged adults (slightly younger ages for dermoids). Most epidermoids are asymptomatic, although they can also show mass effect symptoms. Dermoids usually present with pain. Macroscopically, epidermoids are smooth, lobulated or nodular, white, and pearly masses (**Fig. 19**). The cyst contents are solid cholesterol, keratinaceous debris, and they grow by progressive desquamation from the lining, forming concentric lamellae (like an onion skin) (**Fig. 20**).

Epidermoids are well-defined CSF-like masses that insinuate and surround as well as displace adjacent structures (**Fig. 21**). Calcification in the wall is present in 10% to 25% of cases. They usually do not enhance or only minimally and peripherally in the rim. The contents are nonliving and nonperfused desquamated debris. They may be

Table 1
Epithelial cystic masses

Lesion	Location	Epithelium	Gross Pathology	CT	MR Imaging
Epidermoid	CPA >> middle fossa	Squamous only	Dry flaky waxy lamellar keratin, pearly	Homogeneous water-like attenuation	Lamellar, do not suppress on FLAIR or DWI
Dermoid	Retroclival suprasellar	Squamous, hair follicles, sebaceous gland, sweat glands	Mixture of hair, sebaceous grummus, buttery or cheesy	Fluid-fluid level, lipid top layer, hairball	Lipid layer bright on T1W
Colloid	Anterior third ventricle	Ciliated Cuboidal, low columnar, Goblet cells	Gelatinous, hyaline	Round sharply demarcated, some hyperdense	Round sharply demarcated some bright on T1W, some bright on T2W, some with black hole on T2W
Arachnoid	Middle fossa	Subarachnoid, cistern	CSF	CSF isoattenuation	CSF Isointense
Rathke cleft	Intrasellar, suprasellar, anterior to pituitary stalk	Ciliated cuboidal — columnar, goblet cells		Water like	Bright on T1W and dark on T2W rim enhancement in residual pituitary
Craniopharyngioma — child	Suprasellar above and anterior to stalk	Squamous (stratified and palisading) and adamantinomatous tissue with connective tissue	Wet nodular keratin, "machine oil" with cholesterol	Ca++, mixed cystic and solid, solid enhances	May be bright on T1W, solid regions enhance
Craniopharyngioma — adult	Suprasellar above and anterior to stalk	Squamous (sheets, no palisading) and forming (pseudo) papillary structures	Solid masses without cholesterol, no wet keratin, no Ca++	Solid mass	solid regions enhance

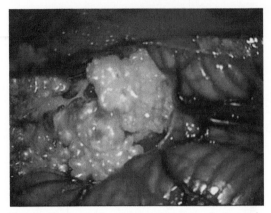

Fig. 19. Epidermoid cyst operative gross photograph. Suprasellar location — there is a shiny mother-of-pearl appearance to the lesion — from the waxy flakey keratin of this suprasellar epidermoid cyst.

differentiated from normal CSF and arachnoid cysts (its major differential diagnosis) by not suppressing completely on FLAIR images and showing high signal on DWIs (Fig. 22). In contrast to epidermoid cysts, arachnoid cysts typically displace, rather than surround, adjacent structures. Rarely, an epidermoid cyst may be bright on T1W (white epidermoid) (Fig. 23).

Dermoid cysts are usually unilocular inclusion cysts, with a thicker wall compared with epidermoids. They may have wall calcifications and vascularization — distinct from epidermoids. Dermoids contain multiple dermal elements, sebaceous lipids, hair, and cholesterol floating on proteinaceous material (Fig. 24). They may be

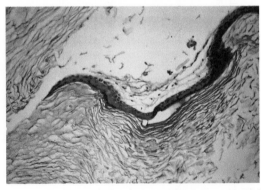

Fig. 20. Epidermoid cyst hematoxylin-eosin, original magnification ×200 photomicrograph, high power. The dark purple is the living squamous epithelium, which produces the dry keratin material forming multiple layers within the cyst lumen.

associated with calvarial defects and fibrous tract or sinus that communicates with the skin surface. The latter creates risk for infection in the dermoid cyst.

The radiologic appearance (Box 4) depends on whether it has ruptured. Unruptured cysts present as midline nonenhancing unilocular cystic lesions — sometimes with a fluid-fluid level — and associated with supernatant lipid signal: T1W hyperintense and heterogeneous on T2W, best demonstrated using fat-saturation sequences. If the cyst is ruptured, however, there are subarachnoid lipid, or fatty, droplets — often dispersed in the sulci and cisterns. Secondary chemical meningitis may produce extensive pial enhancement and vasospasm with ischemia may cause neurologic complications, including seizure and infarction (Fig. 25).

Epidermoid and dermoid cysts are benign slow-growing masses. Rare malignant transformation of the lining into squamous cell carcinoma is possible. In the case of dermoids, larger lesions have higher rupture rate, which is a rare but threatening situation that may lead to seizures, coma, vasospasm, infarction, or death. Retroclival dermoid cysts are more prone to rupture than infracerebellar or suboccipital locations.

Treatment is usually surgical. Incomplete resections have high rates of recurrence. Subarachnoid dissemination of contents may cause chemical meningitis.

ARACHNOID CYSTS

Arachnoid cysts are benign, congenital, intra-arachnoidal space-occupying lesions that are filled with clear CSF and do not communicate with either the ventricular system or the greater extra-axial CSF spaces. They represent approximately 1% of all intracranial masses.

They are usually located in the supratentorial subarachnoid space, most commonly found anterior to the temporal lobe in the middle fossa, and/or invaginating into the sylvian fissure. They can occur anywhere though, including CPA and suprasellar cisterns. They are slightly more frequent in men. A majority are sporadic.

Arachnoid cysts collapse on incision from CSF escape and surgical specimens are rare. There is neither solid component nor epithelial lining, and the wall consists of a vascular collagenous membrane lined by arachnoid cells.

On imaging (see Box 4), they are usually unilocular, smooth, and expansile lesions that mold the adjacent structures — similar to a water balloon. They are well circumscribed but the wall is imperceptible, and there is no enhancement. Arachnoid

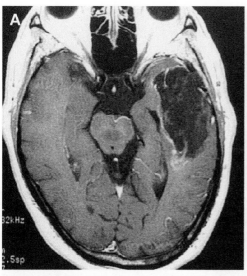 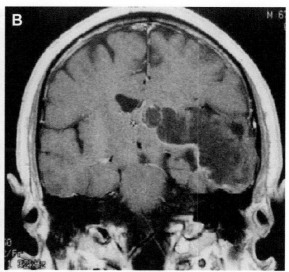

Fig. 21. Epidermoid inclusion cyst. (*A*) Axial and (*B*) coronal — both T1W after gadolinium. The low-intensity lesion has slowly invaginated from extra-axial into the left temporal lobe. Some fine lines of internal structure represent the layers of desquamated keratin. There is some mild reactive gliosis cause wispy linear enhancement around the outside of the lesion.

cysts should show CSF signal on all sequences. Occasionally, they may have protein in the fluid — and their appearance is less specific. Over time they can stimulate remodeling of bone (**Fig. 26**).

Arachnoid cysts are benign lesions, usually asymptomatic, and as so, they do not need any

treatment or follow-up. If symptomatic due to mass-effect, surgery can be through a craniotomy and fenestration.

COLLOID CYSTS

Colloid cysts are congenital benign lesions of the anterior third ventricle. They have also been known as ependymal cyst, endodermal cysts, or choroid cyst. In the past they were described as similar to paraphyseal cysts — which occur in lower animals.

They are thought to originate from abnormal folding of the primitive neuroepithelium. They are lined by a cuboidal to low columnar pseudostratified epithelium — resembling respiratory epithelium — and including goblet cells, which produce mucin. They have scant connective tissue supporting the epithelium, and they enlarge and are filled with mucus and a variable quantity of old blood, cholesterol, and other proteinaceous materials (**Fig. 27**).[31]

They are localized — almost by definition — at the foramen of Monro, attached to the roof of the third ventricle. This situation can potentially convert this benign condition into a devastating problem, from acute and severe hydrocephalus and secondary transtentorial herniation (**Figs. 28** and **29**). The protein concentration in the cyst contents determine the attenuation on CT and the signal intensity on T1W and T2W MR imaging. Highly proteinaceous secretions are

Fig. 22. Epidermoid inclusion cyst axial DWI MR imaging showing increased signal intensity from a mixture of T2W shine-through and restricted diffusion within the cyst.

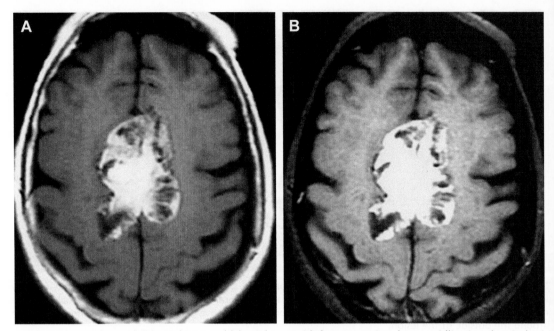

Fig. 23. White epidermoid. (*A*) Axial T1W and (*B*) axial T1W with fat suppression show a midline interhemispheric mass that is hyperintense and does not suppress, which means that it does not contain lipids, but the T1W hyperintensity comes from the water protons associated with keratin debris. (*Courtesy of* Lara Brandão, MD, Rio De Janeiro, Brazil.)

hyperattenuating (white) on CT and often are dark on T2W and sometimes even on T1W.

They present as a sharply demarcated rounded lesion (see **Box 4**), usually hyperdense on CT and with mild enhancement usually limited to the rim.

They are isointense to hyperintense on T1W imaging and hyperintense to hypointense in T2W imaging. Their signal intensity on T2W gives practical information regarding their treatment options, because T2W dark cysts are too thick for

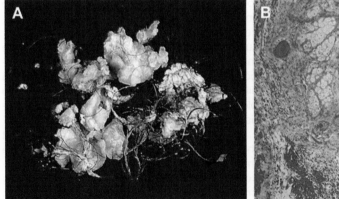
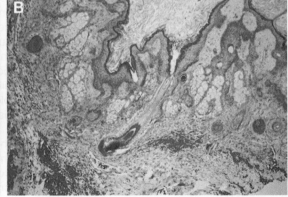

Fig. 24. Dermoid inclusion cyst. (*A*) Gross photograph. Dermoid cysts are ectodermal, just like epidermoid cysts, but in addition to squamous epithelium, they have sebaceous glands and secretions as well as hair and hair follicles and form pilosebaceous units (*B*) Hematoxylin-eosin photomicrograph 50×. There is a heterogeneous mixture of squamous epithelium and keratin debris (*top*) hair shafts (most in cross-section, one prominently in the *center* is longitudinal) and multiple sebaceous glands.

Box 4
Epithelial cystic masses key points

Imaging tips

Best modality: FLAIR and DWI help identify epidermoids. MR imaging with fat saturation may distinguish dermoids.

Diagnostic criteria

Epidermoids: CSF-like density/signal. Insinuates and surrounds vessels, usually off the midline in cerebellopontine cistern.

Dermoids: resemble fat, near midline, clivus, under cerebellum

Differential diagnosis

Inflammatory cysts (ie, neurocysticercosis) or cystic neoplasms for epidermoids: Often enhance, with or without adjacent edema/gliosis.

Craniopharyngioma, teratoma, lipoma for dermoid: nodular calcifications, T2W hyperintense and strong enhancement in cranio, pineal location for teratoma, homogenous lipoma.

Pearls, pitfalls, and variants

Dermoids in midline vs epidermoids lateral/midline

Epidermoids: CSF-like but mild hyperintensity on FLAIR and DWI usually some internal texture (lines)

Chronic subdural hematoma, subdural hygroma, or other nonneoplastic cysts may mimic arachnoid cysts.

Neurocysticercosis, CSF flow artifact, vertebrobasilar dolichoectasia or aneurysm, subependymoma or craniopharyngioma for colloid cyst

What the referring physician needs to know

Colloid cyst: is stereotactic aspiration feasible (T2W bright cysts) vs an endoscopic approach (T2W dark cysts)?

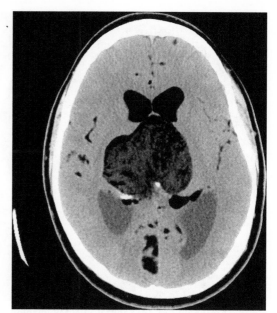

Fig. 25. Dermoid inclusion cyst. CT noncontrast. There is a large midline lesion, which is a mixture of water and lipid attenuation, which has ruptured spilling sebaceous material into the subarachnoid space. There are multiple scattered areas of lipid, including droplets within the sulci of both sylvian fissures, and in the midline of both hemispheres both anterior and posterior to the mass.

stereotactic aspiration, and they need ventricular endoscopic surgery (**Fig. 30**). Although they have been reported to have metallic ions as the cause of this pattern of attenuation and signal (eg, manganese, magnesium, copper, and zinc) the signal may be explained merely by the protein and cholesterol concentration.[32]

Colloid cysts are benign lesions that tend to grow slowly, and if resection is necessary, it is usually performed via transcallosal (more classical approach) or endoscopically/stereotactically depending on the T2W signal (discussed previously).

PINEAL REGION TUMORS

Extra-axial masses also present in the pineal region, where it is helpful to divide lesions into germ cell neoplasms, including germinomas and teratomas (60%), and pineal parenchymal masses, including pineocytomas and pineoblastomas (15%). Common symptoms and signs due to location are: Parinaud syndrome (vertical gaze palsy), precocious puberty, headache, nausea, and vomiting.[33]

GCT subtypes represent the neoplastic correlates of distinct stages of embryonic development from residual primordial ectoderm, mesoderm or endoderm. They are subdivided into germinomas and nongerminomatous GCTs (teratomas, embryonal carcinoma, yolk sac/endodermal sinus tumor, choriocarcinoma, and mixed GCTs).

Intracranial germinomas are morphologic homologues of germinal neoplasms but arising in extragonadal sites.[34] The hypothesized cells of origin are intracranial germ cell rests. The remainder of the GCTs may not arise from germ cells but from misplacement of embryonic cells into lateral mesoderm.[35]

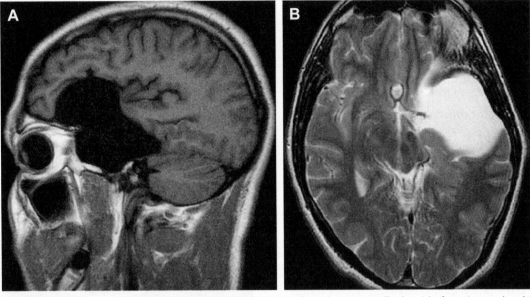

Fig. 26. Arachnoid cyst. (A) Sagittal T1W MR imaging. The arachnoid cyst is totally devoid of any internal architecture and homogenously identical to water signal intensity. The lesion is anterior to the temporal lobe, and forms a sharp margin with the displaced temporal lobe. (B) Axial T2W MR. Nicely shown is how the flow-void of the middle cerebral artery is displaced and does not enter the lesion. The arachnoid cyst is homogeneous and nearly isointense to CSF on T2W.

Pure germinoma is considered WHO grade 2; germinomas with syncytiotrophoblastic giant cells range from WHO grade 1 to grade 3.

The WHO classification of GCTs distinguishes mature and immature teratomas as well as teratomas with malignant transformation.

Synonyms for intracranial germinoma include Pinealoma, extragonadal seminoma, dysgerminoma, and atypical teratoma.

Intracranial germinomas may be sporadic, but several associated abnormalities to CNS include Klinefelter syndrome (47XXY) and Down syndrome.[36,37]

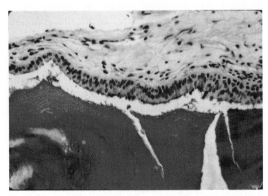

Fig. 27. Colloid cyst (wall). Photomicrograph hematoxylin-eosin medium power (100×). There is a cuboidal to low-columnar epithelium. Some cilia are clearly seen facing the lumen — which is filled with amorphous acellular material, secreted by the lining.

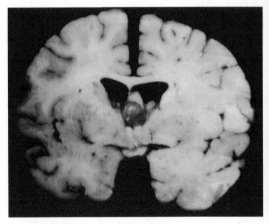

Fig. 28. Colloid cyst. Coronal gross autopsy photograph. This young woman died from acute hydrocephalus, caused by the colloid cyst shown here, impacted in the foramen of Monro. The cyst is very round and sharply demarcated.

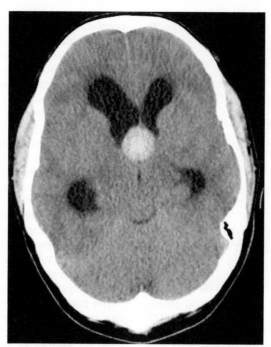

Fig. 29. Colloid cyst. Noncontrast CT. There is an almost 2-cm diameter, very round, hyperattenuating mass in the anterior third ventricle — at the foramen of Monro. The third ventricle is collapsed, whereas the frontal and inferior horns of the lateral ventricle are dilated by obstructive hydrocephalus. The high attenuation is due to the protein concentration of the cyst contents.

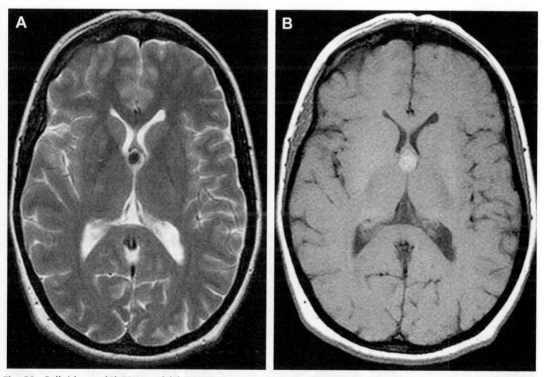

Fig. 30. Colloid cyst. (*A*) T2W and (*B*) T1W MR imaging. The colloid cyst is in the anterior third ventricle, at the foramen of Monro. (*A*) The cyst is hyperintense on T1W and (*B*) it has a bright rim with a dark center on the T2W image. These signal changes are related to the protein concentration of the cyst contents. The fresh mucoid secretions are on the outside — where the secreting epithelium is located — and the older, drier, often inspissated high-protein material is in the center.

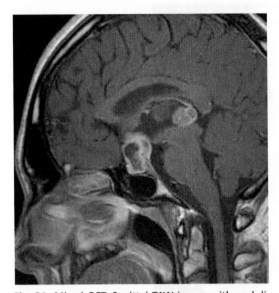

Fig. 31. Mixed GCT. Sagittal T1W image with gadolinum. There are 2 lesions — 1 in the posterior third ventricle/quadrigeminal cistern and the larger 1 extra-axial in the suprasellar cistern, extending into the pituitary fossa. Although either may be primary, with the other a CSF dissemination, it is far more likely for a pineal region mass to spread downward than for a suprasellar lesion to spread upward.

CNS germinomas have a propensity for midline: pineal region (50%–65%), suprasellar (25%–35%), and basal ganglia/thalami (**Fig. 31**).

Intracranial GCTs usually present between ages of 5 and 35 years, with a clear male predominance: male-to-female ratio 2:7. Suprasellar germinomas, however, that account for the 22% of all the germinomas, have been reported to have a weak female predilection. The prevalence of intracranial GCT is approximately 0.3% to 3.4% of all CNS tumors, far more common in Asians. Germinomas represent a majority of these neoplasms (representing 50% of all pineal tumors), but teratoma is the leading perinatal brain tumor — presenting within the first 2 months after birth.

Macroscopically, germinomas are well-circumscribed, soft, and friable white masses that can present a variable grade of necrosis. Microscopically they are tumors composed by sheets of large polygonal primitive germ cells with mitosis, prominent nuclei and nucleoli, and periodic acid–Schiff–positive cytoplasm. Lymphocytic infiltrates along fibrovascular septa are abundant. Germinomas can be divided into 2 subtypes with different WHO classification due to its prognostic implications: pure germinoma and germinoma with syncytiotrophoblastic cells.

The pathologic and histologic features of teratomas depend on their grade of maturity: mature teratomas reveal a lobulated neoplasm with a complex mixture of adult-type tissues, whereas inmature teratomas contain incompletely differentiated tissue elements that resemble fetal tissue (**Fig. 32**).

Intracranial germinomas usually appear as sharply circumscribed midline masses that surround or engulf the pineal gland (or its calcifications) (**Box 5, Fig. 33**). They are homogenous and hyperdense on nonenhanced CT, presenting a homogenous enhancement in contrast-enhanced CT. In MR imaging they are usually isointense to gray matter in all sequences. Restricted diffusion is typically demonstrated due to high cell density. It is recommended to

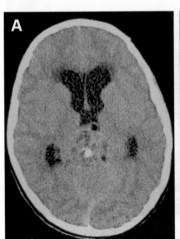
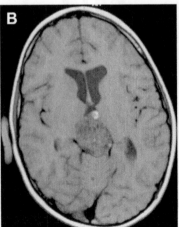
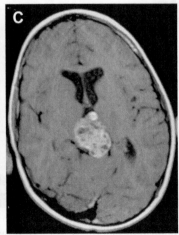

Fig. 32. Pineal region teratoma. (*A*) NECT, note the small peripheral focus of very low attenuation (less than water), and (*B*) T1W, corresponding T1W-shortening from lipid. This could be sebaceous (ectodermal) lipid or mesodermal lipid (adipose tissue). The lipid focus does not enhance after contrast (*C*, T1W with gadolinium).

Box 5
Pineal region masses key points

Imaging tips

MR imaging with and without contrast using thin sections (3 mm)

Imaging the entire neuroaxis if germinoma or pineoblastoma are considered. CT can be helpful in some cases.

Differential diagnosis: pineal region tumors

GCTs

    Germinoma: most common (50% pineal tumors)

    Teratoma: second most common

    Others: embryonal carcinoma, yolk sac tumor, choriocarcinoma, and mixed GCTs

Pineal parenchymal tumors: pineoblastoma, pineal parenchymal tumor of intermediate differentiation, pineocytoma

Other: pineal cyst, meningioma, metastases, astrocytoma (intra-axial)

Pearls, pitfalls, and variants

Germinoma vs pineoblastoma: both frequently hyperattenuating on CT (hypointense T2W imaging) and prone to CSF dissemination. Typical central engulfed Ca++ in germinoma vs peripheral exploded Ca++ in pineoblastoma.

What the referring physician needs to know

Mass effect: check aqueduct obstruction-hydrocephalus.

Relation between tumor and deep veins (vein of Galen and basal veins of Rosenthal).

Rule out CSF dissemination (scan entire spine with gadolinium)

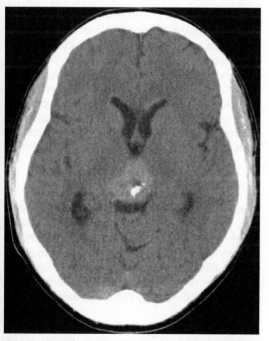

Fig. 33. Pineal region germinoma. Axial CT (non-contrast) The tumor is hyperattenuating compared with brain and surrounds a central region of calcification — representing the normal pineal calcifications surrounded by the neoplasm.

perform a complete evaluation of neuroaxis before treatment, due to its possible CSF seeding and brain invasion.

Pineal region teratomas are also sharply circumscribed and lobulated masses. They are usually heterogeneous in attenuation and signal, however, representing a mixture of watery fluid, lipid (including sebaceous material), soft tissues, and calcium (including possible bone and even teeth). Multiloculated masses with enhancement of the solid areas are typical (**Fig. 34**).

Intracranial GCTs (germinoma) are very radiosensitive and chemosensitive tumors, with a prognosis up to 90% survival after 5 years and a median survival of 19 years.[38]

Pineal parenchymal tumors account for less than 0.2% of intracranial neoplasms and are more common in the pediatric population, although they all can be found at any age. They arise from pineocytes or their precursors and include pineocytoma WHO grade 1, pineal parenchymal tumor with intermediate differentiation WHO grades 2–3, papillary tumor of pineal region WHO grades 2–3, and pineoblastoma WHO grade 4.

Radiologically they may show a pattern of peripheral calcifications that may appear like an exploded pineal gland, with homogenous and

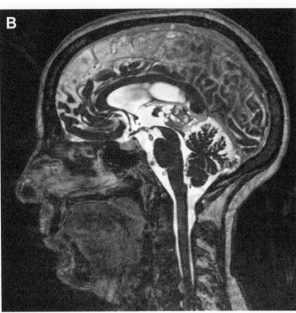

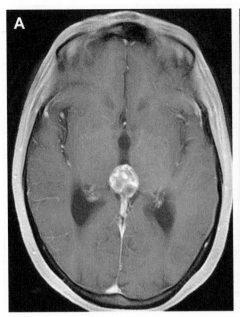

Fig. 34. Papillary tumor of the pineal region (WHO III). Axial T1W MR imaging with gadolinium (A). The lesion extends from the tectal cistern toward the posterior third ventricle (B).

well-demarcated masses for pineocytomas versus heterogeneous enhancement and restricted diffusion seen in pineoblastomas — the latter are usually masses measuring more than 3 cm and showing infiltrative features, including frequent CSF dissemination.

Pineal cysts are common with frequently asymptomatic and incidental findings in patients over 25 years old, with a prevalence of 2% to 8%. Cyst size is similar at all ages, but older patients are more likely than younger to have them.

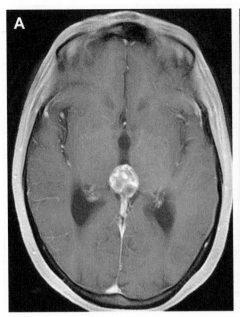

Fig. 35. Pineal (intrapineal) cyst. This lesion is seen clearly within the quadrigeminal (tectal) cistern with a fluid-like central portion within the pineal gland.

They present with homogeneous fluid-like features on imaging and possible thin rim or ring enhancement less than 2 mm.

The natural history of pineal cysts and implications for follow-up have received multiple reviews, and there is general agreement that most pineal cysts do not exhibit radiographic change or clinical symptoms at a mean follow-up interval of 3 to 15 years. Even those cysts that change or grow, however, are likely to remain asymptomatic. Therefore, pineal cysts do not routinely require imaging follow-up, and development of symptoms in these patients is often unrelated to the pineal cyst. The recommendation is to follow-up on a clinical basis alone rather than on imaging (Fig. 35).[39]

SUMMARY

Meningiomas are the most common extra-axial tumor. Their typical — and far less common — differential diagnosis includes HPCs (mesenchymal tumors), dural metastasis, and granulomatous diseases. Masses in the sellar region are most commonly pituitary adenomas and craniopharyngiomas — but watch out for aneurysms of the circle of Willis.

Lesions in the pineal region are most likely consistent with GCTs — especially in young males — and pineal parenchymal tumors. FLAIR/DWI features help in the differential diagnosis for epithelial-lined cystic masses (epidermoid and dermoid) besides their typical localization.

REFERENCES

1. CBTRUS Statistical Report: Primary brain and central nervous system tumors diagnosed in eighteen states in 2004–2008. Central Brain Tumor Registry of the United States, Hisdale. 2012.

2. Joseph E, Sandhyamani S, Rao MB, et al. Atypical meningioma: a clinicopathological analysis. Neurol India 2000;48:338–42.

3. Dezamis E, Sanson M. The molecular genetics of meningiomas and genotypic/phenotypic correlations. Rev Neurol (Paris) 2003;159(8–9):727–38.

4. Niedermaier T, Behrens G, Schmid D, et al. Body mass index, physical activity, and risk of adult meningioma and glioma: a meta-analysis. Neurology 2015;85(15):1342–50.

5. Wiemels J, Wrensch M, Claus EB. Epidemiology and etiology of meningioma. J Neurooncol 2010;99(3):307–14.

6. Buetow MP, Buetow PC, Smirniotopoulos JG. From the archives of the AFIP: typical, atypical and misleading features in meningioma. Radiographics 1991;11:1087–106.

7. Bulakbasi N, Kocaoglu M, Ors F, et al. Combination of single-voxel proton MR spectroscopy and apparent diffusion coefficient calculation in the evaluation of common brain tumors. AJNR Am J Neuroradiol 2003;24(2):225–33.

8. Hsu CC, Pai CY, Kao HW, et al. Do aggressive imaging features correlate with advanced histopathological grade in meningiomas? J Clin Neurosci 2010;17(5):584–7.

9. Jääskeläinen J. Seemingly complete removal of histologically benign intracranial meningioma: late recurrence rate and factors predicting recurrence in 657 patients. A multivariate analysis. Surg Neurol 1986;26(5):461–9.

10. Klinger DR, Flores BC, Lewis JJ, et al. Atypical meningiomas: recurrence, reoperation and radiotherapy. World Neurosurg 2015;84:839–45.

11. Boyd Smith A, Horkanyne-Szakaly I, Schroeder JW, et al. From the radiologic pathology archives. Mass lesions of the dura: beyond meningioma-radiologic-pathologic correlation. Radiographics 2014;34:295–312.

12. Giannini C, Rushing EJ, Hainfellner JA. Haeman-giopericytoma. In: Louis DN, Ohagaki H, Wiestler OD, et al, editors. WHO classification of tu-mours of the central nervous system. Lyon (France): IARC; 2007. p. 178–80.

13. Liu G, Chen ZY, Ma L, et al. Intracranial hemangiopericytoma: MR imaging findings and diagnostic usefulness of minimum ADC values. J Magn Reson Imaging 2013;38(5):1146–51.

14. Barba I, Moreno A, Martínez-Pérez I, et al. Magnetic resonance spectroscopy of brain hemangiopericytomas: high myoinositol concentrations and discrimination from meningiomas. J Neurosurg 2001;94:55–60.

15. Melone AG, D'Elia A, Santoro F, et al. Intracranial hemangiopericytoma—our experience in 30 years: a series of 43 cases and review of the literature. World Neurosurg 2014;81:556–62.

16. Hebel R, Dubaniewicz-Wybieralska M, Dubaniewicz A. Overview of neurosarcoidosis: recent advances. J Neurol 2015;262(2):258–67.

17. Lill H, Kliiman K, Altraja A. Factors signifying gender differences in clinical presentation of sarcoidosis among Estonian population. Clin Respir J 2016;10(3):282–90.

18. Iannuzzi MC, Rybicki BA, Teirstein AS. Sarcoidosis. N Engl J Med 2007;357(21):2153–65.

19. Koyama T, Ueda H, Togashi K, et al. Radiologic manifestations of sarcoidosis in various organs. Radiographics 2004;24(1):87–104.

20. D'Ambrosio N, Soohoo S, Warshall C, et al. Craniofacial and intracranial manifestations of langerhans cell histiocytosis: report of findings in 100 patients. AJR Am J Roentgenol 2008;191(2):589–97.

21. Haimes AB, Zimmerman RD, Morgello S, et al. MR imaging of brain abscesses. AJR Am J Roentgenol 1989;152(5):1073–85.

22. Symss NP, Cugati G, Vasudevan MC, et al. Intracranial Rosai Dorfman Disease: report of three cases and literature review. Asian J Neurosurg 2010;5(2):19–30.

23. Melmed S. Mechanisms for pituitary tumorigenesis: the plastic pituitary. J Clin Invest 2003;112(11):1603–18.

24. Bergsneider M, Mirsadraei L, Yong WH, et al. The pituitary stalk effect: is it a passing phenomenon? J Neurooncol 2014;117(3):477–84.

25. Kinoshita M, Tanaka H, Arita H, et al. Pituitary-targeted dynamic contrast-enhanced multisection CT for detecting MR imaging-occult functional pituitary microadenoma. AJNR Am J Neuroradiol 2015;36(5):904–8.

26. Friedman TC, Zuckerbraun E, Lee ML, et al. Dynamic pituitary MRI has high sensitivity and specificity for the diagnosis of mild Cushing's syndrome and should be part of the initial workup. Horm Metab Res 2007;39(6):451–6.

27. Haupt R, Magnani C, Pavanello M, et al. Epidemiological aspects of craniopharyngioma. J Pediatr Endocrinol Metab 2006;19(Suppl 1):289–93.

28. Zacharia BE, Bruce SS, Goldstein H, et al. Incidence, treatment and survival of patients with craniopharyngioma in the surveillance, epidemiology and end results program. Neuro Oncol 2012;14(8):1070–8.

29. Ettinger RL, Manderson RD. Implantation keratinizing epidermoid cysts. A review and case history. Oral Surg Oral Med Oral Pathol 1973;36:225–30.

30. Park MH, Cho TG, Moon JG, et al. Iatrogenic intraspinal epidermoid cyst. Korean J Spine 2014;11:195–7.

31. Osborn AG, Preece MT. Intracranial cysts: radiologic-pathologic correlation and imaging approach. Radiology 2006;239(3):650–64.

32. Armao D, Castillo M, Chen H, et al. Colloid cyst of the third ventricle: imaging-pathologic correlation. AJNR Am J Neuroradiol 2000;21:1470–7.

33. Smith AB, Rushing EJ, Smirniotopoulos JG. From the archives of the AFIP lesions of the pineal region: radiologic- pathologic correlation. Radiographics 2010;30:2001–20.

34. Echevarría ME, Fangusaro J, Goldman S. Pediatric central nervous system germ cell tumors: a review. Oncologist 2008;13(6):690–9.

35. Sano K. Pathogenesis of intracranial germ cell tumors reconsidered. J Neurosurg 1999;90:258–64.

36. Nakata Y, Yagishita A, Arai N. Two patients with intraspinal germinoma associated with Klinefelter syndrome: case report and review of the literature. AJNR Am J Neuroradiol 2006;27:1204–10.

37. Matsumura N, Kurimoto M, Endo S, et al. Intracranial germinoma associated with Down's syndrome. Report of 2 cases. Pediatr Neurosurg 1998;29: 199–202.

38. Kawabata Y, Takahashi JA, Arakawa Y, et al. Long term outcomes in patients with intracranial germinomas: a single institution experi-ence of irradiation with or without chemotherapy. J Neurooncol 2008; 88(2):161–7.

39. Al-Holou WN, Maher CO, Muraszko KM, et al. The natural history of pineal cysts in children and young adults. J Neurosurg Pediatr 2010;5(2):162–6.

Advanced MR Imaging Techniques in Daily Practice

Marc C. Mabray, MD[a],*, Soonmee Cha, MD[b]

KEYWORDS

- MR imaging • Diffusion-weighted imaging • Diffusion-tensor imaging
- Susceptibility-weighted imaging • Functional imaging • MR spectroscopy • Perfusion imaging

KEY POINTS

- Areas of postoperative reduced diffusion representing cytotoxic edema may be expected to enhance on subsequent follow-up imaging as a subacute infarct would and should not be mistaken for recurrent/residual tumor.
- Diffusion-tensor imaging currently is mainly applicable for tractography, in which the corticospinal tracts, optic radiations, and potentially other tracts of interest are displayed in commercially available surgical navigational packages.
- Foci of susceptibility that develop following radiation therapy represent microhemorrhages or induced small vascular malformations; a delayed toxicity of radiation therapy.
- Higher relative cerebral blood volume can be useful to suggest residual/recurrent tumor as opposed to treatment effect.
- A perfusion curve that does not return close to baseline is suggestive of leaky capillaries, such as those found in metastasis, or an extra-axial tumor as opposed to a glioma.

INTRODUCTION

Advanced MR imaging techniques have become an integral part of the evaluation of patients with brain tumors. Although structural imaging provides the primary foundation of an MR examination, advanced MR imaging techniques can potentially provide valuable insight into the physiology, histology, genetics, hemodynamics, and chemistry of a patient's tumor and brain. These techniques are being applied to diagnose and grade tumors preoperatively, to plan and navigate surgery intraoperatively, to monitor and assess treatment response, and to understand the effects of treatment on the patients' brains.[1,2] Advanced imaging techniques include techniques that are routine and fairly quick, such as diffusion-weighted imaging (DWI), frequently used problem-solving techniques such as dynamic susceptibility contrast-enhanced (DSC) perfusion imaging and MR spectroscopy (MRS), and currently less frequently used techniques such as functional MR (fMR) imaging (Table 1).

This article reviews the following techniques: DWI, diffusion-tensor imaging (DTI), susceptibility-weighted imaging (SWI), MRS, perfusion imaging, and fMR imaging (see Table 1). It emphasizes the clinical applications of these techniques as they

Disclosures: No relevant disclosures.
[a] Department of Radiology, University of New Mexico School of Medicine, MSC 10 5530, 1 University of New Mexico, Albuquerque, NM 87131, USA; [b] Department of Radiology and Biomedical Imaging, University of California San Francisco, 505 Parnassus Avenue, L325, San Francisco, CA 94143, USA
* Corresponding author. Department of Radiology, University of New Mexico School of Medicine, MSC 10 5530, 1 University of New Mexico, Albuquerque, NM 87131.
E-mail addresses: marccm7@gmail.com; mamabray@salud.unm.edu

Neuroimag Clin N Am 26 (2016) 647–666
http://dx.doi.org/10.1016/j.nic.2016.06.010
1052-5149/16/© 2016 Elsevier Inc. All rights reserved.

Table 1
Imaging protocols

Technique	Basics	When Used
DWI	Echo-planar imaging technique B = 1000, at least 3 orthogonal directions	Routine in all MR brain protocols
DTI	Echo-planar imaging technique B = 2000, numerous (ie, 55) directions. Long acquisition	Preoperative navigation MR for tractography
DSC perfusion	Echo-planar imaging; negative contrast technique; radiologist selects level, processes, and draws regions of interest to measure rCBV	Initial evaluation of brain tumors and follow-up for progression
DCE perfusion	T1-based positive contrast technique, main measure of interest is permeability (endothelial transfer coefficient K^{trans})	In general, only in some research protocols
ASL	Noncontrast perfusion technique based on inflow spin tagging. Processed CBF map	Stroke, vascular malformations, tumors (increasing experience)
MRS	$20 \times 20 \times 20$ mm for single voxel, smaller for multivoxel techniques In general, with echo time = 288 ms; 144 ms if trying to flip lactate. Short echo time in certain situations (eg, myo-inositol)	Problem solving when evaluating unknown lesions or in follow-up
Susceptibility-sensitive imaging	T2* gradient echo–based sequences (eg, SWI) Magnitude and phase information available	Routine in most MR brain protocols
fMR imaging	BOLD echo-planar imaging technique with a standardized administered paradigm for functional localization	Select cases for preoperative functional localization
RS-fMR imaging	BOLD echo-planar imaging technique while at rest for approximately 8 min. Heavy postprocessing to identify resting-state networks	Research use

apply to brain tumor imaging. An in-depth discussion of the underlying physics of these techniques is beyond the scope of this article and is only reviewed where relevant.

NORMAL ANATOMY AND IMAGING TECHNIQUE
Diffusion-weighted Imaging and Related Techniques (Tagging: Diffusion-weighted Imaging, Diffusion-tensor Imaging)

DWI has become a routine sequence in brain imaging but nonetheless offers valuable insight into the diffusion of water molecules in tissues beyond traditional structural MR imaging. This quick sequence uses applied gradients usually with an echo-planar imaging technique to measure the brownian motion of water molecules.[3,4] An apparent diffusion coefficient (ADC) is derived for each voxel and is displayed as a calculated ADC map. DWI has become indispensable in the evaluation of stroke but also offers significant value in the evaluation of brain tumors and is routinely used in daily practice in this role (**Figs. 1C, D and 2C**).

DTI and related techniques can be considered more complex versions of standard DWI. DTI involves the interrogation of the motion of water with numerous gradient directions, which allows the measurement of directional diffusion.[5,6] This technique provides additional abilities compared with standard isotropic DWI. Anisotropic diffusion measured by DTI is characterized by eigenvectors (direction) and eigenvalues (magnitude), which can

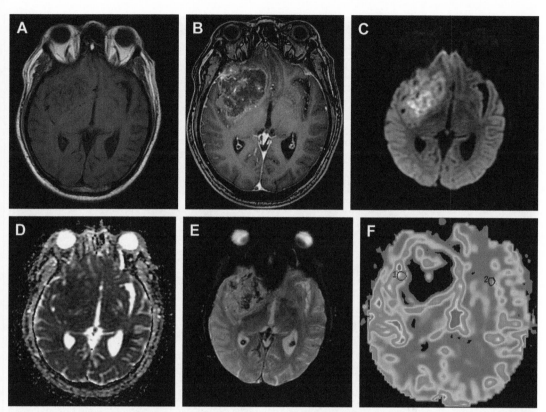

Fig. 1. Right insular glioblastoma. Axial T1 (*A*), axial T1 postgadolinium (*B*), axial DWI (*C*), axial ADC (*D*), axial T2* (*E*), color DSC perfusion cerebral blood volume map (*F*), DSC curves (*G*), right corticospinal tracts superimposed on axial T1 postgadolinium (*H*), and on sagittal reformat of high-resolution T2 (*I*), for operative navigation. This large infiltrative mass shows irregular enhancement, areas of hemorrhage on T2*, areas of mildly reduced diffusion, and increased relative cerebral blood volume (Green ROI (*F*) and curve (*G*) correspond to tumor/peritumoral region and purple ROI and curve correspond to contralateral side).

be used to derive numerous parameters.[7] DTI and other similar advanced (predominately research) techniques such as diffusion-spectrum imaging, diffusion-kurtosis imaging, and tract-density imaging provide additional insight beyond DWI into the microstructure and integrity of the white matter.[3] Fractional anisotropy (FA), mean diffusivity, track density, neuronal density, and multiple other measures derived from these techniques all offer additional means to study brain tumors and the effects of treatment, which may be further realized in the future. DTI is currently most relevant clinically as tractography, whereby white matter fiber tracts are derived from the DTI data based on fiber tracking of anisotropy from anatomic seed points. These white matter tracts are then displayed three-dimensionally for navigational purposes.[8,9] At our institution, tractography of the corticospinal tracts and optic radiations is routinely displayed superimposed on high-resolution three-dimensional (3D) T2-weighted and postgadolinium spoiled gradient echo recalled images for intraoperative navigational purposes with additional

tracts of interest, such as the arcuate fasciculus, produced in certain cases (**Fig. 1H, I, 3D**).

T2* Susceptibility-sensitive Sequences (Tagging: Susceptibility-weighted Imaging, T2*, Susceptibility, Microhemorrhage)

High-resolution 3D T2* gradient echo sequences such as SWI offer high sensitivity to small regions of magnetic susceptibility,[10,11] which includes susceptibility from iron, making susceptibility-sensitive sequences excellent for the depiction of hemorrhage and microhemorrhage (**Figs. 1E, 3B and 4D**).[10,11] The magnitude images depict hemorrhage, blood vessels, and calcification/mineralization as dark lack of signal from susceptibility (see **Figs. 1E; 3B, 4D**). However, phase images can potentially be useful to distinguish iron and deoxygenated blood products (paramagnetic and dark on a right-handed system) from calcium (diamagnetic and bright on a right-handed system).[10,11] Minimum intensity projection images can also be reviewed to more clearly differentiate

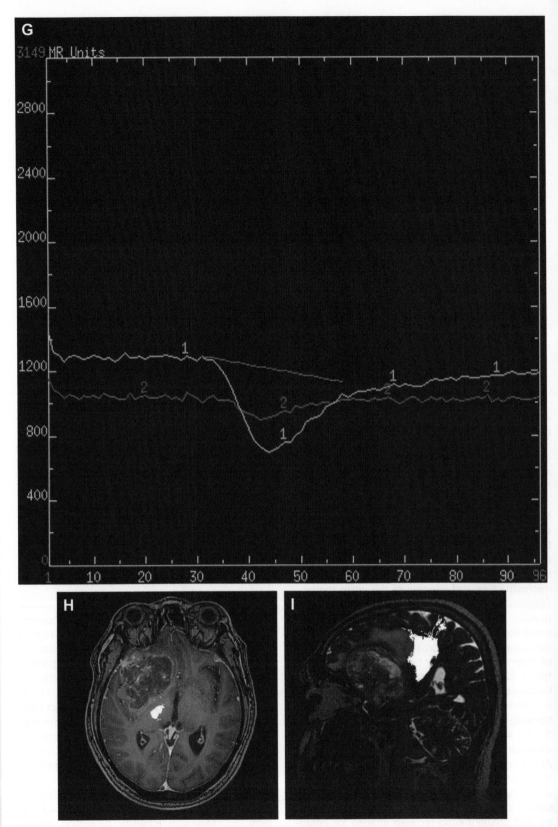

Fig. 1.

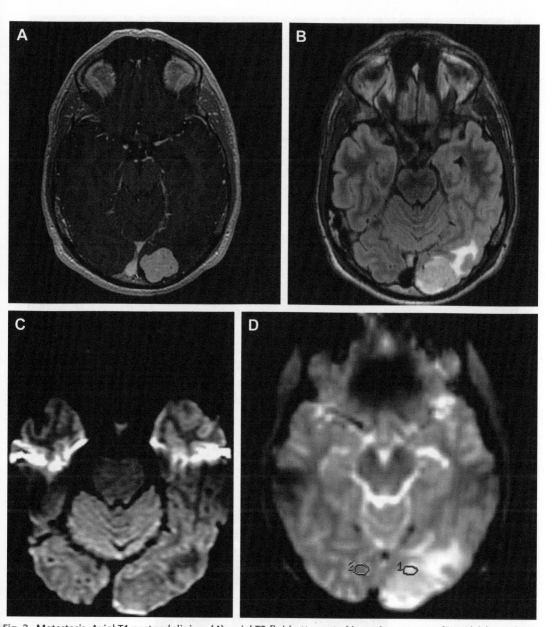

Fig. 2. Metastasis. Axial T1 postgadolinium (*A*), axial T2 fluid-attenuated inversion recovery (FLAIR) (*B*), axial DWI (*C*), axial DSC perfusion (*D*), DSC perfusion curves (*E*), and color DSC perfusion cerebral blood volume map (*F*). This solitary enhancing lesion with surrounding vasogenic edema was a fibrolamellar hepatocellular carcinoma metastasis. Although there is increased relative cerebral blood flow (Purple ROI (*D*) and curve (*E*) correspond to tumor and green ROI and curve correspond to contralateral side), the curve (*top purple curve in E*) does not return close to baseline, consistent with a metastasis with leaky capillaries.

normal venous structures from parenchymal foci of susceptibility.[10,11]

Magnetic Resonance Spectroscopy (Tagging: Magnetic Resonance Spectroscopy)

MRS provides insight into the chemical profile of interrogated brain tissue. Proton (^{1}H) MRS is the most clinically relevant technique. The most

recognizable peaks on long-echo ^{1}H-MRS, which are of interest in the evaluation of brain tumors, include *N*-acetylaspartate (NAA) at approximately 2.0 parts per million (ppm), creatine (Cr) at approximately 3.0 ppm, and choline (Cho) at approximately 3.2 ppm.[12] NAA is considered a neuronal marker, Cr a marker for cellular metabolism, and Cho a marker for cell membrane turnover. Additional metabolites of interest include lipid and

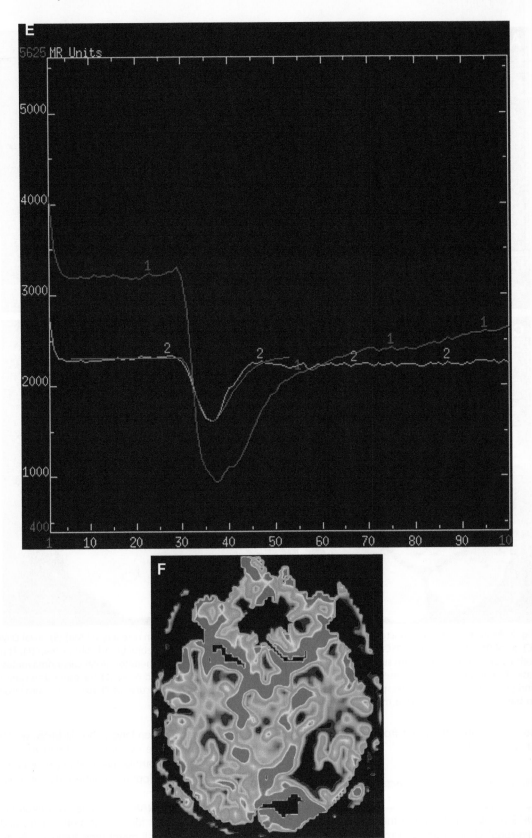

Fig. 2.

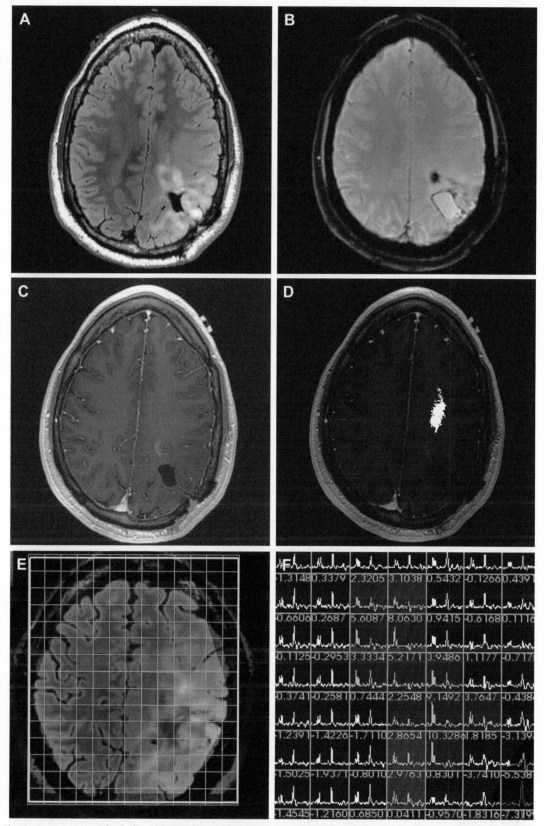

Fig. 3. Recurrent/residual oligodendroglioma. Axial T2 FLAIR (*A*), axial T2* (*B*), axial T1 postgadolinium (*C*), axial T1 postgadolinium with superimposed left corticospinal tracts for surgical navigation (*D*), and multivoxel long-echo MRS with color overlay on axial T2 FLAIR (*E*) and spectra (*F*). Choline/NAA ratios of greater than 2 are color coded with ratios greater than 4 red. Increased choline/NAA is shown in voxels corresponding with the infiltrative masslike T2 FLAIR hyperintensity surrounding the left parietal resection cavity.

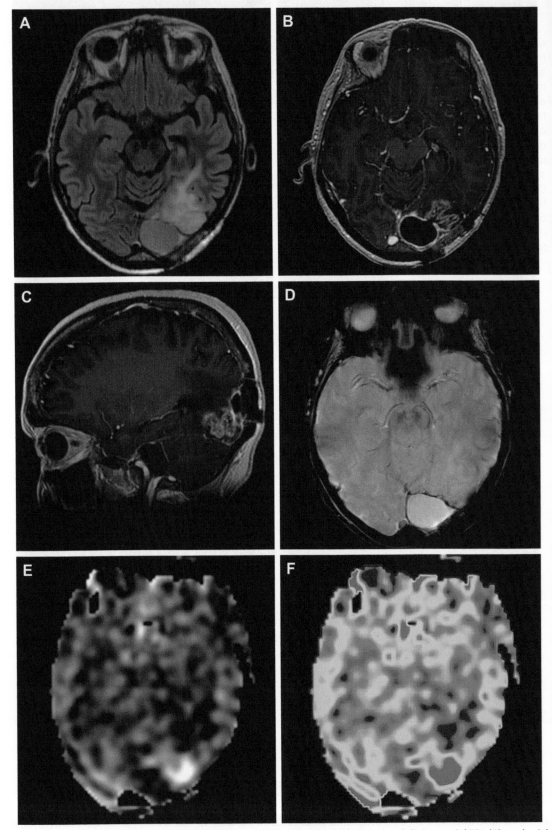

Fig. 4. Recurrent glioblastoma. Axial T2 FLAIR (*A*), axial (*B*) and sagittal (*C*) T1 postgadolinium, axial T2* (*D*), and axial ASL perfusion CBF map in greyscale (*E*) and color (*F*). This masslike T2 FLAIR hyperintense, irregularly enhancing lesion showing increased CBF located just anterior to the left occipital resection cavity was recurrent glioblastoma.

lactate peaks at approximately 1.3 ppm and myo-inositol at approximately 3.5 ppm. Lipids and lactate are considered markers of necrosis and hypoxia, respectively, and myo-inositol is considered to be related to astrocytic integrity and regulation of brain osmosis.[12–15] Clinically, MRS is performed with a single-voxel technique to a targeted region of interest or with a multivoxel or 3D technique in order to cover a broader area and evaluate regional differences (Figs. 3E, F and 5C, D). In general, long-echo MRS is performed for the evaluation of brain tumors (288 milliseconds or 144 milliseconds if trying to invert a lactate peak). A short-echo technique can be used if trying to show myo-inositol. A related emerging method

currently confined to research use is hyperpolarized ^{13}C MR. Hyperpolarized ^{13}C agents have a greatly increased signal, which provides the opportunity to follow a substance such as pyruvate through its biochemical pathways as it is converted to alanine, lactate, and bicarbonate.[16,17]

Perfusion Imaging (Tagging: Perfusion, Dynamic Susceptibility Contrast Enhanced, Dynamic Contrast Enhanced, Arterial Spin Labeling)

The 2 main established contrast-based methods of MR perfusion imaging in brain tumors are T2*-weighted DSC perfusion and T1-weighted

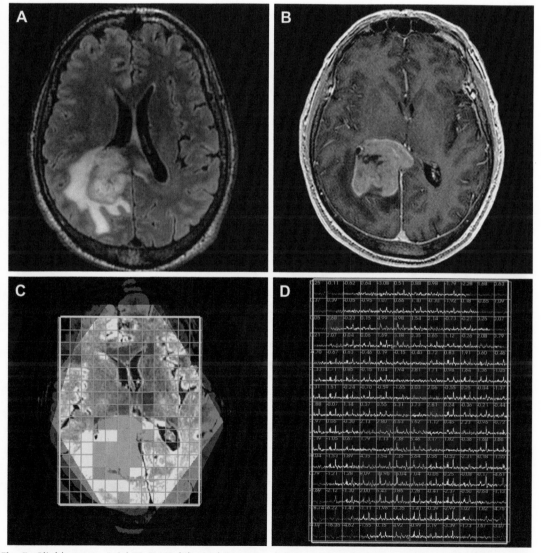

Fig. 5. Glioblastoma. Axial T2 FLAIR (A), axial T1 postgadolinium (B), and multivoxel long-echo MRS with color overlay on axial T2 FLAIR (C) and spectra (D). Choline/NAA ratios of greater than 2 are color coded with ratios greater than 4 red. Increased choline/NAA is shown in voxels corresponding with the infiltrative mass.

dynamic contrast-enhanced (DCE) perfusion.[18–21] DSC (Figs. 1F, G and 2D, E, F) is a negative-contrast first-pass bolus tracking blood volume technique and DCE is a positive-contrast steady-state permeability technique. Both can be used to derive multiple perfusion parameters, such as cerebral blood volume (CBV) and endothelial transfer coefficient (K^{trans}).[22] Relative CBV (rCBV), which is the calculated CBV relative to the contralateral side, is the most widely used parameter derived from DSC and is considered a marker of angiogenesis. The main metric derived from DCE perfusion MR imaging is K^{trans}, considered a measure of microvascular permeability. Arterial spin labeling (ASL) is a more recently

clinically available noncontrast perfusion technique that quantitatively measures cerebral blood flow (CBF) with applicability to a broad range of disease states (Figs. 4E, F, 6C, D, 7E, F).[23–25] We have recently converted our brain tumor protocols to use ASL as the preferred perfusion method because ASL is quick, images the whole brain, and has little postprocessing. In ASL, an inversion pulse is used to tag or label inflowing blood proximal to the area of imaging and these labeled spins are imaged along with control images. Pairwise subtraction of labeled and control images yields CBF maps with normal increased CBF in gray matter compared with white matter (see Figs. 4E, F, 6C, D, 7E, F).[23]

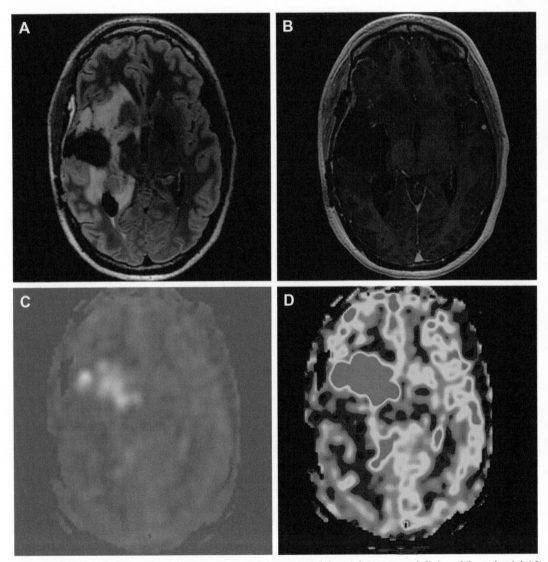

Fig. 6. Residual grade III anaplastic astrocytoma. Axial T2 FLAIR (A), axial T1 postgadolinium (B), and axial ASL perfusion CBF map in grayscale (C) and color (D). There is increased CBF corresponding with the residual infiltrative tumor anterior to the resection cavity.

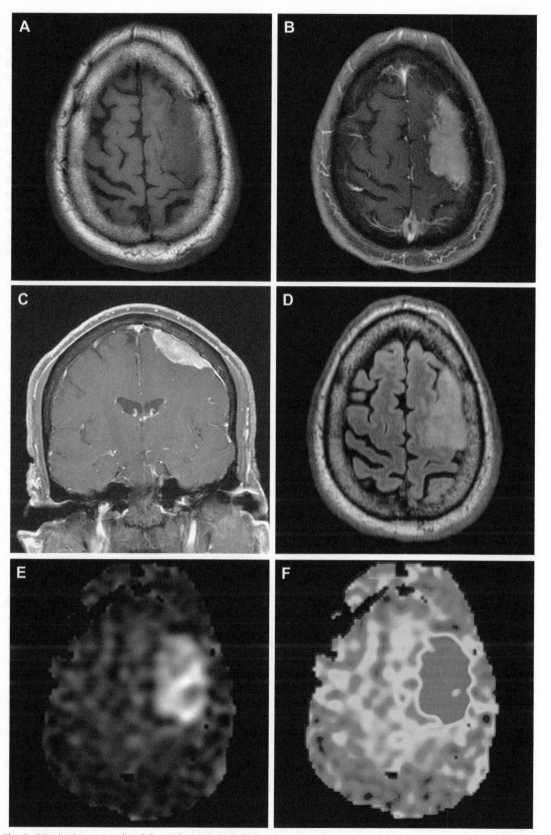

Fig. 7. Meningioma. Axial T1 (*A*), axial T1 postgadolinium (*B*), coronal T1 postgadolinium (*C*), axial T2 FLAIR (*D*), and axial ASL perfusion CBF map in grayscale (*E*) and color (*F*). This large homogeneously enhancing extra-axial meningioma overlying the left frontal lobe shows markedly increased cerebral blood flow, consistent with a highly vascular tumor.

Functional MR Imaging (Tagging: Blood Oxygen Level Dependent, Functional MR Imaging, Resting-state Functional MR Imaging)

fMR imaging uses relative changes in the blood oxygen level–dependent (BOLD) signal to infer brain activity because activity correlates with blood flow and blood flow with BOLD signal.[26] During task-based fMR imaging the BOLD sequence is performed during the performance of a task administered as a standardized paradigm (Fig. 8). Non–task-based imaging, in which the sequence is performed at rest, is known as resting-state fMR imaging (RS-fMR imaging). RS-fMR imaging uses spontaneous low-frequency fluctuations (<0.1 Hz) in the BOLD signal to pick out areas of correlation and anticorrelation, which form the basis for defining resting-state networks, the most widely studied of which is the default mode network.[26–29] RS-fMR imaging has some distinct advantages compared with task-based fMR imaging, including not having to administer a paradigm, the ability to study patients who may not be able to fully cooperate with a paradigm (eg, children, patients with altered mental status), and the ability to detect many networks retrospectively. Vascular tumors can potentially affect the BOLD signal; however, both task-based and RS-fMR imaging have been effectively applied in patients with brain tumors (see Table 1).

IMAGING FINDINGS/PATHOLOGY
Diffusion-weighted Imaging and Related Techniques (Tagging: Diffusion-weighted Imaging, Diffusion-tensor Imaging)

DWI offers valuable insight into the diffusion of water molecules in tissues and is of value in the evaluation of patients with brain tumors. ADC values derived from DWI are generally decreased in highly cellular tumors such as central nervous system (CNS) lymphoma, medulloblastoma, and high-grade glioma (see Fig. 1C, D) and in highly viscous materials such as within cerebral abscesses.[30–37] In primary CNS lymphoma, patients with lower tumor ADC values have also been reported to have poorer survival than patients with higher tumor ADC values.[30,38] In patients with glioma, lower ADC values have been associated with higher-grade gliomas and lower ADC values have been associated with a poorer prognosis independent of tumor grade.[39–41] ADC values may also provide insight into T2/fluid-attenuated inversion recovery (FLAIR) signal abnormality surrounding an enhancing lesion. Although this has not been found consistently in all studies, ADC values

have been reported to be higher in vasogenic peritumoral edema T2/FLAIR abnormality surrounding enhancing metastases than in the more cellular infiltrative peritumoral edema T2/FLAIR abnormality seen in glioblastoma.[41–44]

On immediate postoperative imaging, it is common to see small areas of reduced ADC surrounding the surgical bed, indicating areas of devitalized tumor tissue or devitalized ischemic brain tissue related to surgery.[45] These areas may be expected to evolve as a cerebral infarction would and develop contrast enhancement and normalization of ADC on subsequent imaging; contrast enhancement that develops in the appropriate time course and corresponds with these areas should not be mistaken for tumor progression.[45]

DWI is also helpful in the follow-up imaging of patients with brain tumors, particularly in the settings of antiangiogenic treatment and in distinguishing treatment effect from true tumor progression. The antiangiogenic effects of bevacizumab may markedly decrease the contrast enhancement of a tumor; however, DWI may be useful to show persistent or progressive nonenhancing tumor despite the lack of contrast enhancement.[46] However, interpretation of new areas of reduced diffusion in patients on bevacizumab is complex and currently incompletely understood; reduced diffusion can develop in tumor and in ischemic areas of normal brain and can persist over time, possibly related to ischemic necrosis.[47,48] Interpretation of these diffusion abnormalities in patients on bevacizumab requires follow-up over time and consideration of additional advanced imaging sequences such as perfusion and spectroscopy. With regard to the question of treatment effect versus true tumor progression, lower ADC values have been reported in true tumor progression than in the setting of pseudoprogression, likely because of the cellular nature of true progressive tumor and the edema associated with the inflammatory response in treatment-related pseudoprogression.[49,50]

As mentioned, DTI is currently most relevant clinically as tractography for surgical planning and navigational purposes (see Figs. 1H, I and 3D).[8,9] FA derived from DTI has been used as a marker of white matter integrity in multiple conditions and although primarily of research interest it may offer insight into the effects of radiation damage to the brains of patients with brain tumors. FA has been shown to decrease in normal-appearing white matter following radiation therapy, showing white matter injury and likely decreased structural connectivity.[51,52] FA may also offer some insight into the T2/FLAIR

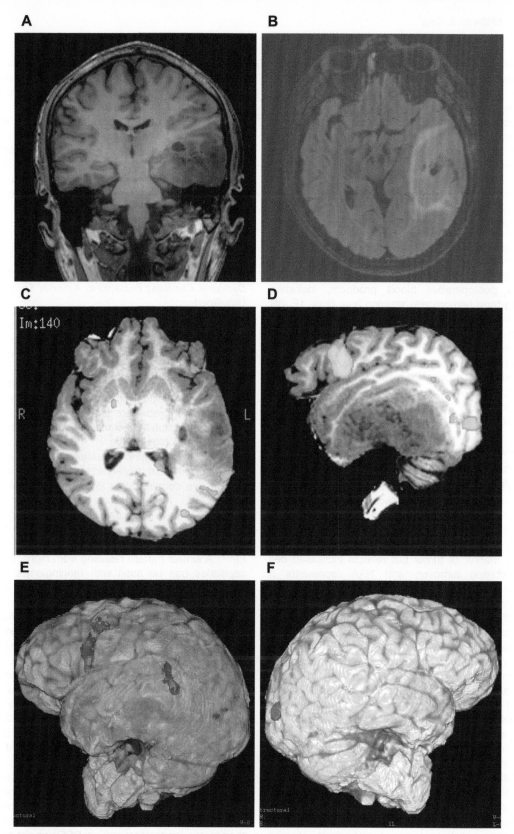

Fig. 8. Coronal T1 (*A*), axial T2 FLAIR (*B*), and fMR imaging showing functional activation during a semantic language paradigm represented on axial T1 (*C*), left sided sagittal T1 (*D*), surface rendering of the left side of the brain (*E*), and surface rendering of the right side of the brain (*F*), showing left language dominance with activation predominantly on the left side; the side of the infiltrative left temporal lobe mass.

signal abnormality surrounding enhancing lesions; FA has been reported to be increased in the infiltrative peritumoral edema surrounding high-grade gliomas compared with the vasogenic edema surrounding metastases, presumably because of the more ordered nature of the more cellular edema associated with gliomas.[53]

T2* Susceptibility–sensitive Sequences (Tagging: Susceptibility-weighted Imaging, SWAN, T2*, Susceptibility, Microhemorrhage)

In general T2*-based susceptibility-sensitive sequences such as SWI are useful to depict hemorrhage and calcification associated with tumors and postoperative blood products, including long-term hemosiderin staining (see **Figs. 1E, 3B and 4D**). These sequences are also useful to depict small microhemorrhages or small vascular malformations that develop over time in patients who have received radiation therapy.[54–56] These small foci of susceptibility likely indicate a delayed toxicity of radiation on the microvasculature of the brain and are well depicted by T2*-based susceptibility sensitive sequences.

Magnetic Resonance Spectroscopy (Tagging: Magnetic Resonance Spectroscopy)

The MRS profile of gliomas is generally considered to be increased Cho and decreased NAA, creating a characteristic downsloping appearance compared with the normal upsloping appearance (see **Figs. 3E, F and 5C, D**).[57–59] Cho is not a specific marker of tumor but reflects increased cell membrane turnover, and NAA represents a neuronal marker, decreased in the setting of tumor as well as many other conditions. Absolute heights of these peaks are generally not used and the metabolic peaks can be analyzed as ratios, including Cho/NAA and Cho/Cr. MRS can potentially be useful to differentiate high-grade gliomas from low-grade gliomas because high-grade gliomas have been found to have higher Cho/NAA and Cho/Cr ratios than lower-grade gliomas.[59,60] Lower-grade gliomas have been associated with an increased myo-inositol/Cr ratio (myo-inositol is best identified with a short echo time of 35 milliseconds).[13]

MRS can also be useful in the evaluation of the T2/FLAIR signal abnormality surrounding an enhancing lesion; increased Cho/NAA and Cho/Cr ratios have been reported in the peritumoral infiltrative cellular edema of high-grade gliomas compared with the peritumoral vasogenic edema surrounding metastases.[61,62] MRS may also be useful in the ongoing posttreatment evaluation of

patients with brain tumors. Although this may be challenging to apply in daily practice, in the situation of possible treatment effect or radiation necrosis, higher Cho/NAA or Cho/Cr ratios have been reported in true progressive tumor compared with treatment effect or radiation necrosis (see **Fig. 3E, F**).[63–67] Some overlap may be seen in the ^{1}H-MRS of tumors and radiation change. An increase in Cho-containing compounds after radiation therapy as a result of cell damage and astrogliosis may be seen in radiation necrosis misclassified as tumors.[68,69]

Perfusion Imaging (Tagging: Perfusion, Dynamic Susceptibility Contrast Enhanced, Dynamic Contrast Enhanced, Arterial Spin Labeling)

DSC perfusion is the most studied and widely applied perfusion technique in the evaluation of patients with brain tumors, with rCBV being the main parameter of interest (see **Figs. 1F, G and 2D–F**).[18–21] rCBV may help distinguish glioma grade, because high-grade gliomas generally have higher rCBV than low-grade gliomas; however, this should be used with caution because oligodendrogliomas can also have high rCBVs.[18,70–74] rCBV may also be useful in distinguishing tumefactive demyelinating lesions from high-grade gliomas because tumefactive demyelinating lesions generally have lower rCBV.[75] Metastasis can have high rCBV, but they tend to have leaky capillaries with leakage of contrast, resulting in a signal intensity curve that does not return close to baseline (see **Fig. 2D–F**).[2,76] A similar pattern resulting from highly leaky capillaries can be seen with meningiomas and choroid plexus tumors.[2,18,77,78] rCBV has also been reported to be more increased within the infiltrative cellular peritumoral T2/FLAIR abnormality surrounding the enhancing portions of high-grade gliomas compared with the vasogenic peritumoral T2/FLAIR abnormality surrounding metastases.[61,79] DSC may also be helpful in the ongoing evaluation of patients with known brain tumors and the question of tumor versus treatment effect or radiation necrosis. Tumor has been shown to have higher rCBV than radiation necrosis and, although there may be more overlap, higher rCBV than in treatment effect/pseudoprogression.[18,80–82]

K^{trans}, the main metric derived from DCE, may potentially be used to distinguish glioma grade, with higher K^{trans} presumably caused by the greater capillary permeability seen in higher-grade gliomas than in low-grade gliomas.[83–86] DCE has not been as extensively studied as DSC in the evaluation of treatment response and the question of treatment effect versus true progression but has been reported to be able to distinguish recurrent or progressive tumor from pseudoprogression using the maximum slope of initial enhancement.[87]

ASL perfusion imaging has not been extensively studied in the setting of brain tumor but has been found to show increased CBF in vascular tumors such as meningiomas and many metastases and high-grade gliomas (see Figs. 4E, F, 6C, D, 7E, F).[25,88] Although the experience is limited, ASL has been used to predict glioma grade, with higher-grade tumors showing higher perfusion.[88] The authors have found ASL to be a very helpful and easily applied technique with distinct feasibility advantages compared with other perfusion techniques. Limited early experience suggests that increased CBF is likely to be predictive of residual/recurrent tumor as opposed to treatment effect (see Figs. 4E, F, 6C, D).

Functional MR Imaging (Tagging- Blood Oxygen Level–Dependent, Functional MR Imaging, Resting-state Functional MR Imaging)

Task-based fMR imaging can be used for preoperative localization of eloquent cortex with identification of language and somatomotor function with similar accuracy to more invasive techniques (see Fig. 8).[89–91] Task-based fMR imaging is one of several measures that are useful for preoperative planning to identify the relationship of a brain tumor to important functional cortex.[92] The distance from the functional area depicted on task-based fMR imaging to a tumor to be resected has been correlated with the degree of postoperative loss of function, with a small margin (<1 cm) predicting a poorer outcome.[92]

RS-fMR imaging has also been used to identify eloquent cortex as part of presurgical planning in patients with brain tumors.[93] Although the experience is more limited, several studies have shown the ability to localize somatosensory cortex in relationship to brain tumors.[94,95] RS-fMR imaging offers the ability to study functional connectivity of the brain and is thus a potentially powerful research sequence for studying the brains of patients with tumors and the effects of treatment. To date there have been several small studies that have shown decreased functional connectivity in resting-state networks in patients with brain tumors but this is expected to be an ongoing area of active research in the future.[96–98]

Diagnostic criteria
Technique
DWI
Low ADC: cellular tumor such as lymphoma, high-grade gliomas often with areas of mildly reduced diffusion
Postoperative cytotoxic edema in devitalized tissues
Higher ADC: surrounding vasogenic edema as opposed to cellular infiltrative edema. Treatment effect may have higher ADC values than true progression, but difficult to distinguish in daily clinical practice
DTI
Infiltrative tumors may infiltrate as opposed to displace functional tracts, complicating and likely precluding surgical resection
DSC perfusion
Perfusion curves in gliomas should return close to baseline
Perfusion curves with leaky capillaries (metastases, choroid plexus tumors, extra-axial tumors) generally do not return close to baseline
Higher rCBV is suggestive of higher-grade as opposed to lower-grade glioma and in the setting of follow-up is suggestive of true progression as opposed to treatment effect
DCE perfusion
Higher permeability suggestive of higher-grade glioma as opposed to lower-grade glioma. Within a tumor may potentially identify areas of higher grade

ASL

Higher blood flow may be useful to identify areas of recurrent tumor

Although experience is limited, higher blood flow may be seen in higher-grade as opposed to lower-grade gliomas

MRS

Gliomas generally characterized by increased choline (3.2 ppm) and decreased NAA (2.0 ppm) levels, although this is nonspecific

Higher-grade gliomas show higher choline/NAA and choline/creatine ratios than lower-grade gliomas

Higher choline ratios are also suggestive of true progressive tumor compared with treatment effect/necrosis

Susceptibility-sensitive imaging

Useful to show/identify tumor mimics such as cavernous malformations

Identify blood products and calcifications. Identify radiation-induced microhemorrhages/induced vascular malformations

fMR imaging

Select cases for preoperative functional localization

RS-fMR imaging

Research use for identifying resting-state networks and evaluating changes in functional connectivity

---

Differential diagnosis

Pearls, pitfalls, variants: bulleted list

- Areas of low ADC signifying postoperative cytotoxic edema immediately following a tumor resection can be expected to enhance on subsequent follow-up imaging as a subacute stroke would. Review the initial immediate postoperative MR imaging on follow-up.

- Lower ADC values, higher rCBV, and higher choline/NAA ratio are all suggestive of higher-grade as opposed to lower-grade glioma and in follow-up are all suggestive of residual/progressive tumor as opposed to treatment effect/necrosis. This distinction can be difficult to implement in daily practice but can be useful in problem solving.

- A brain mass with a DSC perfusion curve that does not return close to baseline is likely a metastasis or extra-axial tumor.

What referring physicians need to know

- On initial evaluation, could it be a tumor mimic? Make a phone call and discuss whether there is something that makes you question whether this is truly a tumor. A small initial biopsy and frozen pathology may be warranted.

- On follow-up, is there convincing progressive tumor or could a progressive abnormality be treatment related? Multiple imaging sequences suggesting true progression are useful to communicate degree of certainty. Time should help clarify.

- It may be useful to communicate to neuro-oncologists in terms of grading a follow-up MR imaging as −2 (convincing/definite tumor progression), −1 (possible tumor progression), 0 (not significantly changed), +1 (possible improvement of tumor burden), +2 (definite improvement of tumor burden).

SUMMARY

The evaluation of patients with brain tumors with imaging continues to evolve and many advanced imaging techniques that evaluate physiologic information are now routine parts of the MR imaging examination. These advanced imaging techniques are all invaluable tools for the evaluation of patients with brain tumors and may all positively affect patient care. Their use is not always straightforward, but they all form a part of the armamentarium of the modern neuroradiologist that can be used as important problem-solving tools. Understanding of these techniques and their clinical application may make the difference in the interpretation of subtle/difficult cases because many of these sequences offer insight into physiologic information beyond standard structural imaging. Ongoing research is needed to clarify and define the roles of all of these techniques, and may offer additional insight into genetic, prognostic, and predictive information that may be further elucidated in the future.

REFERENCES

1. Mabray MC, Barajas RF Jr, Cha S. Modern brain tumor imaging. Brain Tumor Res Treat 2015;3:8–23.
2. Cha S. Update on brain tumor imaging: from anatomy to physiology. AJNR Am J Neuroradiol 2006; 27:475–87.
3. Hagmann P, Jonasson L, Maeder P, et al. Understanding diffusion MR imaging techniques: from scalar diffusion-weighted imaging to diffusion tensor imaging and beyond. Radiographics 2006; 26(Suppl 1):S205–23.
4. Poustchi-Amin M, Mirowitz SA, Brown JJ, et al. Principles and applications of echo-planar imaging: a review for the general radiologist. Radiographics 2001;21:767–79.
5. Mukherjee P, Berman JI, Chung SW, et al. Diffusion tensor MR imaging and fiber tractography: theoretic underpinnings. AJNR Am J Neuroradiol 2008;29: 632–41.
6. Mukherjee P, Chung SW, Berman JI, et al. Diffusion tensor MR imaging and fiber tractography: technical considerations. AJNR Am J Neuroradiol 2008;29: 843–52.
7. Le Bihan D, Mangin JF, Poupon C, et al. Diffusion tensor imaging: concepts and applications. J Magn Reson Imaging 2001;13:534–46.
8. Elhawary H, Liu H, Patel P, et al. Intraoperative real-time querying of white matter tracts during frameless stereotactic neuronavigation. Neurosurgery 2011; 68:506–16 [discussion: 516].
9. Okada T, Mikuni N, Miki Y, et al. Corticospinal tract localization: integration of diffusion-tensor tractography at 3-T MR imaging with intraoperative white matter stimulation mapping–preliminary results. Radiology 2006;240:849–57.
10. Haacke EM. Susceptibility weighted imaging (SWI). Z Med Phys 2006;16:237.
11. Haacke EM, Mittal S, Wu Z, et al. Susceptibility-weighted imaging: technical aspects and clinical applications, part 1. AJNR Am J Neuroradiol 2009; 30:19–30.
12. Horska A, Barker PB. Imaging of brain tumors: MR spectroscopy and metabolic imaging. Neuroimaging Clin North Am 2010;20:293–310.
13. Castillo M, Smith JK, Kwock L. Correlation of myo-inositol levels and grading of cerebral astrocytomas. AJNR Am J Neuroradiol 2000;21:1645–9.
14. Howe FA, Barton SJ, Cudlip SA, et al. Metabolic profiles of human brain tumors using quantitative in vivo 1H magnetic resonance spectroscopy. Magn Reson Med 2003;49:223–32.
15. Haris M, Cai K, Singh A, et al. In vivo mapping of brain myo-inositol. Neuroimage 2011;54:2079–85.
16. Nelson SJ, Vigneron D, Kurhanewicz J, et al. DNP-hyperpolarized C magnetic resonance metabolic imaging for cancer applications. Appl Magn Reson 2008;34:533–44.
17. Park I, Larson PE, Zierhut ML, et al. Hyperpolarized 13C magnetic resonance metabolic imaging: application to brain tumors. Neuro Oncol 2010; 12:133–44.
18. Welker K, Boxerman J, Kalnin A, et al. ASFNR recommendations for clinical performance of MR dynamic susceptibility contrast perfusion imaging of the brain. AJNR Am J Neuroradiol 2015;36: E41–51.
19. Essig M, Nguyen TB, Shiroishi MS, et al. Perfusion MRI: the five most frequently asked clinical questions. AJR Am J Roentgenol 2013;201:W495–510.
20. Petrella JR, Provenzale JM. MR perfusion imaging of the brain: techniques and applications. AJR Am J Roentgenol 2000;175:207–19.
21. Wong JC, Provenzale JM, Petrella JR. Perfusion MR imaging of brain neoplasms. AJR Am J Roentgenol 2000;174:1147–57.
22. Zaharchuk G. Theoretical basis of hemodynamic MR imaging techniques to measure cerebral blood volume, cerebral blood flow, and permeability. AJNR Am J Neuroradiol 2007;28:1850–8.
23. Deibler AR, Pollock JM, Kraft RA, et al. Arterial spin-labeling in routine clinical practice, part 1: technique and artifacts. AJNR Am J Neuroradiol 2008;29: 1228–34.
24. Deibler AR, Pollock JM, Kraft RA, et al. Arterial spin-labeling in routine clinical practice, part 2: hypoperfusion patterns. AJNR Am J Neuroradiol 2008;29: 1235–41.
25. Deibler AR, Pollock JM, Kraft RA, et al. Arterial spin-labeling in routine clinical practice,

part 3: hyperperfusion patterns. AJNR Am J Neuro-radiol 2008;29:1428–35.

26. Lee MH, Smyser CD, Shimony JS. Resting-state fMRI: a review of methods and clinical applications. AJNR Am J Neuroradiol 2013;34:1866–72.

27. Fox MD, Snyder AZ, Vincent JL, et al. The human brain is intrinsically organized into dynamic, anticor-related functional networks. Proc Natl Acad Sci U S A 2005;102:9673–8.

28. De Luca M, Beckmann CF, De Stefano N, et al. fMRI resting state networks define distinct modes of long-distance interactions in the human brain. Neuro-image 2006;29:1359–67.

29. Biswal B, Yetkin FZ, Haughton VM, et al. Functional connectivity in the motor cortex of resting human brain using echo-planar MRI. Magn Reson Med 1995;34:537–41.

30. Barajas RF Jr, Rubenstein JL, Chang JS, et al. Diffu-sion-weighted MR imaging derived apparent diffu-sion coefficient is predictive of clinical outcome in primary central nervous system lymphoma. AJNR Am J Neuroradiol 2010;31:60–6.

31. Guo AC, Cummings TJ, Dash RC, et al. Lymphomas and high-grade astrocytomas: comparison of water diffusibility and histologic characteristics. Radiology 2002;224:177–83.

32. Herneth AM, Guccione S, Bednarski M. Apparent diffusion coefficient: a quantitative parameter for in vivo tumor characterization. Eur J Radiol 2003; 45:208–13.

33. Tung GA, Evangelista P, Rogg JM, et al. Diffusion-weighted MR imaging of rim-enhancing brain masses: is markedly decreased water diffusion spe-cific for brain abscess? AJR Am J Roentgenol 2001; 177:709–12.

34. Stadnik TW, Chaskis C, Michotte A, et al. Diffusion-weighted MR imaging of intracerebral masses: comparison with conventional MR imaging and histo-logic findings. AJNR Am J Neuroradiol 2001;22:969–76.

35. Ebisu T, Tanaka C, Umeda M, et al. Discrimination of brain abscess from necrotic or cystic tumors by diffusion-weighted echo planar imaging. Magn Re-son Imaging 1996;14:1113–6.

36. Desprechins B, Stadnik T, Koerts G, et al. Use of diffusion-weighted MR imaging in differential diag-nosis between intracerebral necrotic tumors and ce-rebral abscesses. AJNR Am J Neuroradiol 1999;20: 1252–7.

37. Rumboldt Z, Camacho DL, Lake D, et al. Apparent diffusion coefficients for differentiation of cerebellar tumors in children. AJNR Am J Neuroradiol 2006; 27:1362–9.

38. Valles FE, Perez-Valles CL, Regalado S, et al. Combined diffusion and perfusion MR imaging as biomarkers of prognosis in immunocompetent pa-tients with primary central nervous system lym-phoma. AJNR Am J Neuroradiol 2013;34:35–40.

39. Hilario A, Sepulveda JM, Perez-Nunez A, et al. A prognostic model based on preoperative MRI pre-dicts overall survival in patients with diffuse gliomas. AJNR Am J Neuroradiol 2014;35:1096–102.

40. Bulakbasi N, Guvenc I, Onguru O, et al. The added value of the apparent diffusion coefficient calculation to magnetic resonance imaging in the differentiation and grading of malignant brain tumors. J Comput Assist Tomogr 2004;28:735–46.

41. Kono K, Inoue Y, Nakayama K, et al. The role of diffusion-weighted imaging in patients with brain tu-mors. AJNR Am J Neuroradiol 2001;22:1081–8.

42. Lee EJ, terBrugge K, Mikulis D, et al. Diagnostic value of peritumoral minimum apparent diffusion co-efficient for differentiation of glioblastoma multiforme from solitary metastatic lesions. AJR Am J Roent-genol 2011;196:71–6.

43. Oh J, Cha S, Aiken AH, et al. Quantitative apparent diffusion coefficients and T2 relaxation times in char-acterizing contrast enhancing brain tumors and re-gions of peritumoral edema. J Magn Reson Imaging 2005;21:701–8.

44. Server A, Kulle B, Maehlen J, et al. Quantitative apparent diffusion coefficients in the characteriza-tion of brain tumors and associated peritumoral edema. Acta Radiol 2009;50:682–9.

45. Smith JS, Cha S, Mayo MC, et al. Serial diffusion-weighted magnetic resonance imaging in cases of glioma: distinguishing tumor recurrence from post-resection injury. J Neurosurg 2005;103:428–38.

46. Jain R, Scarpace LM, Ellika S, et al. Imaging response criteria for recurrent gliomas treated with bevacizumab: role of diffusion weighted imaging as an imaging biomarker. J Neurooncol 2010;96: 423–31.

47. Mong S, Ellingson BM, Nghiemphu PL, et al. Persistent diffusion-restricted lesions in bevacizumab-treated malignant gliomas are asso-ciated with improved survival compared with matched controls. AJNR Am J Neuroradiol 2012; 33:1763–70.

48. Rieger J, Bahr O, Muller K, et al. Bevacizumab-induced diffusion-restricted lesions in malignant gli-oma patients. J Neurooncol 2010;99:49–56.

49. Lee WJ, Choi SH, Park CK, et al. Diffusion-weighted MR imaging for the differentiation of true progression from pseudoprogression following concomitant radiotherapy with temozolomide in patients with newly diagnosed high-grade gliomas. Acad Radiol 2012;19:1353–61.

50. Matsusue E, Fink JR, Rockhill JK, et al. Distinction between glioma progression and post-radiation change by combined physiologic MR imaging. Neuroradiology 2010;52:297–306.

51. Haris M, Kumar S, Raj MK, et al. Serial diffusion tensor imaging to characterize radiation-induced changes in normal-appearing white matter following

radiotherapy in patients with adult low-grade gliomas. Radiat Med 2008;26:140–50.

52. Kitahara S, Nakasu S, Murata K, et al. Evaluation of treatment-induced cerebral white matter injury by using diffusion-tensor MR imaging: initial experience. AJNR Am J Neuroradiol 2005;26:2200–6.

53. Lu S, Ahn D, Johnson G, et al. Peritumoral diffusion tensor imaging of high-grade gliomas and metastatic brain tumors. AJNR Am J Neuroradiol 2003;24:937–41.

54. Bian W, Hess CP, Chang SM, et al. Susceptibility-weighted MR imaging of radiation therapy-induced cerebral microbleeds in patients with glioma: a comparison between 3T and 7T. Neuroradiology 2014;56:91–6.

55. Gaensler EH, Dillon WP, Edwards MS, et al. Radiation-induced telangiectasia in the brain simulates cryptic vascular malformations at MR imaging. Radiology 1994;193:629–36.

56. Lupo JM, Chuang CF, Chang SM, et al. 7-Tesla susceptibility-weighted imaging to assess the effects of radiotherapy on normal-appearing brain in patients with glioma. Int J Radiat Oncol Biol Phys 2012;82:e493–500.

57. Tien RD, Lai PH, Smith JS, et al. Single-voxel proton brain spectroscopy examination (PROBE/SV) in patients with primary brain tumors. AJR Am J Roentgenol 1996;167:201–9.

58. McKnight TR, von dem Bussche MH, Vigneron DB, et al. Histopathological validation of a three-dimensional magnetic resonance spectroscopy index as a predictor of tumor presence. J Neurosurg 2002;97:794–802.

59. Fountas KN, Kapsalaki EZ, Vogel RL, et al. Noninvasive histologic grading of solid astrocytomas using proton magnetic resonance spectroscopy. Stereotact Funct Neurosurg 2004;82:90–7.

60. Huang Y, Lisboa PJ, El-Deredy W. Tumour grading from magnetic resonance spectroscopy: a comparison of feature extraction with variable selection. Stat Med 2003;22:147–64.

61. Law M, Cha S, Knopp EA, et al. High-grade gliomas and solitary metastases: differentiation by using perfusion and proton spectroscopic MR imaging. Radiology 2002;222:715–21.

62. Server A, Josefsen R, Kulle B, et al. Proton magnetic resonance spectroscopy in the distinction of high-grade cerebral gliomas from single metastatic brain tumors. Acta Radiol 2010;51:316–25.

63. Plotkin M, Eisenacher J, Bruhn H, et al. 123I-IMT SPECT and 1H MR-spectroscopy at 3.0 T in the differential diagnosis of recurrent or residual gliomas: a comparative study. J Neurooncol 2004;70:49–58.

64. Traber F, Block W, Flacke S, et al. 1H-MR Spectroscopy of brain tumors in the course of radiation therapy: Use of fast spectroscopic imaging and single-voxel spectroscopy for diagnosing recurrence. Rofo 2002;174:33–42 [in German].

65. Ando K, Ishikura R, Nagami Y, et al. Usefulness of Cho/Cr ratio in proton MR spectroscopy for differentiating residual/recurrent glioma from non-neoplastic lesions. Nihon Igaku Hoshasen Gakkai Zasshi 2004;64:121–6 [in Japanese].

66. Hygino da Cruz LC Jr, Rodriguez I, Domingues RC, et al. Pseudoprogression and pseudoresponse: imaging challenges in the assessment of posttreatment glioma. AJNR Am J Neuroradiol 2011;32:1978–85.

67. Henry RG, Vigneron DB, Fischbein NJ, et al. Comparison of relative cerebral blood volume and proton spectroscopy in patients with treated gliomas. AJNR Am J Neuroradiol 2000;21:357–66.

68. Hourani R, Brant LJ, Rizk T, et al. Can proton MR spectroscopic and perfusion imaging differentiate between neoplastic and nonneoplastic brain lesions in adults? AJNR Am J Neuroradiol 2008;29:366–72.

69. Brandao LA, Castillo M. Adult brain tumors: clinical applications of magnetic resonance spectroscopy. Neuroimaging Clin North Am 2013;23:527–55.

70. Aronen HJ, Gazit IE, Louis DN, et al. Cerebral blood volume maps of gliomas: comparison with tumor grade and histologic findings. Radiology 1994;191:41–51.

71. Knopp EA, Cha S, Johnson G, et al. Glial neoplasms: dynamic contrast-enhanced T2*-weighted MR imaging. Radiology 1999;211:791–8.

72. Lev MH, Ozsunar Y, Henson JW, et al. Glial tumor grading and outcome prediction using dynamic spin-echo MR susceptibility mapping compared with conventional contrast-enhanced MR: confounding effect of elevated rCBV of oligodendrogliomas [corrected]. AJNR Am J Neuroradiol 2004;25:214–21.

73. Cha S, Tihan T, Crawford F, et al. Differentiation of low-grade oligodendrogliomas from low-grade astrocytomas by using quantitative blood-volume measurements derived from dynamic susceptibility contrast-enhanced MR imaging. AJNR Am J Neuroradiol 2005;26:266–73.

74. Law M, Yang S, Babb JS, et al. Comparison of cerebral blood volume and vascular permeability from dynamic susceptibility contrast-enhanced perfusion MR imaging with glioma grade. AJNR Am J Neuroradiol 2004;25:746–55.

75. Cha S, Pierce S, Knopp EA, et al. Dynamic contrast-enhanced T2*-weighted MR imaging of tumefactive demyelinating lesions. AJNR Am J Neuroradiol 2001;22:1109–16.

76. Cha S, Lupo JM, Chen MH, et al. Differentiation of glioblastoma multiforme and single brain metastasis by peak height and percentage of signal intensity recovery derived from dynamic

susceptibility-weighted contrast-enhanced perfusion MR imaging. AJNR Am J Neuroradiol 2007; 28:1078–84.

77. Cha S, Knopp EA, Johnson G, et al. Intracranial mass lesions: dynamic contrast-enhanced susceptibility-weighted echo-planar perfusion MR imaging. Radiology 2002;223:11–29.

78. Saloner D, Uzelac A, Hetts S, et al. Modern meningioma imaging techniques. J Neurooncol 2010;99: 333–40.

79. Chiang IC, Kuo YT, Lu CY, et al. Distinction between high-grade gliomas and solitary metastases using peritumoral 3-T magnetic resonance spectroscopy, diffusion, and perfusion imagings. Neuroradiology 2004;46:619–27.

80. Kong DS, Kim ST, Kim EH, et al. Diagnostic dilemma of pseudoprogression in the treatment of newly diagnosed glioblastomas: the role of assessing relative cerebral blood flow volume and oxygen-6-methylguanine-DNA methyltransferase promoter methylation status. AJNR Am J Neuroradiol 2011; 32:382–7.

81. Barajas RF, Chang JS, Sneed PK, et al. Distinguishing recurrent intra-axial metastatic tumor from radiation necrosis following gamma knife radiosurgery using dynamic susceptibility-weighted contrast-enhanced perfusion MR imaging. AJNR Am J Neuroradiol 2009;30:367–72.

82. Barajas RF Jr, Chang JS, Segal MR, et al. Differentiation of recurrent glioblastoma multiforme from radiation necrosis after external beam radiation therapy with dynamic susceptibility-weighted contrast-enhanced perfusion MR imaging. Radiology 2009; 253:486–96.

83. Roberts HC, Roberts TP, Ley S, et al. Quantitative estimation of microvascular permeability in human brain tumors: correlation of dynamic Gd-DTPA-enhanced MR imaging with histopathologic grading. Acad Radiol 2002;9(Suppl 1):S151–5.

84. Roberts HC, Roberts TP, Bollen AW, et al. Correlation of microvascular permeability derived from dynamic contrast-enhanced MR imaging with histologic grade and tumor labeling index: a study in human brain tumors. Acad Radiol 2001;8:384–91.

85. Roberts HC, Roberts TP, Brasch RC, et al. Quantitative measurement of microvascular permeability in human brain tumors achieved using dynamic contrast-enhanced MR imaging: correlation with histologic grade. AJNR Am J Neuroradiol 2000;21: 891–9.

86. Patankar TF, Haroon HA, Mills SJ, et al. Is volume transfer coefficient (K(trans)) related to histologic grade in human gliomas? AJNR Am J Neuroradiol 2005;26:2455–65.

87. Narang J, Jain R, Arbab AS, et al. Differentiating treatment-induced necrosis from recurrent/progressive brain tumor using nonmodel-based semiquantitative indices derived from dynamic contrast-enhanced T1-weighted MR perfusion. Neuro Oncol 2011;13: 1037–46.

88. Kim HS, Kim SY. A prospective study on the added value of pulsed arterial spin-labeling and apparent diffusion coefficients in the grading of gliomas. AJNR Am J Neuroradiol 2007;28:1693–9.

89. Binder JR, Swanson SJ, Hammeke TA, et al. Determination of language dominance using functional MRI: a comparison with the Wada test. Neurology 1996;46:978–84.

90. Adcock JE, Wise RG, Oxbury JM, et al. Quantitative fMRI assessment of the differences in lateralization of language-related brain activation in patients with temporal lobe epilepsy. Neuroimage 2003;18: 423–38.

91. Vlieger EJ, Majoie CB, Leenstra S, et al. Functional magnetic resonance imaging for neurosurgical planning in neurooncology. Eur Radiol 2004;14:1143–53.

92. Haberg A, Kvistad KA, Unsgard G, et al. Preoperative blood oxygen level-dependent functional magnetic resonance imaging in patients with primary brain tumors: clinical application and outcome. Neurosurgery 2004;54:902–14 [discussion: 914–5].

93. Shimony JS, Zhang D, Johnston JM, et al. Resting-state spontaneous fluctuations in brain activity: a new paradigm for presurgical planning using fMRI. Acad Radiol 2009;16:578–83.

94. Zhang D, Johnston JM, Fox MD, et al. Preoperative sensorimotor mapping in brain tumor patients using spontaneous fluctuations in neuronal activity imaged with functional magnetic resonance imaging: initial experience. Neurosurgery 2009;65:226–36.

95. Kokkonen SM, Nikkinen J, Remes J, et al. Preoperative localization of the sensorimotor area using independent component analysis of resting-state fMRI. Magn Reson Imaging 2009;27:733–40.

96. Mickevicius N, Sabsevitz D, Bovi J, et al. Effects of whole-brain radiation therapy on resting state connectivity: a case study. Int J Radiat Oncol Biol Phys 2014;90:S325.

97. Sours C, Mistry N, Zhang H, et al. Feasibility study testing the incorporation of resting state fMRI data in radiation therapy planning to limit dose to cognitive function networks in patients with primary brain tumors. Int J Radiat Oncol Biol Phys 2013;87:S254–5.

98. Harris RJ, Bookheimer SY, Cloughesy TF, et al. Altered functional connectivity of the default mode network in diffuse gliomas measured with pseudo-resting state fMRI. J Neurooncol 2014;116:373–9.

Adult Brain Tumors and Pseudotumors
Interesting (Bizarre) Cases

Lazaro D. Causil, MD[a],*, Romy Ames, MD[a],
Paulo Puac, MD[a], Mauricio Castillo, MD[b]

KEYWORDS

- Bizarre tumors • Adult brain tumors • Tumor histology • Prognosis • Imaging findings
- Differential diagnosis • Treatment

KEY POINTS

- The most likely diagnosis of a hemorrhagic pineal lesion associated with elevated serum β-HCG levels in CSF is pineal choriocarcinoma (PCCC).
- Meningioangiomatosis (MA) is a rare epileptogenic pseudotumor that in a majority of the cases shows calcifications and cortical invasion mimicking a malignant meningioma.
- Diffuse midline glioma (DMG) comprises 80% of all brain stem tumors in children and 80% of them are malignant.
- Papillary glioneuronal tumor (PGNT) is a rare cystic mass with an enhancing mural nodule located in the temporal lobes.
- Diffuse leptomeningeal glioneuronal tumor (DLGNT) is a very rare and aggressive disease with fatal outcome.

INTRODUCTION

This article discusses the most important features regarding epidemiology, prevailing location, clinical presentation, histopathology, and imaging findings of cases that the authors consider interesting due to their rarity. New nomenclature related to these tumors is included, according to the 2016 World Health Organization (WHO) central nervous system (CNS) tumor classification.[1] A review of the most recent literature dealing with these unusual tumors and pseudotumors is presented, highlighting key points related to the diagnosis, treatments, outcomes, and differential diagnosis.

PINEAL CHORIOCARCINOMA

PCCC is a rare malignant nongerminomatous germ cell tumor (GCT) and most aggressive form of the gestational trophoblastic disease that has an exceedingly low survival rate when compared with other GCTs.[2,3] PCCC is always mixed with other elements of GCTs and because they contain syncytiotrophoblasts (β-HCG–producing cells) they result in high levels of HCG in blood and CSF.[3,4] Due to their location, they cause hydrocephalus despite a small size.[5,6] A key imaging feature of PCCCs is the presence of intratumoral hemorrhage, which correlates with a poor prognosis.[3]

Funding Sources: None.

Disclosures: The authors have nothing to disclose.

Conflict of Interests: None.

[a] Neuroradiology Section, Department of Radiology, University of North Carolina School of Medicine, Room 3326, Old Infirmary Building, Manning Drive, Chapel Hill, NC 27599-7510, USA; [b] Department of Radiology, University of North Carolina School of Medicine, Room 3326, Old Infirmary Building, Manning Drive, Chapel Hill, NC 27599-7510, USA

* Corresponding author.

E-mail addresses: Lazaro_causil@med.unc.edu; Lazaroc66@gmail.com

1052-5149/16/© 2016 Elsevier Inc. All rights reserved.

Epidemiology

Most patients with primary intracranial PCCC are young men (3–22 years of age) who experience precocious puberty.[7] Mean age of presentation is 11.8 years with a male-to-female ratio of 74:19.

Location

Choriocarcinoma arising within or outside the uterus after pregnancy is referred to as gestational choriocarcinoma. Nongestational choriocarcinoma arises from germ cells in gonadal or extragonadal locations (mediastinum, retroperitoneum, and pineal gland), generally in the midline.

Clinical Presentation

In the majority of patients, the clinical presentation depends on the tumor location. There are no specific symptoms related to this tumor. However, headache, vomiting, nausea, visual impairment, polydipsia, polyuria, and endocrinologic abnormalities are among the most common reported symptoms.[6,8]

Imaging Findings

Most nongerminomatous GCTs reported are case reports with nonspecific imaging findings. Intracranial choriocarcinomas and specifically PCCC, however, tend to appear on CT as ovoid, heterogeneous, slightly hyperdense, and relatively well-defined lesions with lobulated margins centered in the pineal gland region (Fig. 1). At the time of diagnosis, tumor size ranges from 2.0 cm to 4.5 cm. MRI offers better characterization of the tumor than CT. Tumors and their metastases are highly vascular and intratumoral hemorrhage is typical.[6,9] On T1-weighted images, they demonstrate high signal due to presence of subacute blood. As a result, multiple areas of heterogeneous hypointensity and hyperintensity are seen on T2-weighted images. Susceptibility-weighted imaging (SWI) demonstrates blooming artifact within the tumor due to presence of hemoglobin products.[6]

Histopathology

PCCCs are characterized by presence of stromal vascular channels that form blood lakes and

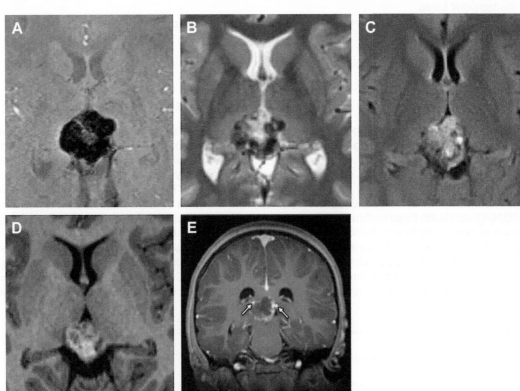

Fig. 1. PCCC. An 18-year-old man presenting with precocious puberty, headaches, and vomiting. There is a mass centered in the pineal gland region that measures approximately 2.5 cm. The mass is heterogeneous (*C*), but note the increased signal on T1WI (*D*) and low signal on T2 (*B*) with striking susceptibility artifact on SWI (*A*) compatible with hemorrhage. The lesion demonstrates faint peripheral enhancement after the intravenous administration of gadolinium (*Arrows* in *E*). There is no hydrocephalus.

hemorrhagic necrosis.[10] Recent publications suggest that the connections between tumor-formed sinusoids and blood vessels might be a cause of hemorrhage in PCCC.

Treatment

PCCC is highly resistant to standard treatments. The first option is total tumor resection even in absence of hydrocephalus. In the recent years, many investigators[3,11,12] have used a combination of total tumor removal, chemotherapy, and radiation therapy with satisfactory results.[5,13] Despite these therapeutic strategies, the disease is usually fatal.

Differential Diagnosis

Because hemorrhage is a key feature of PCCC and hemorrhagic lesions centered in the pineal region are exceptional, the differential diagnosis can be narrowed to a few entities, including hemorrhagic metastasis, vascular malformation, cavernous malformation, and hemorrhagic pineal cyst. In addition, other tumors in the pineal region with intratumoral hemorrhage include pineocytoma, meningioma, hemangiopericytoma, embryonal carcinoma, and ganglioglioma.[14] Nevertheless, the presence of elevated β-HCG level in serum and/or CSF favors the diagnosis of choriocarcinoma.

Prognosis

When the diagnosis is confirmed before the lesion develops hemorrhage, gross total resection has been demonstrated to improve hydrocephalus and prognosis. In the presence of hemorrhage, rebleeding rate is high as is the risk of massive hemorrhage and, for this reason, prompt and total tumor resection followed by radiotherapy and chemotherapy is recommended to prevent fatal outcomes.[3,14,15]

EXTRAVENTRICULAR NEUROCYTOMA

CNs are rare benign tumors usually located in the lateral ventricles near the foramina of Monro but can also occur in the third and fourth ventricles.[16] The name CN reflects its midline location within the ventricular system, but when these tumors arise in the brain parenchyma they are called EVNs.[17] EVN shares similar biological behavior and histopathologic characteristics with CN.[18] These neurocytomas were included in the 2000 WHO classification of tumors of the CNS but it was not until 2007 when they were classified as separate entities.[19] EVNs have a more aggressive biological behavior and a poorer outcome

than CNs.[20] CNs as well as EVNs may mimic several entities, such as oligodendrogliomas, ependymomas, and astrocytomas.[16] For this reason, they can pose a diagnostic challenge. Immunohistochemistry, however, has greatly improved diagnostic accuracy.[21]

Epidemiology

EVN occur with almost equal sex distribution with a slight female predominance.[16,22] Their exact incidence is unclear, with fewer than 100 cases reported in the literature to date. EVN typically affects children and young adults during the third to fourth decades.[23] Mean age of presentation is approximately 27 years.[24]

Location

EVNs have been reported in most of the nervous system but they tend to arise in the periventricular regions. In adults, EVNs occur in the frontal lobes, followed by temporal, parietal, and occipital lobes.[25] In children, the spine is a common location after the frontal and temporal lobes.[26]

Clinical Presentation

Most common symptoms include increased intracranial pressure, seizures, gait disturbances, vision changes, headaches, and vomiting.[17,24] Symptom onset varies from 3 months to 10 years.

Imaging Findings

EVNs do not have specific imaging characteristics and appear as solid well-circumscribed lesions involving the deep white matter or the cortical gray matter of the cerebral hemispheres.[22] EVNs demonstrate a wide range of appearances, including perilesional edema and heterogeneous contrast enhancement (**Fig. 2**).[23] They contain areas of calcification, cystic degeneration, and hemorrhage. Even though nonenhancing EVNs resembling low-grade gliomas have been described, the former generally are hypointense or slightly hyperintense on T1-weighted images.[20] Magnetic resonance spectroscopy (MRS) shows a nonspecific pattern with prominent choline and decreased or absent NAA.[27,28] Perfusion is usually increased in the solid components of the tumor, which may indicate atypical features.

Histopathology

Histologic features of EVNs are small round neoplastic cells with round, regular nuclei embedded in a matrix of fine neuronal processes.[16,24] Unlike the uniform morphologic pattern of CNs, EVNs show sheetlike patterns,

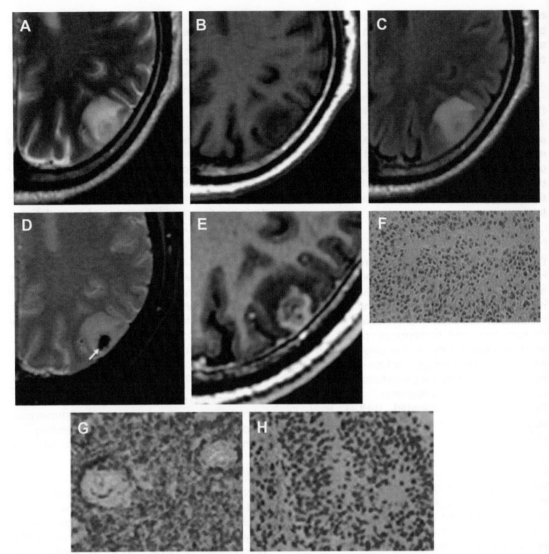

Fig. 2. EVN. A 46-year-old man with history of seizures. There is a cortical-based mass with surrounding vasogenic edema in the left parietal lobe. The lesion is hypointense on T1WI (*B*) and hyperintense on T2WI and FLAIR (*A, C*) with a focal area of susceptibility in the center (*arrow* [*D*]) probably representing hemorrhage and/or calcification. On T1 postgadolinium, a peripheral rim of enhancement is noted (*E*). No other lesions are visualized. Hematoxylin-eosin 400× (*F*) shows monomorphic proliferation of cells with clear cytoplasm and round nuclei and presence of occasional mitoses. (*F*) Immunohistochemical staining (*G, H*) shows a strong, diffuse in immuno-reaction for synaptophysin (*G*), and immunoreaction of nuclei with NeuN (*H*). (*Courtesy of* Francisco Sepulveda, MD, Fundación para la Lucha de Enfermedades Neurológicas de la Infancia [FLENI].)

clusters, ribbon-like appearance, or Homer-Wright rosettes.[29] EVNs differ from CNs in their pronounced tendency for astrocytic, typically pilocytic features and/or ganglionic differentiation, which can be seen in 50% to 60% of cases.[20,30] It may be difficult to differentiate EVN from oligodendroglioma, but, unlike the latter, EVNs are strongly immunoreactive for synaptophysin, both in the neuropil and in perinuclear cytoplasm. EVNs that have an MIB-1 index greater than 2%,

focal necrosis, increased vascularity, and mitoses are called "atypical neurocytomas," resulting in higher rates of mortality and recurrences than typical EVNs.[17,20]

Treatment

Extent of resection is the key determinant of recurrence and gross total excision is the best prognostic indicator leading to better local control and survival rates, but total excision is often limited by proximity to eloquent areas.[31] Radiotherapy has demonstrated good results in local control but no improvement of overall survival.[25]

Differential Diagnosis

Oligodendrogliomas comprise the most challenging differential diagnosis due to their similar appearances and histopathologic features. Immunohistochemistry has improved the differentiation of oligodendrogliomas from EVNs. Although a specific genetic profile has not been found in EVNs, some investigators have described the presence of codeletion of 1p19q in approximately 25% of EVNs with atypical features and infiltrative growth patterns.[32] Recent studies have demonstrated that EVNs lack p53 overexpression, α-internexin positivity, O6-methylguanine DNA methyltransferase (MGMT) promotor methylation, and isocitrate dehydrogenase (IDH)1/IDH2 mutation.[33]

Other differential diagnoses include pilocytic astrocytoma, PXA, and ganglioglioma. A diagnosis of EVNs can be aided by imaging features that demonstrate well-demarcated borders rather than infiltrating edges.[22]

Prognosis

EVNs are benign neoplasms in nature, except for atypical neurocytomas, which display an aggressive behavior and have overall a poor prognosis with a high rate of recurrence. According to some reports, extreme age, especially younger age, is associated with atypical features and higher risk for recurrence with a worse outcome.[24]

PLEOMORPHIC XANTHOASTROCYTOMA WITH INTRAVENTRICULAR EXTENSION

PXA is an uncommon, generally benign astrocytic neoplasm first described as a variant of cerebral astrocytomas that demonstrates extensive involvement of the leptomeninges.[34–36] PXA is a WHO grade II neoplasm. However, 9% to 20% of PXAs undergo malignant transformation when they recur after resection and some show anaplastic features at diagnosis.[35,37] Moreover, several investigators suggest the existence of high-grade PXA or at least the existence of a PXA with aggressive presentation.[38] Recently, the 2016 WHO classification included a different type of PXA with aggressive behavior, numerous recurrences, shorter survival times, and poor outcome compared with the more benign variant.[39] Anaplastic PXA (aPXA) WHO grade III is the nomenclature given to this entity, as an alternative to PXA with anaplastic features.[1] To date,

more than 20 cases that fulfill the criteria for aPXA have been reported. Primary meningeal aPXAs and leptomeningeal dissemination of intraparenchymal aPXA have also been described.[37,40] A parenchymal mass with intraventricular extension is an exceedingly rare presentation of PXA, with only a few case reports in the English literature.[41] The following discussion focuses on the classic presentation of PXA.

Epidemiology

PXA generally arises in children and young adults with an incidence rate of 0.07:100,000.[39] PXAs can arise at any decade of life with a mean age of 26 years.[38,42] Most data about these tumors come from case reports and small series, reflecting their rarity.[43] Currently, there are not enough cases to determine gender or racial predilection.

Location

The classic presentation is that of mass with a dominant intra-axial component, localized superficially in the cerebral hemispheres.[37] Approximately 98% of cases reported are supratentorial. The most common location is the temporal lobes, followed by the parietal, frontal, and occipital lobes. It is typically superficial, consistently involving the leptomeninges, infiltrating the underlying parenchyma, and extending into the perivascular spaces.[38] Less common locations include the cerebellum, spinal cord, retina, and sellar region.[44]

Clinical Presentation

The most common presentation is chronic epilepsy.[42,45] There are few reports of PXAs with CSF dissemination at the time of diagnosis.[46]

Imaging Findings

Although PXA is associated with a wide range of imaging appearances due to its inherent "pleomorphic" histopathology, presence of a cystic tumor with an enhancing mural nodule and adjacent inner skull table scalloping are common findings. Perilesional edema and intratumoral hemorrhage have also been reported (Fig. 3).[44,47] Scarce data on diffusion-weighted MRI suggest that relatively low apparent diffusion coefficient (ADC) values are found in PXA compared with other peripheral low-grade supratentorial neoplasms.[44]

Differential Diagnosis

PXA should be included in the differential diagnosis of cortical-based cystic lesions with a solid

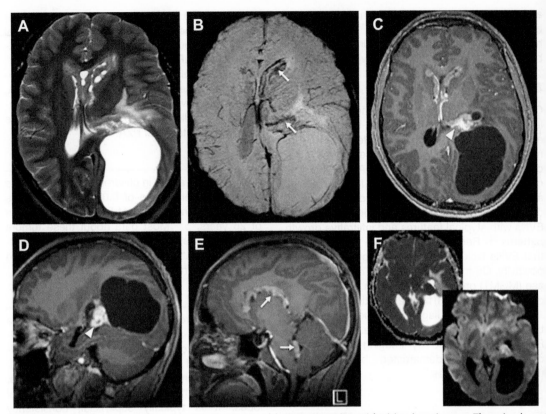

Fig. 3. PXA with intraventricular extension. A 16-year-old man presenting with vision impairment. There is a large cystic mass (*A*) within the left temporal/occipital region with a peripheral solid enhancing nodule (*arrowheads* [*C*, *D*]). Immediately anterior to the solid portion, there is nodular enhancement along the lining of the lateral ventricles extending to the fourth ventricle (*arrows* [*E*]). Note presence of microhemorrhages within the enhancing nodules in the lateral ventricles on SWI (*arrows* [*B*]). Histopathology revealed PXAA (WHO grade II). Note the low ADC values (*F*).

enhancing mural nodule or neoplasms with extensive involvement of the leptomeninges in young patients. Differential includes ganglioglioma, pilocytic astrocytoma, glioblastoma (GB), oligodendroglioma, and dysembrioblastic neuroepithelial tumor (DNET). Most DNETs and oligodendrogliomas do not enhance. Occasionally, different entities may mimic a cortical-based enhancing mass and could be considered in the differential (eg, meningioma, sarcoid, or lymphoproliferative mass).

Histopathology

Hallmarks of PXAs include pleomorphism with dense reticulin network and lipid deposits in neoplastic cells. Almost every PXA shows glial fibrillary acid protein (GFAP)-positive cells and S100 immunoreactivity. aPXA shows malignant histologic features with aggressive clinical behavior. A PXA can be considered anaplastic if 5 or more mitoses per 10 high-power fields and necrosis are present.[40]

Treatment

Treatment of choice is gross total resection, which is the most important predictor of recurrence but not of overall survival.[40] Although PXA has a benign behavior, there is a tendency to recur if incompletely excised. Because of the rarity of the tumor, the role of adjuvant radiotherapy or chemotherapy remains uncertain.

Prognosis

Despite their highly pleomorphic cytology, PXA has a relatively favorable prognosis.[38,39] Nevertheless, advanced patient age and CSF dissemination at presentation are poor prognostic factors.[34] A significant decrease in overall survival is seen with aPXA compared with PXA.[40]

MENINGIOANGIOMATOSIS

MA is a rare meningovascular malformation of the CNS first described as an incidental autopsy finding in a patient with neurofibromatosis (NF type 2.[48] It is characterized by presence of an epileptogenic plaque-like or nodular mass in the leptomeningeal and cortex.[48–50] Approximately 25% to 50% of MAs are associated with NF type 2 whereas the remaining cases occur sporadically.[51,52] Multiple lesions have also been reported.[53,54] Several publications report MA in association with oligodendroglioma, cerebral hemorrhage, arteriovenous malformations, and meningeal hemangiopericytoma, with meningiomas the most commonly associated neoplasms. It does not become malignant or recur. Its pathogenesis remains unclear. Consequently, MA is usually misdiagnosed and occasionally mistreated by unsuccessful methods.[54–56]

Epidemiology

MA occurs in children and young adults with no gender predilection.[54,55]

Location

Most MAs are supratentorial and involve the cerebral cortex (90%), particularly in the frontal or temporal lobes. Other locations, including third ventricle, thalamus, cerebral peduncles, and brainstem, have been reported.[54] Some publications suggest that when MA is associated with NF type 2 there is a frontal lobe tendency.[55]

Clinical Presentation

Patients with meningioangiomatosis typically present with seizure disorders, which are the exclusive clinical problem in the majority of cases. Seizures are usually simple or complex partial, and tend to be refractory to treatment. Persistent headache is the second most common symptom and usually disappears after surgical resection of the lesion.[53]

Imaging Findings

Imaging findings vary according to the histopathologic components. Gliosis and edema can be seen in the periphery of the lesion on CT and MRI.[54] Regardless of location, MA is always well defined intra-axially or extra-axially but occasionally may have ill-defined margins as a result of cortical invasion. The utility of CT is to detect calcifications, which have been reported in up to 89.6% of cases.[55] On MRI, the lesion is classically isointense to hypointense on T1-weighted imaging (T1WI) and hypointense to hyperintense on T2-weighted imaging (T2WI). A most striking characteristic of MA is presence of a gyriform hyperintensity on fluid-attenuated inversion recovery (FLAIR), which corresponds to thickened cortex with proliferating leptomeningeal vessels interwoven with bands of fibrous connective tissue.[57] SWI identifies calcifications missed on CT. Occasionally, MA can be divided into 2 imaging patterns: solid and a cystic appearances (the solid variant being more common).[55] On T1 postcontrast sequences, various patterns of enhancement have been reported, including avid, mild, or no enhancement. Most of cases, however, demonstrate prominent homogenous contrast enhancement (Fig. 4).[58]

Histopathology

The hallmark of MA is leptomeningeal calcification and meningovascular proliferation intermingled with fine bands of fibrous connective tissue.[53,55] MA involves the cerebral cortex and subcortical white matter.[59]

MA has a low MIB-1 index.[60] Neurofibrillary tangles are not unusual.[30,53,61] Its pathogenesis is controversial but a hamartoma with degenerative changes, leptomeningeal meningioma with invasion in adjacent brain tissue, and cortical vascular malformation have been proposed. Kim and colleagues[62] found that the meningiomatosis portions of meningiomatosis-meningioma have loss of heterozygosity at the 22q12 locus in 28.6% of coexisting cases of meningiomatosis-meningioma, whereas each pure meningiomatosis harbors 1 loss of heterozygosity at either 22q12 or 9p21. Approximately 90% of cases show cortical invasion, but findings like atypia, mitoses, and necrosis are not found. Immunohistochemical staining of MA shows markers, such as epithelial membrane antigen, S-100 protein, and GFAP.[63]

Treatment

Treatment of choice is total surgical removal, which is important for seizure control and pathologic diagnosis. An accurate diagnosis is important, especially when MA is associated with an underlying meningioma because a misinterpretation of atypical or malignant meningioma may result in incorrect treatment.[54,55]

Differential Diagnosis

Differential diagnosis includes oligodendroglioma, ganglioglioma, dysembryoplastic neuroepithelial tumor, low-grade astrocytoma, meningioma, granulomatous meningitis, and parasitic diseases.[64] The main differential diagnosis of MA-associated meningioma to be considered is a malignant meningioma with an invasion of the brain.[65]

Prognosis

Excellent results are obtained after total surgical removal because most patients became free of

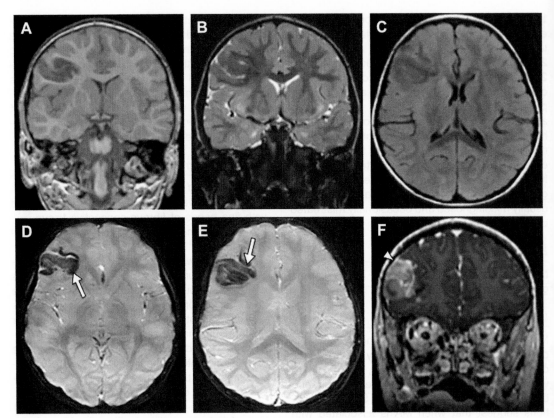

Fig. 4. MA. A 3-year-old boy presenting with seizures. There is a cortical lesion involving the right frontal lobe that demonstrates low signal on T1, T2, and FLAIR (*A–C*), gyriform blooming artifact on SWI (*arrows [D, E]*). T1W coronal image after Gd-based contrast material injection (*F*) shows diffuse irregular enhancement. Additionally, there is minimal dural enhancement adjacent to the lesion (*arrowhead [F]*). (*Courtesy of* Francisco Sepulveda, MD, Fundación para la Lucha de Enfermedades Neurológicas de la Infancia [FLENI].)

seizure and recurrence after surgical treatments.[54] Antiepileptic drug administration, however, is required in greater than 70% of patients.

INTRAVENTRICULAR GLIOBLASTOMA

GB is the most common and most malignant primary brain tumor of adults.[43,66,67] Despite the different locations and patterns, IVGB is extremely rare.[68–75] GB is classified as WHO grade IV due to the presence of hypercellularity, nuclear polymorphism, brisk mitotic activity, prominent microvascular proliferation, and/or necrosis.[67–69,75] IVGB is thought to arise from the neuroglial cells of the septum pellucidum or fornix or may be secondary to an abnormal healing process in the subependymal zone.[69,70]

Epidemiology

In the United States, GB accounts for 15.1% of all primary brain tumors and for 46.1% of primary malignant brain tumors. It is more common in older adults (65–84 years), 1.6 times more common in

men than in women, and has prevalence 2 times higher among whites compared with blacks.[43] IVGBs are found in younger patients (19–47 years).[68,69]

Location

IVGBs are rare, with only 30 cases reported to date.[68] Most IVGBs are located in the frontal horns or ventricular bodies (Fig. 5B, C). The third ventricle is an extremely rare location.[68–75]

Clinical Presentation

Symptoms are vague, including headaches, urinary incontinence, gait disturbances, blurred vision, vomiting, and confusion.[68–75] Symptoms do not develop until the tumor reaches a size large enough to cause obstructive hydrocephalus or compression of surrounding structures.[69]

Imaging Findings

Imaging features of IVGB are similar to those located in extraventricular locations. On CT they present as

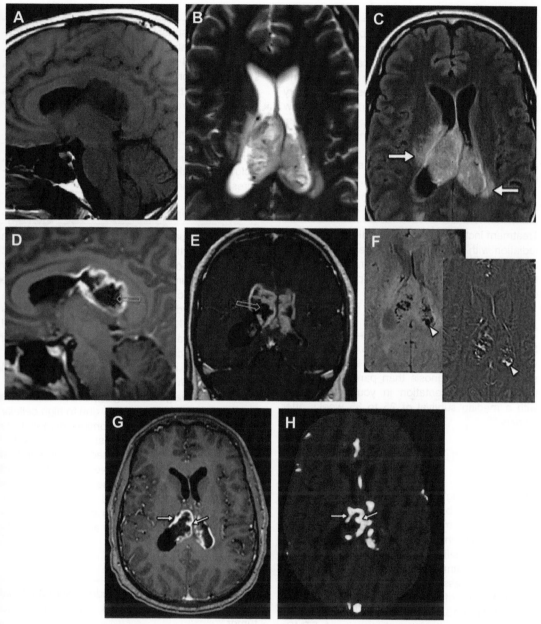

Fig. 5. IVGB: a 40-year-old man with a history of headaches. There is an intraventricular mass attached to the septum pellucidum with extension into the atria. The lesion is hypointense on T1 (*A*) and hyperintense on T2/FLAIR (*B, C*). Infiltrative pattern affecting the bilateral corona radiata on FLAIR (*arrows* in *C*) is present. Hemorrhagic components are seen centrally within the mass and depicted on SWI and corroborated on phase images (*arrowheads* [*F*]). Postcontrast sagittal and coronal T1 images (*D, E*) show a ring-enhancing pattern surrounding a central core of necrosis (*empty arrows*). High rCBV is present in the nodular enhancing areas (*arrows* [*G, H*]).

mixed density masses with contrast enhancement of the non-necrotic areas.[68] On MRI, T1WIs shows an infiltrative mass with irregular borders and mixed signal intensity. T2 sequences show surrounding edema. T1 postcontrast images show heterogeneous or ringlike contrast enhancement surrounding the necrosis. On perfusion images, high rCBV could be seen within the solid portions of the tumor

(see **Fig. 5**).[68–75] One case of IVGB with minimal enhancement has been reported.[76]

Differential Diagnosis

Differential diagnosis includes ependymoma, subependymoma, subependymal giant cell astrocytoma, and choroid glioma.

Histopathology

GBs are classified into IDH wild-type (90%) or IDH mutant (10%) and non-otherwise-specified (NOS) GBs in which IDH evaluation cannot be performed.[1] Presence of extensive necrosis and endothelial cell proliferation raises the category to WHO grade IV. Microscopic features show pleomorphic fibrillary astrocytes, gemistocytes, and bipolar bland-appearing but mitotically active small cells. High proliferation index (MIB-1) exceeding 10% is typical.[67] IVGB shares all these features.

Treatment

Treatment includes surgical resection followed by radiation with a total dose of at least 54 Gy and thereafter chemotherapy.[77] Transcallosal and transcortical are the surgical approaches most commonly used.[68]

Prognosis

Survival for GB is low, with only 5% of patients surviving 5 years postdiagnosis.[43] IVGBs have a slightly better prognosis than parenchymal GBs due to their presentation in younger patients, with a median survival of 25 to 35 weeks after surgery.[69]

EMBRYONAL TUMOR WITH MULTILAYERED ROSETTES

ETMRs are thought to originate from primitive or undifferentiated brain cells.[67,78,79] Embryonal tumors other than medulloblastoma had undergone some changes in their terminology in the 2016 CNS WHO classification. The term, primitive neuroectodermal tumor (PNET), has been removed and they are classified according to the presence of amplification of the C19MC region on chromosome 19 (19q 13.42). The presence of C19 MC amplification results in a diagnosis of ETMRs (ETMR-C19MC-altered). In its absence, the tumor is called ETMR-NOS.[1]

Epidemiology

The incidence of ETMRs peaks between 0 and 4 years.[43] They account for less than 1% of brain tumors in children.[80] ETMRs are rare, with an incidence less than 5% of all supratentorial tumors in children.[81] Only 20% to 30% of these tumors occur in adults, with fewer than 100 ETMRs reported in the literature among this group.[82] In adults the age of presentation is between the second and third decades.[82,83]

Location

Cerebral hemispheres are the most common location with equal distributions among the frontal, temporal, and parietal lobes. Other locations, such as suprasellar region, have been reported.[83,84] At the time of presentation, the tumors usually measure more than 5 cm.[67,82]

Clinical Presentation

Symptoms are related to the size and location, including weakness, headache, vomiting, seizures, and changes in personality.[79,85]

Imaging Findings

ETMRs are usually large masses, more than 5 cm in size at the time of presentation (Fig. 6A).[67,81] They are well-delineated masses with absent or minimal peritumoral edema despite their large size.[79–81] Typically they are heterogeneous isodense to hyperdense masses on CT. Calcifications are seen in 70% of cases.[80,84] On MRI, the signal on T1/T2 is variable due to presence of blood products, calcifications, and cystic changes. FLAIR shows areas of necrosis (hyperintense) and cystic components (hypointense) (Fig. 6).[81] On diffusion-weighted imaging, the tumor shows high signal and reduced ADC, due to high cellular density.[81,84] The solid components demonstrate avid heterogeneous contrast enhancement.[80] Perfusion MRI shows increased relative cerebral blood volume.[80] ETMRs develop subarachnoid dissemination in 40% of cases; thus, the entire neuroaxis should be imaged (see Fig. 6G, H). The presence of metastases changes management, requiring chemotherapy and increased radiation dose.[80,81,84]

Differential Diagnosis

Differential diagnosis includes supratentorial ependymoma and atypical teratoid/rhabdoid tumor.[67,80,81]

Histopathology

ETMRs are composed of poorly differentiated cells with small round to oval hyperchromatic nuclei surrounded by scant cytoplasm with elevated nuclear to cytoplasmatic ratios. Mitotic activity is elevated.[67,82]

Treatment

Treatment is not well established because of poorly understood pathologic mechanisms.[82] Maximal tumor reduction by surgery is the main treatment followed by radiation therapy. Chemotherapy is

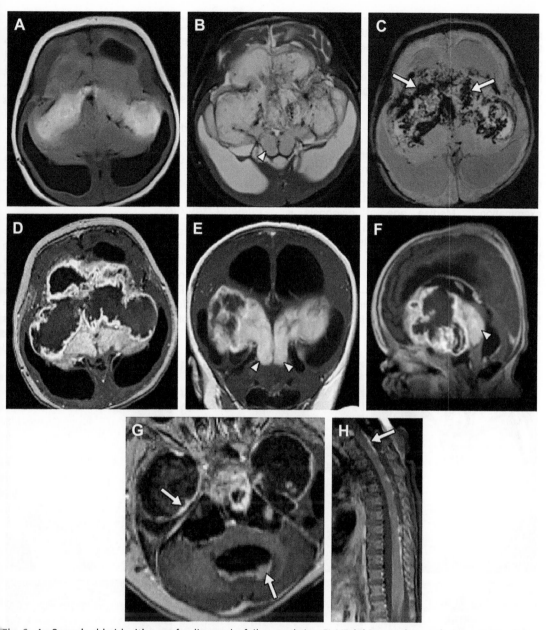

Fig. 6. An 8-week-old girl with poor feeding and a failure to thrive. FLAIR (*A*) image shows a heterogeneous lobulated mass causing obstructive hydrocephalus. On T2-weighted image (*B*), the mass is hyperintense with low signal intensities corresponding to hemorrhagic components identified on SWI (*arrows* in *C*). Postcontrast axial, coronal, and sagittal T1 images (*D–F*) show avid ring enhancement; notice the posterior infiltration into the midbrain and superior aspect of the pons (*arrowheads* in *B* and *C*). Subarachnoid seeding is seen at the roof of the fourth ventricle, posterior surface of the spinal cord and bilateral medial temporal fossa (*arrows* [*G, H*]).

controversial given the poor prognosis of patients especially those with extensive disease.[79,86,87]

Prognosis

Survival improves with increasing age at presentation. Prognosis is related to extent of disease and tumor bulk reduction. Survival estimates for

ETMRs are low, with a 42.1% survival at 10 years. Peripheral ETMRs have a better prognosis than central ones.[88]

DIFFUSE MIDLINE GLIOMA

Diffuse intrinsic pontine gliomas, now called DMGs, are a disease primarily of children characterized by rapid onset of symptoms in previously healthy patients and because of their location and infiltrative nature these tumors are not amenable to surgical resection.[87–89] DMGs are classified according to their pattern of growth as diffuse (astrocytoma) or focal (pilocytic astrocytoma). DMGs generally range from WHO grade II to IV.

Epidemiology

Tumors within the brainstem represent 10% to 15% of all pediatric CNS tumors.[90] DMGs comprise 80% of all brain stem tumors in children and 80% of them are malignant on histologic examination.[91] Median age at diagnosis is 7.5 years.[92] Metastatic disease in the neuroaxis is reported in 5% to 30% of patients generally leptomeningeal and subependymal.[91,92]

Location

DMGs expand and diffusely infiltrate the pons. Supratentorial extension and leptomeningeal spread have been reported.[91,93]

Clinical Presentation

Symptom onset is acute with rapid progression over days or weeks. The most frequent clinical presentation is ataxia, pyramidal tract signs, and cranial nerve palsies.[92] Accepted criteria for making the diagnosis include symptom duration less than 6 months, at least 2 or 3 symptoms related to brainstem dysfunction, and pontine enlargement with the presence of a diffusely infiltrative tumor involving greater than 50% to 66% of the pons.[92,94]

Imaging Findings

Diagnosis is based on a combination of neurologic signs, symptoms, and neuroimaging findings. On MRI, DMGs infiltrate the pons, presenting diffuse bright signal on FLAIR/T2WIs, and hypointensity on T1 (Fig. 7A, B). There is compression but not invasion of the fourth ventricle and engulfment or displacement of the basilar artery by the engorged pons (see Fig. 7B).[90,92] The medulla is generally

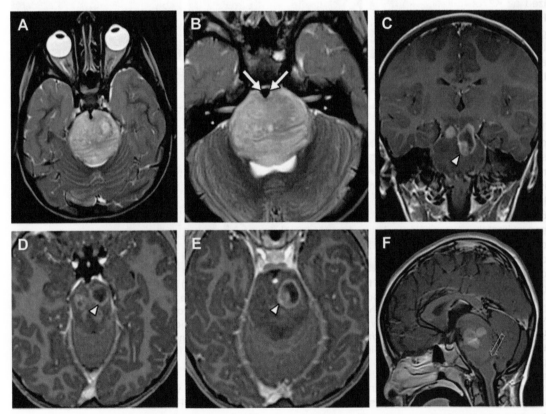

Fig. 7. DMG. An 8-year-old boy who presented with a 2-week history of headache, early morning nausea, and vomiting. There is T2 hyperintense (A, B) infiltrative lesion expanding the brainstem and extending superiorly into the midbrain with mass effect on the fourth ventricle. Postcontrast T1 images (C–E) show nodular and ring-enhancing areas within the mass (arrowheads). Note the clear pontomedullary demarcation on the sagittal image (arrow [F]), a common finding at the initial presentation. Additionally, there is encasement of the basilar artery on T2 axial (arrows [B]).

not involved at presentation resulting in a clear pontomedullary demarcation on sagittal MRI (**Fig. 7F**).[92] After contrast administration, the majority does not enhance, but in some cases, necrosis with ring-enhancement may be seen (**Fig. 7C–E**). Leptomeningeal and subventricular dissemination is rare.[92,93]

Differential Diagnosis

Brainstem embryonal tumors should also be included in the differential.[92] Nontumoral considerations include brainstem encephalitis, demyelinating disease, NF type 1 areas of dysplastic myelination, and osmotic demyelination.

Histopathology

Distinct underlying genetic abnormalities of these tumors allow them to be separated from their brain adult counterparts.[1,89,95] The 2016 WHO classification now uses the term, DMG, H3 K27M-mutant, for the previously called diffuse intrinsic brainstem glioma.[1] These tumors are characterized by K27M mutations in the histone H3 gene H3F3A and less commonly in the HIST1H3B gene.[1,89] Gliomas carrying the K27M mutation in the H3F3A gene are almost exclusively midline and also include rare tumors in basal ganglia, thalami and spinal cord.[95]

Treatment

There has been no improvement in survival for children with DMGs for more than 50 years.[92] Aggressive chemotherapeutic and radiation therapies regimes are not effective.[89,91,96] Radiation therapy is the primary treatment modality and standard treatment consists of a total dose of 54 Gy over 6 weeks.[96] Without radiation, median survival is approximately 4 months.[92] Due to the poor outcome of patients with DMGs, improved quality of life may be obtained by shortening the duration of radiation therapy given as hypofractionated radiotherapy in lesser number of sessions.[96]

Currently, there are several trials developing vaccines to reactive the immune system against brainstem gliomas by using different components, such as imiquimod and antigen-peptides with poly-ICLC, after the completion of radiation therapy or within it.[97,98]

Prognosis

DMGs are devastating tumors with no effective therapy and tumor progression is the rule.[89,92] Median survival is less than 1 year and only 10% of patients survive more than 2 years.[89,96] Long-term survival has been reported and is usually associated with atypical imaging and clinical features.[91,92] Finding the K27M-H3.3 mutation is correlated with poor outcome.[89,95]

PAPILLARY GLIONEURONAL TUMOR

PGNT is a rare cerebral neoplasm.[99] To date, at least 83 cases have been reported.[100,101] PGNT is a WHO grade I neuronal-glial tumor.

Epidemiology

PGNT often affects younger individuals (mean age at diagnosis: 26 years) without gender predominance.[102]

Location

PGNT is exclusively an intraparenchymal intracerebral lesion involving, in decreasing order of frequency, the temporal, parietal, frontal, and occipital lobes usually near the lateral ventricles.[103]

Clinical Manifestations

Clinical manifestations of PGNT are not specific, but declining vision, headache and/or cognition, and motor weakness are the most common ones.[103]

Imaging Findings

Most PGNTs involve the white matter and adjacent lateral ventricles (64%).[102] Size of the tumor may range from 1 cm to 7 cm.[99] The lesion can be a cystic or solid mass with ringlike contrast enhancement.[103] It may have focal calcifications and edema surrounding the tumor, mass effect is generally mild and hemorrhage is rare (**Fig. 8**).[103]

Differential Diagnosis

Differential diagnosis includes ganglioglioma (much more common). PGNT is a histologic diagnosis.[104]

Histopathology

PGNTs are biphasic tumors with both astrocytic and neuronal elements. The hallmark of PGNT is presence of hyalinized vascular pseudopapilla, low MIB labeling index, absence of necrosis and vascular hyperplasia reflecting a benign nature (WHO grade I), pseudopapillary architecture, and a variety of cellular constituents that set this tumor apart from other mixed glioneuronal tumors. Histogenesis of PGNT is uncertain and an origin from multipotent precursor cells capable of divergent glioneuronal differentiation has been suggested. Komori and colleagues[99] believe that it possibly derives from 2 locations: the subependymal plate and cortical plate.[103] Expression of

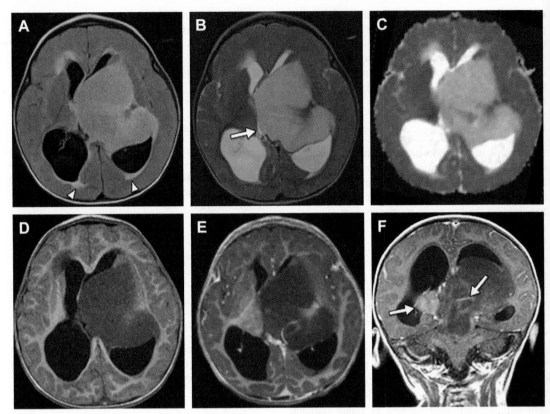

Fig. 8. PGNT. A 4 year-old girl presents with headache and acute motor weakness. There is a large solid mass in the left basal ganglia with well-defined borders compressing the third ventricle (*arrow* [*B*]) with secondary dilatation of the lateral ventricles and transependymal edema (*arrowheads* in *A*). The mass extends caudally infiltrating the midbrain. The tumor is homogeneously hypointense on T1WI (*D*) and hyperintense on FLAIR and T2WI (*A, B*). No restricted diffusion is visualized (*C*). On T1 postgadolinium (*E, F*), there is homogeneous enhancement of a peripheral nodule and subtle enhancement of internal septa (*arrows* [*F*]).

PDGF Ra, Olig2, and Nestin indicates an origin from subependymal progenitor cells. MIB-1 labeling rates are usually in the range of 1.0% to 2.0% and if higher suggest atypical or aggressive forms.[103,105]

Treatment

Treatment is gross total resection. Adjuvant chemotherapy, radiotherapy, or a combination has been used in few cases with high MIB-1 labeling index (4%–26%) and/or subtotal resection.[103]

Prognosis

Recurrence or tumor progression is unusual and leads to an unfavorable prognosis. Most cases, however, have a benign outcome with no evidence of recurrence.[102]

ROSETTE-FORMING GLIONEURONAL TUMOR

RGNT of the fourth ventricle is a rare, benign, mixed neuronal-glial primary brain tumor although

RGNT variant with aggressive behavior has been described.[106] It is recognized as a distinct entity since the 2007 WHO Classification of Tumors of the Central Nervous System.[107] was first described in the posterior fossa, specifically in the fourth ventricle.[99] No fewer than 55 RGNTs have been described in the English literature to date.[107,108]

Epidemiology

RGNT preferentially affects young women with a mean age of 31 (range 6–79) years. There is a female-to-male predilection of 1.6:1.[107]

Location

RGNT often occupies the fourth ventricle but occasionally it shows cerebellar (vermian) invasion or may involve the aqueduct.[109] Rare extraventricular locations have been reported, including the cerebellar hemispheres, cerebellopontine angles, pineal gland, tectum, thalami, third ventricle, optic chiasm, spinal cord, and a recent case in the septum pellucidum.[106]

Clinical Presentation

Patients usually present with hydrocephalus and increased intracranial pressure. Symptoms are nonspecific and include headache, gait disturbances, vertigo, and visual disturbances, which develop over months to years. The tumor may be incidentally discovered.[109]

Imaging Findings

Most RGNTs appear as well-circumscribed, solid (40%), mixed solid and cystic (34%), or only cystic (26%) masses (**Fig. 9**). A majority show variable gadolinium enhancement (70%).[107] Lesion size ranges from 5 mm to 96 mm.[107] Contrast enhancement may be focal (50%), heterogeneous (19%), minimal (13%), or ring and nodular (9%). Intratumoral hemorrhage and calcifications (25%) may occur.[109] The diagnosis of RGNT should be considered when a cystic neoplasm of the fourth ventricle/superior vermis is encountered in an adult.

RGNT may expand the cortex and involve underlying white matter or be deeply situated abutting the ventricles. One case of RGNT in a NF type 1 patient has been reported but no genetic link was identified.[110]

Histopathology

RGNT has 2 separate histologic components: glial and neurocytic. Site of origin may be periventricular germinal matrix and its neurocytic component consists of small cells with round hyperchromatic nuclei in a background of mucinous matrix-forming rosettes around central aggregates of fibrillary material with positive synaptophysin staining, whereas the glial component resembles that of low-grade gliomas with positive immunostaining for GFAP and S-100 protein. MIB-1 proliferation index is typically low (0.35%–3.07%). The nature of the tumor is indolent as evidenced by

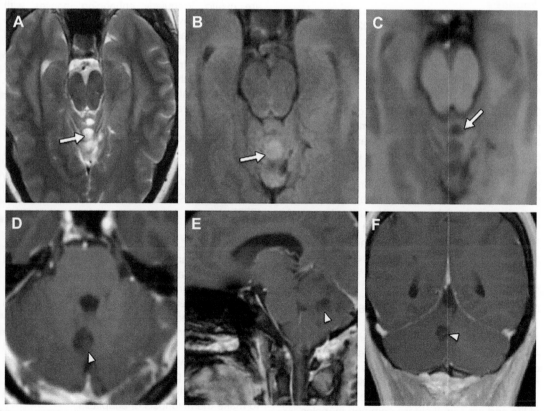

Fig. 9. RFGT. A 34-year-old woman presents with balance difficulty, headache, and vision disturbance. MRI reveals multiple lesions involving the cerebellar vermis with cystic appearance (*arrows A–C*). Most of them are hypointense on T1WI (*C*) and hyperintense on T2WI (*A*). There is no suppression of signal on FLAIR sequence (*B*) and after Gd-DTPA administration there is no evidence of contrast enhancement within the lesion (*arrowheads*) (*D–F*). There is no mass effect or perilesional edema associated.

the absence of aggressive histologic features and low MIB-1 proliferative index.[106]

Treatment

RGNT is treated with gross total resection or subtotal resection and radiotherapy or only with ventriculostomy. The optimal management is surgical resection mainly in symptomatic patients where the tumor causes mass effect. Due to its intimate relationship to key neural structures in cerebellum and brainstem, however, gross total resection is not always possible.[107] Adjuvant treatments, like chemotherapy and radiotherapy, are not typically used. Radiation therapy has been used in cases of progression or progressive symptoms.

Differential Diagnosis

Differential diagnosis includes dysembryoplastic neuroepithelial tumor, pilocytic astrocytoma, medulloblastoma, ependymoma, choroid plexus papilloma, ETMRs, and metastases.[111]

Prognosis

After surgical resection at least 92% of the patients do not demonstrate tumor recurrence or growth of residual tumor.[107]

ANAPLASTIC GANGLIOGLIOMA

Gangliogliomas are classified as glioneural neoplasms WHO grade I and are composed of variable proportions of glial (mainly astrocytic) cells and mature or dysplastic neurons, usually benign. Anaplastic changes, however, have been reported. Most malignant transformation, WHO grade III (anaplastic ganglioglioma), is related to radiation therapy, often occurring several years after treatment, and most malignant changes arise from their glial cells.[112,113] Nevertheless, de novo anaplastic gangliogliomas have been reported.[114]

Epidemiology

Gangliogliomas comprise 0.4% to 6.25% of all primary brain tumors in adults and approximately 10% of all primary brain tumors in children. Anaplastic gangliogliomas represent 3% to 5% of all gangliogliomas and usually develop after radiotherapy for a benign ganglioglioma.[114,115]

Gangliogliomas often occur in the first 3 decades of life and are slightly more common in males.[113] Average age of patients with WHO grade III anaplastic ganglioglioma is 35 years; for WHO grade IV tumors, 32 years; and for WHO grade I and II tumors, 22 to 24 years.[116,117]

Location

Gangliogliomas are frequently found in the temporal lobe. Frontal and parietal lobes are the second most frequent sites. Posterior fossa gangliogliomas are infrequent and affect mostly patients younger than 30 years of age.[118] Supratentorial gangliogliomas are mostly found in the temporal lobes (79%).[118] Between 30% and 46% of the anaplastic gangliogliomas are located in the temporal lobes and the remainder are located in other parts of the cerebral hemispheres or unusual locations, such as the brainstem, pineal region, and optic nerves, and spinal cord.[114]

Clinical Presentation

Seizures are the most common presenting symptom (75%–100%). Ganglioglioma is found in 15% to 25% of patients undergoing surgery for chronic temporal lobe epilepsy.

Imaging Findings

WHO 1 gangliogliomas are typically well defined, cystic, and/or calcified. Anaplastic gangliogliomas are cystic, irregularly enhancing masses with edema and have an appearance consistent with that of malignant gliomas but they may be solid or partially cystic, have focal calcifications (35%), and show contrast enhancement (50%). They are heterogeneously hyperintense on T2WIs and isointense or hypointense on T1WIs (**Fig. 10**). Nevertheless, there are too few cases of anaplastic ganglioglioma to establish imaging parameters that can be used to differentiate low-grade from high-grade tumors.[112] MRS of WHO grade I and II gangliogliomas shows reduced ratios of choline to creatine and of N-acetyl aspartate to creatine with increased choline-to–N-acetyl aspartate ratios.[119]

Histopathology

Anaplastic gangliogliomas show a neuronal component characterized by neoplastic neurons. The CD34 neuronal stem cell marker is typically present in neurons but is less common in anaplastic tumors. Immunoreactivity to synaptophysin and neurofilament is positive. The astrocyte component is malignant, GFAP negative, and vimentin positive. The Ki-67 index and MIB-1 labeling index is greater than 10% in the anaplastic areas and the tumor is required to have necrosis to make the diagnosis of anaplasia.[117]

Treatment

Treatment of choice for all grades of gangliogliomas is gross total resection. Adjuvant radiotherapy

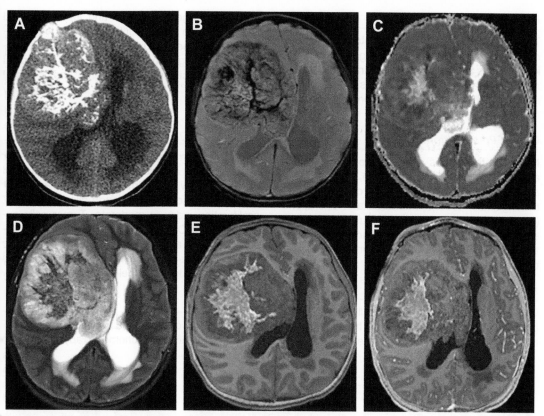

Fig. 10. Anaplastic ganglioglioma. An 8-year-old boy presenting with acute motor weakness. There is a large partially calcified mass in the right frontal lobe (*A*, *B*). Its medial portion shows an infiltrative pattern extending into the right lateral ventricle causing midline shift and hydrocephalus. The mass is predominantly hypointense on T1 (*E*), has heterogeneous signal intensity on T2 (*D*), and demonstrates partial restricted diffusion on the ADC map (*C*). In comparison with noncontrast T1 (*E*), a subtle internal enhancement is seen on T1 post-Gd and DTPA (*F*).

and/or chemotherapy generally are not recommended after gross or subtotal resection of WHO grade I and II gangliogliomas.[114] Brainstem gangliogliomas generally require alternative or additional treatments, such as radiation therapy or chemotherapy.[118]

Differential Diagnosis

Anaplastic ganglioglioma should be included in the differential diagnosis of a cortical-based solid or partially cystic mass, with focal calcifications and heterogeneous enhancement. Thus, the differential includes oligodendroglioma, where calcifications are common; PXA shows prominent contrast enhancement and a dural tail sign; desmoplastic infantile ganglioglioma occurs in young children and has prominent dural involvement; and most embryonal tumors with multilayered rosettes are found in children between 0 and 4 years of age.

Prognosis

Outcome in anaplastic ganglioglioma is worse than for WHO grades I and II gangliogliomas and

32% of patients with anaplastic gangliogliomas who underwent surgery plus radiation and/or chemotherapy died an average of 13 months after diagnosis.[114]

DIFFUSE LEPTOMENINGEAL GLIONEURONAL TUMOR

DLGNT (also known as primary diffuse leptomeningeal gliomatosis or disseminated oligodendroglial-like leptomeningeal tumor of childhood) is a rare and aggressive disease that has a fatal outcome and is characterized by diffuse meningeal infiltration by glial tumor cells without involvement of the brain or spinal cord.[120]

Epidemiology

Age range of presentation of DLGNT varies widely (1–84 years) with no gender predilection but most primary disseminated oligodendroglial-like tumors reported have occurred in the first decade of life.[121]

Location

The tumor derives from heterotopic nests of neuroglial tissue in the leptomeninges. Heterotopic glial nests are found in the subarachnoid space in approximately 1% of autopsies with a higher incidence (25%) in patients with congenital malformations of the CNS.[120]

Clinical Presentation

Most common signs and symptoms are headaches (75%), papilledema (56%), cranial nerve palsies (53%), nausea (47%), vomiting (47%), meningismus (44%), mental state alterations (44%), progressive hydrocephalus, and cauda equina findings[122] but symptoms and signs similar to those of chronic infectious meningitis have also been described.[120]

Imaging Findings

On MRI, these tumors cause nodular leptomeningeal enhancement with or without hydrocephalus. In the early stages of the disease, MRI may be normal. Enlarged ventricles and leptomeningeal thickening with focal or diffuse contrast enhancement are frequent findings (Fig. 11). Leptomeningeal thickening can be confined to the spinal cord, basal cisterns, brainstem, and cerebral hemispheres.[122] Calcifications are infrequently reported.

Histopathology

Pathology demonstrates a moderately cellular neoplasm with a nodular component and marked desmoplasia with uniform round nuclei and clear cytoplasm typical of oligodendroglioma. The ki67 proliferation index is moderate. Tumor cells express mutant IDH1 (IDH1 R132H) by immunohistochemistry and are positive for glial fibrillary acidic protein. Fluorescence in situ hybridization analysis demonstrates 1p19q codeletion.[123]

Treatment

A combination of craniospinal irradiation and intrathecal/intraventricular chemotherapy has been

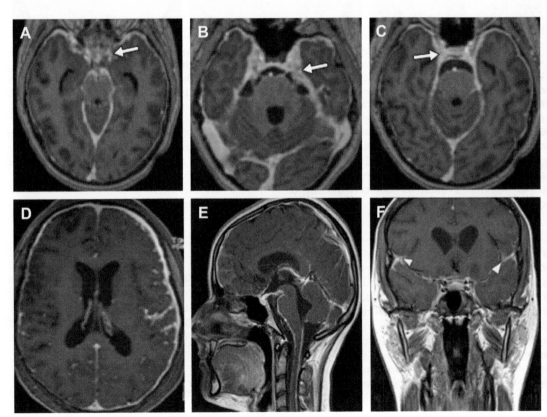

Fig. 11. DLGNT. An 11-year-old boy presenting with headache, papilledema, and cranial nerve palsy. Axial postcontrast T1-weighted images show extensive leptomenigeal thickening (A–F) and nodular enhancement along the basal cisterns (arrow on A), cavernous sinuses (arrows on B and C), cerebral convexities (D and E) and Silvian fissures (arrowheads on F).

reported to prolong the life expectancy in some patients and there are reports that describe that a combination of temozolomide and craniospinal irradiation slow down the progression of disease.[122,124] A study that examined 67 patients found a mean survival rate of 4 months in adults who did not receive any treatment as opposed to 15.6 months in patients who received radiotherapy and/or chemotherapy. In children, mean survival rates are 4 months and 23 months, respectively.[120,122]

Differential Diagnosis

Differential diagnosis includes tuberculous meningitis and antituberculosis treatment is generally initiated before establishing a definitive diagnosis of DLGNT in many patients because the clinical and CSF findings may resemble those of chronic infectious meningitis. Other tumors with secondary malignant dissemination, subacute/chronic meningitis, and autoimmune and inflammatory diseases should also be considered.[122]

Prognosis

Longer survival after chemotherapy and craniospinal radiation has been reported. Patients with DLGNT may experience periods of stability or slow progression. Approximately one-third, however, progress to anaplasia, leading to death in months after diagnosis. The presence of p19q codeletion is not associated with better overall survival.[99,125]

REFERENCES

1. Louis DN, Perry A, Reifenberger G, et al. The 2016 World Health Organization classification of tumors of the central nervous system: a summary. Acta Neuropathol 2016;131(6):1–18.
2. Matsutani M, Sano K, Takakura K, et al. Primary intracranial germ cell tumors: a clinical analysis of 153 histologically verified cases. J Neurosurg 1997;86:446–55.
3. Shinoda J, Sakai N, Yano H, et al. Prognostic factors and therapeutic problems of primary intracranial choriocarcinoma/germ-cell tumors with high levels of HCG. J Neurooncol 2004;66(1–2):225–40.
4. Cheung AN, Zhang HJ, Xue WC, et al. Pathogenesis of choriocarcinoma: clinical, genetic and stem cell perspectives. Future Oncol 2009;5:217–31.
5. Qi ST, Zhang H, Song Y, et al. Tumor cells forming sinusoids connected to vasculature are involved in hemorrhage of pineal choriocarcinoma. J Neurooncol 2014;119(1):159–67.
6. Lv XF, Qiu YW, Zhang XL, et al. Primary intracranial choriocarcinoma: MR imaging findings. AJNR Am J Neuroradiol 2010;31(10):1994–8.
7. Blümel P, Grümayer ER, Machacek E, et al. Beta-HCG-producing choriocarcinoma of the pineal area as a cause of precocious puberty. Helv Paediatr Acta 1985;40(6):473–9 [in German].
8. Wass JA, Jones AE, Rees LH, et al. hCG beta producing pineal choriocarcinoma. Clin Endocrinol (Oxf) 1982;17(5):423–31.
9. Smirniotopoulos JG, Rushing EJ, Mena H. Pineal region masses: differential diagnosis. Radiographics 1992;12(3):577–96.
10. Sato K, Takeuchi H, Kubota T. Pathology of intracranial germ cell tumors. Prog Neurol Surg 2009; 23:59–75.
11. Kageji T, Nagahiro S, Matsuzaki K, et al. Successful neoadjuvant synchronous chemo- and radiotherapy for disseminated primary intracranial choriocarcinoma: case report. J Neurooncol 2007; 83(2):199–204.
12. Kyritsis AP. Management of primary intracranial germ cell tumors. J Neurooncol 2010;96(2):143–9.
13. Ogawa K, Toita T, Nakamura K, et al. Treatment and prognosis of patients with intracranial nongerminomatous malignant germ cell tumors: a multiinstitutional retrospective analysis of 41 patients. Cancer 2003;98(2):369–76.
14. Kim DS, Shim KW, Kim TG, et al. Pineal cavernous malformations: report of two cases. Yonsei Med J 2005;46(6):851–8.
15. Park SA, Kim TY, Choi SS, et al. 18F-FDG PET/CT imaging for mixed germ cell tumor in the pineal region. Clin Nucl Med 2012;37(3):e61–3.
16. Ahmad Z, Din NU, Memon A, et al. Central, extraventricular and atypical neurocytomas: a clinicopathologic study of 35 cases from Pakistan plus a detailed review of the published literature. Asian Pac J Cancer Prev 2016;17(3):1565–70.
17. Sweiss FB, Lee M, Sherman JH. Extraventricular neurocytomas. Neurosurg Clin N Am 2015;26(1): 99–104.
18. Kamboj M, Gandhi J, Mehta A, et al. Atypical extraventricular neurocytoma: a report of two cases. J Cancer Res Ther 2015;11(4):1022.
19. Louis DN, Ohgaki H, Wiestler OD, et al. The 2007 WHO classification of tumours of the central nervous system. Acta Neuropathol 2007; 114(2):97–109.
20. Brat DJ, Scheithauer BW, Eberhart CG, et al. Extraventricular neurocytomas: pathologic features and clinical outcome. Am J Surg Pathol 2001;25(10): 1252–60.
21. Conrad MD, Morel C, Guyotat J, et al. Central nervous system neurocytomas: clinicopathological analysis of tree cases. Arq Neuropsiquiatr 2000; 58:1100–6.

22. Yang GF, Wu SY, Zhang LJ, et al. Imaging findings of extraventricular neurocytoma: report of 3 cases and review of the literature. AJNR Am J Neuroradiol 2009;30:581–5.

23. Tortori-Donati P, Fondelli MP, Rossi A, et al. Extraventricular neurocytoma with ganglionic differentiation associated with complex partial seizures. AJNR Am J Neuroradiol 1999;20(4):724–7.

24. Patil AS, Menon G, Easwer HV, et al. Extraventricular neurocytoma, a comprehensive review. Acta Neurochir (Wien) 2014;156(2):349–54.

25. Kane AJ, Sughrue ME, Rutkowski MJ, et al. Atypia predicting prognosis for intracranial extraventricular neurocytomas. J Neurosurg 2012;116(2):349–54.

26. Han L, Niu H, Wang J, et al. Extraventricular neurocytoma in pediatric populations: a case report and review of the literature. Oncol Lett 2013;6(5):1397–405.

27. Möller-Hartmann W, Krings T, Brunn A, et al. Proton magnetic resonance spectroscopy of neurocytoma outside the ventricular region–case report and review of the literature. Neuroradiology 2002;44(3):230–4.

28. Ueda F, Suzuki M, Matsui O, et al. Automated MR spectroscopy of intra- and extraventricular neurocytomas. Magn Reson Med Sci 2007;6(2):75–81.

29. Furtado A, Arantes M, Silva R, et al. Comprehensive review of extraventricular neurocytoma with report of two cases, and comparison with central neurocytoma. Clin Neuropathol 2010;29(3):134–40.

30. Giangaspero F, Cenacchi G, Losi L, et al. Extraventricular neoplasms with neurocytoma features. A clinicopathological study of 11 cases. Am J Surg Pathol 1997;21(2):206–12.

31. Rades D, Fehlauer F, Schild SE. Treatment of atypical neurocytomas. Cancer 2004;100(4):814–7.

32. Rodriguez FJ, Mota RA, Scheithauer BW, et al. Interphase cytogenetics for 1p19q and t(1;19)(q10;p10) may distinguish prognostically relevant subgroups in extraventricular neurocytoma. Brain Pathol 2009;19(4):623–9.

33. Myung JK, Cho HJ, Park CK, et al. Clinicopathological and genetic characteristics of extraventricular neurocytomas. Neuropathology 2013;33(2):111–21.

34. Okazaki T, Kageji T, Matsuzaki K, et al. Primary anaplastic pleomorphic xanthoastrocytoma with widespread neuroaxis dissemination at diagnosis - a pediatric case report and review of the literature. J Neurooncol 2009;94(3):431–7.

35. Lubansu A, Rorive S, David P, et al. Cerebral anaplastic pleomorphic xanthoastrocytoma with meningeal dissemination at first presentation. Childs Nerv Syst 2004;20(2):119–22.

36. Crespo-Rodríguez AM, Smirniotopoulos JG, Rushing EJ. MR and CT imaging of 24 pleomorphic xanthoastrocytomas (PXA) and a review of the literature. Neuroradiology 2007;49(4):307–15.

37. Usubalieva A, Pierson CR, Kavran CA, et al. Primary meningeal pleomorphic xanthoastrocytoma with anaplastic features: a report of 2 cases, one with BRAFV600E mutation and clinical response to the BRAF inhibitor dabrafenib. J Neuropathol Exp Neurol 2015;74(10):960–9.

38. Giannini C, Scheithauer BW, Burger PC, et al. Pleomorphic xanthoastrocytoma: what do we really know about it? Cancer 1999;85(9):2033–45.

39. Kahramancetin N, Tihan T. Aggressive behavior and anaplasia in pleomorphic xanthoastrocytoma: a plea for a revision of the current WHO classification. CNS Oncol 2013;2(6):523–30.

40. Ida CM, Rodriguez FJ, Burger PC, et al. Pleomorphic xanthoastrocytoma: natural history and long-term follow-up. Brain Pathol 2015;25(5):575–86.

41. Rodriguez-Mena R, Joanes-Alepuz V, Barbella-Aponte R, et al. Xantoastrocitoma pleomorfico con extension intraventricular y transformacion anaplasica en paciente adulto: caso clinico. Neurocirugia (Astur) 2012;23(5):203–10.

42. Perkins SM, Mitra N, Fei W, et al. Patterns of care and outcomes of patients with pleomorphic xanthoastrocytoma: a SEER analysis. J Neurooncol 2012;110(1):99–104.

43. Ostrom QT, Gittleman H, Fulop J, et al. CBTRUS statistical report: primary brain and central nervous system tumors diagnosed in the United States in 2008-2012. Neuro Oncol 2015;17(Suppl 4):iv1–62.

44. Fu YJ, Miyahara H, Uzuka T, et al. Intraventricular pleomorphic xanthoastrocytoma with anaplastic features. Neuropathology 2010;30(4):443–8.

45. Tien R, Cardenas C, Rajagopalan S. Pleomorphic xanthoastrocytoma of the brain: MR findings in six patients. Am J Roentgenol 1992;159(6):1287–90.

46. Asano K, Miyamoto S, Kubo O, et al. A case of anaplastic pleomorphic xanthoastrocytoma presenting with tumor bleeding and cerebrospinal fluid dissemination. Brain Tumor Pathol 2006;23(1):55–63.

47. Moore W, Mathis D, Gargan L, et al. Pleomorphic xanthoastrocytoma of childhood: MR imaging and diffusion MR imaging features. AJNR Am J Neuroradiol 2014;35(11):2192–6.

48. Bassoe P, Nuzum F. Report of a case of central and peripheral neurofibromatosis. J Nerv Ment Dis 1915;42(2):785–96.

49. Worster-drought C, Dickson WEC, Mcmenemey WH. Multiple meningeal and perineural tumours with analogous changes in the glia and ependyma (neurofibroblastomatosis): with report of two cases. Brain 1937;60(1):85–117.

50. Aw-Zoretic J, Burrowes D, Wadhwani N, et al. Teaching neuro images: meningioangiomatosis. Neurology 2015;84:9–11.

51. Zhang C, Wang Y, Wang X, et al. Sporadic meningioangiomatosis with and without meningioma: analysis of clinical differences and risk factors for poor seizure outcomes. Acta Neurochir (Wien) 2015;157(5):841–53.

52. Tien RD, Osumi A, Oakes JW, et al. Meningioangiomatosis: CT and MR findings. J Comput Assist Tomogr 1992;16(3):361–5.

53. Halper J, Scheithauer BW, Okazaki H, et al. Meningio-angiomatosis: a report of six cases with special reference to the occurrence of neurofibrillary tangles. J Neuropathol Exp Neurol 1986;45(4):426–46.

54. Park MS, Suh DC, Choi WS, et al. Multifocal meningioangiomatosis: a report of two cases. AJNR Am J Neuroradiol 1999;20(4):677–80.

55. Sun Z, Jin F, Zhang J, et al. Three cases of sporadic meningioangiomatosis with different imaging appearances: case report and review of the literature. World J Surg Oncol 2015;13:89.

56. Feng R, Hu J, Che X, et al. Diagnosis and surgical treatment of sporadic meningioangiomatosis. Clin Neurol Neurosurg 2013;115(8):1407–14.

57. Yao Z, Wang Y, Zee C, et al. Computed tomography and magnetic resonance appearance of sporadic meningioangiomatosis correlated with pathological findings. J Comput Assist Tomogr 2009;33(5):799–804.

58. Kashlan ON, Laborde DV, Davison L, et al. Meningioangiomatosis: a case report and literature review emphasizing diverse appearance on different imaging modalities. Case Rep Neurol Med 2011;2011:361203.

59. Jeon TY, Kim JH, Suh YL, et al. Sporadic meningioangiomatosis: imaging findings with histopathologic correlations in seven patients. Neuroradiology 2013;55(12):1439–46.

60. Prayson RA. Meningioangiomatosis: a clinicopathologic study including MIB1 immunoreactivity. Arch Pathol Lab Med 1995;119(11):1061–4.

61. Paulus W, Peiffer J, Roggendorf W, et al. Meningio-angiomatosis. Pathol Res Pract 1989;184(4):446–54.

62. Kim WY, Kim IO, Kim WS, et al. Meningioangiomatosis: MR imaging and pathological correlation in two cases. Pediatr Radiol 2002;32(2):96–8.

63. Wiebe S, Munoz DG, Smith S, et al. Meningioangiomatosis. A comprehensive analysis of clinical and laboratory features. Brain 1999;122(Pt 4):709–26.

64. Aizpuru RN, Quencer RM, Norenberg M, et al. Meningioangiomatosis: clinical, radiologic, and histopathologic correlation. Radiology 1991;179(3):819–21.

65. Chen YY, Tiang XY, Li Z, et al. Sporadic meningioangiomatosis-associated atypical meningioma mimicking parenchymal invasion of brain: a case report and review of the literature. Diagn Pathol 2010;5:39.

66. Agnihotri S, Burrell KE, Wolf A, et al. Glioblastoma, a brief review of history, molecular genetics, animal models and novel therapeutic strategies. Arch Immunol Ther Exp (Warsz) 2013;61(1):25–41.

67. Osborn AG. Osborn's Brain: Imaging, Pathology, and Anatomy. 1st edition. Salt Lake City (UT): Amirsys Inc; 2012.

68. Ben Nsir A, Gdoura Y, Thai QA, et al. Intraventricular glioblastomas. World Neurosurg 2016;88:126–31.

69. Secer HI, Dinc C, Anik I, et al. Glioblastoma multiforme of the lateral ventricle: report of nine cases. Br J Neurosurg 2008;22(3):398–401.

70. Kim YJ, Lee SK, Cho MK, et al. Intraventricular glioblastoma multiforme with previous history of intracerebral hemorrhage: a case report. J Korean Neurosurg Soc 2008;44(6):405–8.

71. Lee TT, Manzano GR. Third ventricular glioblastoma multiforme: case report. Neurosurg Rev 1997;20(4):291–4.

72. Mandour C, El Mostarchid B. Intraventricular glioblastoma. Pan Afr Med J 2014;18:100.

73. Sarikafa Y, Akçakaya MO, Sarikafa S, et al. Intraventricular glioblastoma multiforme: case report. Neurocirugia 2015;26(3):147–50.

74. Yılmaz B, Ekşi MŞ, Demir MK, et al. Isolated third ventricle glioblastoma. Springerplus 2016;5(1):1–5.

75. Klein O, Marchal JC. Intraventricular glioblastoma: a paediatric case report. Br J Neurosurg 2007;21(4):411–3.

76. Park P, Choksi VR, Gala VC, et al. Well-circumscribed, minimally enhancing glioblastoma multiforme of the trigone: a case report and review of the literature. AJNR Am J Neuroradiol 2005;26(6):1475–8.

77. Stark AM, Nabavi A, Mehdorn HM, et al. Glioblastoma multiforme—report of 267 cases treated at a single institution. Surg Neurol 2005;63(2):162–9.

78. Majós C, Alonso J, Aguilera C, et al. Adult primitive neuroectodermal tumor: proton MR spectroscopic findings with possible application for differential diagnosis. Radiology 2002;225(2):556–66.

79. Prasad AN. Supratentorial PNET in a young child. Indian J Pediatr 2011;78(5):613–5.

80. Borja MJ, Plaza MJ, Altman N, et al. Conventional and advanced MRI features of pediatric intracranial tumors: supratentorial tumors. Am J Roentgenol 2013;200(5):483–503.

81. Chawla A, Emmanuel JV, Seow WT, et al. Paediatric PNET: pre-surgical MRI features. Clin Radiol 2007;62(1):43–52.

82. Lawandy S, Hariri OR, Miulli DE, et al. Supratentorial primitive neuroectodermal tumor in an adult: a case report and review of the literature. J Med Case Rep 2012;6(1):361.

83. Espino Barros Palau A, Khan K, Morgan ML, et al. Suprasellar primitive neuroectodermal tumor in an

adult. J Neuroophthalmol 2015. [Epub ahead of print].

84. Ohba S, Yoshida K, Hirose Y, et al. A supratentorial primitive neuroectodermal tumor in an adult: a case report and review of the literature. J Neurooncol 2008;86(2):217–24.

85. Mueller S, Chang S. Pediatric brain tumors: current treatment strategies and future therapeutic approaches. Neurotherapeutics 2009;6:570–86.

86. Gaffney CC, Sloane JP, Bradley NJ, et al. Primitive neuroectodermal tumours of the cerebrum. Pathology and treatment. J Neurooncol 1985; 3(1):23–33.

87. Timmermann B, Kortmann RD, Kühl J, et al. Role of radiotherapy in the treatment of supratentorial primitive neuroectodermal tumors in childhood: results of the prospective German brain tumor trials hit 88/89 and 91. J Clin Oncol 2002;20(3):842–9.

88. Ostrom QT, de Blank PM, Kruchko C, et al. Alex's Lemonade Stand Foundation Infant and childhood primary brain and central nervous system tumors diagnosed in the United States in 2007-2011. Neuro Oncol 2014;16(10):1–36.

89. Khuong-Quang DA, Buczkowicz P, Rakopoulos P, et al. K27M mutation in histone H3.3 defines clinically and biologically distinct subgroups of pediatric diffuse intrinsic pontine gliomas. Acta Neuropathol 2012;124(3):439–47.

90. Fangusaro J. Pediatric high-grade gliomas and diffuse intrinsic pontine gliomas. J Child Neurol 2009;24(11):1409–17.

91. Gururangan S, McLaughlin CA, Brashears J, et al. Incidence and patterns of neuraxis metastases in children with diffuse pontine glioma. J Neurooncol 2006;77(2):207–12.

92. Robison NJ, Kieran MW. Diffuse intrinsic pontine glioma: a reassessment. J Neurooncol 2014; 119(1):7–15.

93. Caretti V, Bugiani M, Freret M, et al. Subventricular spread of diffuse intrinsic pontine glioma. Acta Neuropathol 2014;128(4):605–7.

94. Hargrave D, Bartels U, Bouffet E. Diffuse brainstem glioma in children: critical review of clinical trials. Lancet Oncol 2006;7(3):241–8.

95. Feng J, Hao S, Pan C, et al. The H3.3 K27M mutation results in a poorer prognosis in brainstem gliomas than thalamic gliomas in adults. Hum Pathol 2015;46(11):1626–32.

96. Hankinson TC, Patibandla MR, Green A, et al. Hypofractionated radiotherapy for children with diffuse intrinsic pontine gliomas. Pediatr Blood Cancer 2016;63(4):716–8.

97. Pollack IF, Jakacki RI, Butterfield LH, et al. Immune responses and outcome after vaccination with glioma-associated antigen peptides and poly-ICLC in a pilot study for pediatric recurrent low-grade gliomas. Neuro Oncol 2016;18(8):1157–68.

98. Masonic Cancer Center, University of Minnesota. Imiquimod/BTIC Lysate-Based Vaccine Immunotherapy for diffuse intrinsic pontine glioma in children and young adults. In: Clinical Trials.gov (internet), editor. Bethesda (MD): National Library of Medicine (US); 2011. NML Identifier: NCT01400672. Available at: https://clinicaltrials.gov/ct2/show/NCT01400672. Accessed June 14, 2016.

99. Komori T, Scheithauer BW, Anthony DC, et al. Papillary glioneuronal tumor: a new variant of mixed neuronal-glial neoplasm. Am J Surg Pathol 1998;22(10):1171–83.

100. Carangelo B, Arrigucci U, Mariottini A, et al. Papillary glioneuronal tumor: case report and review of literature. G Chir 2014;36(2):63–9.

101. Zhao RJ, Zhang XL, Chu SG, et al. Clinicopathologic and neuroradiologic studies of papillary glioneuronal tumors. Acta Neurochir (Wien) 2016; 158(4):695–702.

102. Xiao H, Ma L, Lou X, et al. Papillary glioneuronal tumor: radiological evidence of a newly established tumor entity. J Neuroimaging 2011;21(3): 297–302.

103. Govindan A, Mahadevan A, Bhat DI, et al. Papillary glioneuronal tumor-evidence of stem cell origin with biphenotypic differentiation. J Neurooncol 2009; 95(1):71–80.

104. Osborn AG, Salzman KL, Thurnher MM, et al. The new World Health Organization classification of central nervous system tumors: what can the neuroradiologist really say? AJNR Am J Neuroradiol 2012;33(5):795–802.

105. Preusser M, Ströbel T, Gelpi E, et al. Alzheimer-type neuropathology in a 28 year old patient with iatrogenic Creutzfeldt-Jakob disease after dural grafting. J Neurol Neurosurg Psychiatry 2006;77(3): 413–6.

106. Sharma P, Swain M, Padua MD, et al. Rosette-forming glioneuronal tumors: a report of two cases. Neurol India 2012;59(2):276–80.

107. Hsu C, Kwan G, Lau Q, et al. Rosette-forming glioneuronal tumour: Imaging features, histopathological correlation and a comprehensive review of literature. Br J Neurosurg 2012;26(5):668–73.

108. Cebula H, Chibbaro S, Santin MN, et al. Thalamic rosette-forming a glioneuronal tumor in an elderly patient: case report and literature review. Neurochirurgie 2016;62(1):60–3.

109. Kumar M, Samant R, Ramakrishnaiah R, et al. Radiology case reports Rosette-forming glioneuronal tumor of the fourth ventricle. Radiol Case Rep 2013;8(1):1–4.

110. Kemp S, Kemp S, Achan A, et al. Rosette-forming glioneuronal tumour of the lateral ventricle in a patient with neurofibromatosis 1. J Clin Neurosci 2012;19(8):1180–1.

111. Frelinghuysen M, Luna F, Spencer L, et al. Aggressive Rosette forming glioneuroma: case report and review of the literature. Cancer Clin Oncol 2014; 3(2):10–5.

112. Lucas JT, Huang AJ, Mott RT, et al. Anaplastic ganglioglioma: a report of three cases and review of the literature. J Neurooncol 2015;123(1):171–7.

113. Lee CC, Wang WH, Lin CF, et al. Malignant transformation of supratentorial ganglioglioma. Clin Neurol Neurosurg 2012;114(10):1338–42.

114. DeMarchi R, Abu-Abed S, Munoz D, et al. Malignant ganglioglioma: case report and review of literature. J Neurooncol 2011;101(2):311–8.

115. Čupić H, Sajko T, Sesar N, et al. Malignant transformation of grade II ganglioglioma to glioblastoma: a case report. Transl Neurosci 2012;3(2). http://dx.doi.org/10.2478/s13380-012-0017-x.

116. Blümcke I, Wiestler OD. Gangliogliomas: an intriguing tumor entity associated with focal epilepsies. J Neuropathol Exp Neurol 2002;61(7): 575–84.

117. Schittenhelm J, Reifenberger G, Ritz R, et al. Primary anaplastic ganglioglioma with a small-cell glioblastoma component. Clin Neuropathol 2008; 27(2):91–5.

118. Song JY, Kim JH, Cho YH, et al. Treatment and outcomes for gangliogliomas: a single-center review of 16 patients. Brain Tumor Res Treat 2014;2(2):49.

119. Im SH, Chung CK, Cho BK, et al. Intracranial ganglioglioma: preoperative characteristics and oncologic outcome after surgery. J Neurooncol 2002; 59(2):173–83.

120. Savci Heijink DS, Urgun K, Sav A, et al. A case of primary diffuse leptomeningeal gliomatosis predominantly involving the cervical spinal cord and mimicking chronic meningitis. Turk Neurosurg 2012;22(1):90–4.

121. Rossi S, Rossi S, Rodriguez FJ, et al. Primary leptomeningeal oligodendroglioma with documented progression to anaplasia and t(1;19)(q10;p10) in a child. Acta Neuropathol 2009;118(4):575–7.

122. Kosker M, Sener D, Kilic O, et al. Primary diffuse leptomeningeal gliomatosis mimicking tuberculous meningitis. J Child Neurol 2014;29(12):NP171–5.

123. Leep Hunderfund AN, Zabad RK, Aksamit AJ, et al. Diffuse anaplastic leptomeningeal oligodendrogliomatosis mimicking neurosarcoidosis. Neurol Clin Pract 2013;3(3):261–5.

124. Kim SH, Jun DC, Park JS, et al. Primary diffuse leptomeningeal gliomatosis: report of a case presenting with chronic meningitis. J Clin Neurol 2006;2(3): 202–5.

125. Bourne TD, Mandell JW, Matsumoto JA, et al. Primary disseminated leptomeningeal oligodendroglioma with 1p deletion. Case report. J Neurosurg 2006;105(6 Suppl):465–9.

Index

Note: Page numbers of article titles are in **boldface** type.

Neuroimag Clin N Am 26 (2016) 691–694
http://dx.doi.org/10.1016/S1052-5149(16)30081-8
1052-5149/16/$ – see front matter

UNITED STATES POSTAL SERVICE ® Statement of Ownership, Management, and Circulation
(All Periodicals Publications Except Requester Publications)

1. Publication Title	2. Publication Number	3. Filing Date
NEUROIMAGING CLINICS OF NORTH AMERICA	010 – 548	9/18/2016

4. Issue Frequency	5. Number of Issues Published Annually	6. Annual Subscription Price
FEB, MAY, AUG, NOV	4	$360.00

7. Complete Mailing Address of Known Office of Publication (Not printer) (Street, city, county, state, and ZIP+4®)

ELSEVIER INC.
360 PARK AVENUE SOUTH
NEW YORK, NY 10010-1710

Contact Person
STEPHEN R. BUSHING

Telephone (Include area code)
215-239-3688

8. Complete Mailing Address of Headquarters or General Business Office of Publisher (Not printer)

ELSEVIER INC.
360 PARK AVENUE SOUTH
NEW YORK, NY 10010-1710

9. Full Names and Complete Mailing Addresses of Publisher, Editor, and Managing Editor (Do not leave blank)

Publisher (Name and complete mailing address)

ADRIANNE BRIGIDO, ELSEVIER INC.
1600 JOHN F KENNEDY BLVD. SUITE 1800
PHILADELPHIA, PA 19103-2899

Editor (Name and complete mailing address)

JOHN VASSALLO, ELSEVIER INC.
1600 JOHN F KENNEDY BLVD. SUITE 1800
PHILADELPHIA, PA 19103-2899

Managing Editor (Name and complete mailing address)

PATRICK MANLEY, ELSEVIER INC.
1600 JOHN F KENNEDY BLVD. SUITE 1800
PHILADELPHIA, PA 19103-2899

10. Owner (Do not leave blank. If the publication is owned by a corporation, give the name and address of the corporation immediately followed by the names and addresses of all stockholders owning or holding 1 percent or more of the total amount of stock. If not owned by a corporation, give the names and addresses of the individual owners. If owned by a partnership or other unincorporated firm, give its name and address as well as those of each individual owner. If the publication is published by a nonprofit organization, give its name and address.)

Full Name	Complete Mailing Address
WHOLLY OWNED SUBSIDIARY OF REED/ELSEVIER, US HOLDINGS	1600 JOHN F KENNEDY BLVD. SUITE 1800 PHILADELPHIA, PA 19103-2899

11. Known Bondholders, Mortgagees, and Other Security Holders Owning or Holding 1 Percent or More of Total Amount of Bonds, Mortgages, or Other Securities. If none, check box. ▶ ☐ None

Full Name	Complete Mailing Address
N/A	

12. Tax Status (For completion by nonprofit organizations authorized to mail at nonprofit rates) (Check one)
The purpose, function, and nonprofit status of this organization and the exempt status for federal income tax purposes:
☐ Has Not Changed During Preceding 12 Months
☐ Has Changed During Preceding 12 Months (Publisher must submit explanation of change with this statement)

13. Publication Title	14. Issue Date for Circulation Data Below
NEUROIMAGING CLINICS OF NORTH AMERICA	AUGUST 2016

15. Extent and Nature of Circulation			Average No. Copies Each Issue During Preceding 12 Months	No. Copies of Single Issue Published Nearest to Filing Date
a. Total Number of Copies (Net press run)			564	658
b. Paid Circulation (By Mail and Outside the Mail)	(1)	Mailed Outside-County Paid Subscriptions Stated on PS Form 3541 (include paid distribution above nominal rate, advertiser's proof copies, and exchange copies)	346	433
	(2)	Mailed In-County Paid Subscriptions Stated on PS Form 3541 (include paid distribution above nominal rate, advertiser's proof copies, and exchange copies)	0	0
	(3)	Paid Distribution Outside the Mails Including Sales Through Dealers and Carriers, Street Vendors, Counter Sales, and Other Paid Distribution Outside USPS®	82	97
	(4)	Paid Distribution by Other Classes of Mail Through the USPS (e.g., First-Class Mail®)	0	0
c. Total Paid Distribution (Sum of 15b (1), (2), (3), and (4))		▶	428	530
d. Free or Nominal Rate Distribution (By Mail and Outside the Mail)	(1)	Free or Nominal Rate Outside-County Copies included on PS Form 3541	19	28
	(2)	Free or Nominal Rate In-County Copies Included on PS Form 3541	0	0
	(3)	Free or Nominal Rate Copies Mailed at Other Classes Through the USPS (e.g., First-Class Mail)	0	0
	(4)	Free or Nominal Rate Distribution Outside the Mail (Carriers or other means)	0	0
e. Total Free or Nominal Rate Distribution (Sum of 15d (1), (2), (3) and (4))		▶	19	28
f. Total Distribution (Sum of 15c and 15e)		▶	447	558
g. Copies not Distributed (See Instructions to Publishers #4 (page #3))		▶	117	100
h. Total (Sum of 15f and g)		▶	564	658
i. Percent Paid (15c divided by 15f times 100)		▶	96%	95%

* If you are claiming electronic copies, go to line 16 on page 3. If you are not claiming electronic copies, skip to line 17 on page 3.

16. Electronic Copy Circulation	Average No. Copies Each Issue During Preceding 12 Months	No. Copies of Single Issue Published Nearest to Filing Date
a. Paid Electronic Copies ▶	0	0
b. Total Paid Print Copies (Line 15c) + Paid Electronic Copies (Line 16a) ▶	428	530
c. Total Print Distribution (Line 15f) + Paid Electronic Copies (Line 16a) ▶	447	558
d. Percent Paid (Both Print & Electronic Copies) (16b divided by 16c × 100) ▶	96%	95%

☒ I certify that 50% of all my distributed copies (electronic and print) are paid above a nominal price.

17. Publication of Statement of Ownership
☒ If the publication is a general publication, publication of this statement is required. Will be printed
in the **NOVEMBER 2016** issue of this publication. ☐ Publication not required.

18. Signature and Title of Editor, Publisher, Business Manager, or Owner

STEPHEN R. BUSHING - INVENTORY DISTRIBUTION CONTROL MANAGER

Date 9/18/2016

I certify that all information furnished on this form is true and complete. I understand that anyone who furnishes false or misleading information on this form or who omits material or information requested on the form may be subject to criminal sanctions (including fines and imprisonment) and/or civil sanctions (including civil penalties).

PS Form **3526**, July 2014 [Page 1 of 4 (see instructions page 4)] PSN: 7530-01-000-9931   PRIVACY NOTICE: See our privacy policy on www.usps.com.

PS Form **3526**, July 2014 (Page 3 of 4)   PRIVACY NOTICE: See our privacy policy on www.usps.com.

Moving?

Make sure your subscription moves with you!

To notify us of your new address, find your **Clinics Account Number** (located on your mailing label above your name), and contact customer service at:

Email: journalscustomerservice-usa@elsevier.com

800-654-2452 (subscribers in the U.S. & Canada)
314-447-8871 (subscribers outside of the U.S. & Canada)

Fax number: 314-447-8029

**Elsevier Health Sciences Division
Subscription Customer Service
3251 Riverport Lane
Maryland Heights, MO 63043**

*To ensure uninterrupted delivery of your subscription, please notify us at least 4 weeks in advance of move.

Printed and bound by CPI Group (UK) Ltd, Croydon, CR0 4YY

03/10/2024

01040383-0003